Ophthalmology: Causes, Symptoms and Treatment of Eye Infections

Ophthalmology: Causes, Symptoms and Treatment of Eye Infections

Editor: Terry Bailey

MURPHY & MOORE
www.murphy-moorepublishing.com

www.murphy-moorepublishing.com

MURPHY & MOORE

Cataloging-in-Publication Data

Ophthalmology : causes, symptoms and treatment of eye infections / edited by Terry Bailey.
p. cm.
Includes bibliographical references and index.
ISBN 978-1-63987-411-8
1. Eye--Infections. 2. Eye--Infections--Etiology. 3. Eye--Infections--Treatment. 4. Eye--Diseases.
5. Ophthalmology. I. Bailey, Terry.
RE96 .O64 2022
617.71--dc23

Murphy & Moore Publishing,
1 Rockefeller Plaza,
New York City, NY 10020, USA

ISBN 978-1-63987-411-8 (Hardback)

Contents

Preface

The branch of medicine which is involved in diagnosing, preventing and treating infections which can affect the eye is known as ophthalmology. Eye infections are caused when harmful micro-organisms such as bacteria, viruses and fungi invade a part of the eyeball or surrounding tissues including the cornea and conjunctiva. A few of the major symptoms of eye infections are pain, blurry vision, itching, swelling around the eyes, swollen eyes, light sensitivity, dry eyes, watery eyes, eye discharge and red eyes. Some examples of bacterial, fungal and viral eye infection are pink eye or conjunctivitis, ocular herpes, fungal keratitis, acanthamoeba keratitis, trachoma and endophthalmitis. An eye infection can also affect the interior portions of lower and upper eyelids to create a chalazion or stye. Rubbing or popping a stye can cause a more serious infection known as orbital cellulitis. This book unravels the recent studies on eye infections. The topics covered herein deal with the causes, symptoms and treatment of these infections. This book will serve as a reference to a broad spectrum of readers.

After months of intensive research and writing, this book is the end result of all who devoted their time and efforts in the initiation and progress of this book. It will surely be a source of reference in enhancing the required knowledge of the new developments in the area. During the course of developing this book, certain measures such as accuracy, authenticity and research focused analytical studies were given preference in order to produce a comprehensive book in the area of study.

This book would not have been possible without the efforts of the authors and the publisher. I extend my sincere thanks to them. Secondly, I express my gratitude to my family and well-wishers. And most importantly, I thank my students for constantly expressing their willingness and curiosity in enhancing their knowledge in the field, which encourages me to take up further research projects for the advancement of the area.

Editor

1

Primary Open Angle Glaucoma Surgery in Sub-Saharan African Setting — Benefits and Challenges

Lawan Abdu

Abstract

Background: Primary open angle glaucoma is one of the leading causes of avoidable blindness in Sub-Saharan Africa

Medical therapy: Anti-glaucoma medication pose a special challenge due to high cost, non availability, and presence of sub- standard/ adulterated drugs in the region. With wide spread poverty compliance to medication for life is poor.

Trabeculectomy: Although there are various types of glaucoma surgeries, trabeculectomy with use of anti-fibrotic agent is found to offer good intra ocular pressure control among patients in the region. The use of anti-fibrotic agents like mitomycin-C and 5 Flourouracil becomes necessary due to the tendency of pigmented African eye to form scar that results in bleb failure.

Conclusion: Trabeculectomy with intra operative use of anti metabolite is an acceptable choice in treatment of primary open angle glaucoma in sub-Saharan Africa. The key to success is adequate pre operative patient education on the goal of treatment.

Keywords: POAG, Sub-Sahara, Africa, Trabeculectomy, Anti-metabolite, Counselling

1. Introduction

Glaucoma is a group of disorders manifesting characteristic progressive optic nerve damage and is associated with many risk factors such as central corneal thickness, structure of the optic nerve head, age, genetic factors, race and intraocular pressure (IOP). Primary open angle glaucoma (POAG) is not associated with any other cause. The features include characteristic optic nerve damage, nerve fibre layer loss, visual field changes and an open angle on gonioscopy. The global estimate of glaucomatous optic neuropathy is 60 million and 8.4 million turn blind from the disease. The highest prevalence of POAG occurs in Africans.[1] In the sub-Saharan African (SSA) region there is shortage of population studies on causes of blindness. POAG is under-reported as the mechanism for making a diagnosis is difficult under circumstances in which field surveys are conducted. Local and regional studies have demonstrated the contribution of glaucoma as a major cause of avoidable blindness in SSA.[2-9, 21] There are peculiarities in the way glaucoma is present in the region. These factors are related to the individual, the family, the community and the health-care system. Initially POAG has subtle nature of presentation with symptoms such as pain which is a major driving force for seeking medical help being largely absent. Poor access to health care in general and eye care in particular, superstition and inequity in distribution of human and material resources in eye care result in the largely rural population having minimal access.[10] Even where some level of eye care services are available, basic equipment such as tonometer, visual field analyser, slit lamp and relevant diagnostic lenses are unavailable. The few eye care personnel available are not motivated to work in the rural areas as basic services like good schools; tap water and electricity are not steadily supplied. Patients are left at the mercy of quacks including traditional eye healers (TEH) whose unregulated practices contribute to increase in the burden of avoidable blindness. TEH dispense traditional eye medicine (TEM) of unknown contents, not produced under aseptic conditions and can result in corneal damage and blindness.[11] Patients often present late with advanced optic nerve damage and are visually impaired.[12, 13, 14, 15, 16] One can deduce that only a small fraction of POAG patients make it to the few available centres where quality care can be offered.

2. The argument in favour of POAG surgery

The risk factor most amenable to control is IOP. There are two broad approaches to treatment, which can be surgical or medical. One cannot draw a line between the options, with various permutations and combinations possible in order to achieve success. Even where a decision is reached to do surgery there is need for initial medication to reduce the IOP. Treatment and monitoring is for life. Potent glaucoma medications are expensive with most patients being poor and defendant. Quality and safety is often suspected as adulterated medications float the markets in SSA. Medicines are conveyed in open trucks under the scorching sun or left in the open. Even quality medicine will eventually loose potency before getting to the patients. The few reputable pharmaceutical vendors are located in major cities and townships away from the reach of rural poorPoverty and illiteracy hinder compliance with treatment. The health insurance scheme is for the regular sectors of the economy, accessible to only civil servants and those working for the organized private sector. Bulk of the population has no health insurance cover and need to pay for eye care at the point of service delivery. Inability to pay results in denial of service. Such denial of access to eye care services is against the goals of

Vision 2020: the right to sight. These multitudes of factors make a case for surgery. As clinicians in the SSA region search for better treatment compliance, they move closer to surgery.[17] Considering the unavailability of potent, cost-effective, long-term acceptable medications, surgery can be a worthwhile option.[18] Successful surgery can be a one off expenses alternative. It ensures reduction in IOP round the clock. The patient needs not to remember that it's time to apply the eye drop and is free from local and systemic side effects. The key to surgical success is proper patient's education and counselling. POAG patients are often admitted to the same ward with blind cataract patients. A day after surgery pseudo-phakic patients move around unaided. Glaucoma patient expects the same outcome. Thus, without proper patient education, the seed of discontentment and dissatisfaction is sown. Glaucoma patients need to be educated on the purpose of surgery and its impact on vision. They need to know that the procedure is not free of complications and may accelerate cataract formation resulting in additional surgery at a later date. POAG patients are to be informed that surgery can fail or be partially successful in IOP control warranting reintroduction of eye medications. Penetrating glaucoma surgery mainly trabeculectomy with antimetabolite is the most common procedure performed with encouraging outcome.[19] Trabeculectomy records various success rates at given time intervals after surgery.[19, 20, 21, 22] IOP control appears to be lower when surgery is performed without antimetabolite.[22] Releasable sutures offer additional advantage in reducing IOP in the early post-operative period.[23] Other non-penetrating procedures such as visco-canalostomy and trabeculoplasty are not done routinely. Laser procedures including argon or diode laser trabeculoplasty generally do not give very encouraging outcomes in pigmented African eyes. Where available, laser can be used to augment medical treatment/surgery on a case by case basis.

3. Preoperative management

Patient education is a crucial step in administration of informed consent. Patient and caregiver need to know the status of the patient's vision, the type of procedure to be performed, the goal to be achieved, post-operative medication/management and the possibility that glaucoma drugs may be reinstated after surgery even if partially. The current visual acuity, visual field, tonometry, retinal nerve fibre layer thickness (RNFL) measurements and gonioscopic finding should be available and form frame work of the counselling. Clinicians are often reluctant to do surgery on those with advanced/end-stage glaucoma characterized by 'tunnel visual fields', severe visual impairment and vertical optic disc cupping of 0.9 or worse. Reluctance is related to risk of further sight deterioration which could be attributed to post-operative inflammation, post-operative complications such as endophthalmitis (though rare) or increase in lenticular opacity and the risk of visual wipe out phenomenon. Patients' and caregivers' knowledge of the goal of controlling IOP and by so doing limiting optic nerve damage will reduce complains that 'doctor you have operated my eyes and yet my sight has not improved'. Preoperative routine includes medical treatment to reduce the IOP to lower teens and trimming of the eye lashes. Blood pressure (BP) and fasting blood sugar (FBS) levels are measured to identify undiagnosed hypertension and those with diabetes mellitus. BP and FBS control are essential before, during and after surgery. Physicians managing such conditions are involved in the overall care of the patient. Those with high or minimally responding IOP may benefit from systemic carbonic anhydrase inhibitors or osmotic agents to further reduce the pressure before the procedure is performed. Trabeculectomy can be done as an outpatient procedure in selected cases, but, in most instances, due to the nature of the environment (long distance from eye care facility; hostile, dirty and unhygienic situation of the living environment; and illiteracy), patients often require inpatient care and are discharged within a week. POAG surgery is usually performed under local anaesthesia using lignocaine-containing adrenaline in appropriate dilution. General anaesthesia is administered where there is a need to do so.

4. The procedure: Trabeculectomy with anti-fibrotic agent

This is performed in the operating theatre under complete aseptic condition. The surgeon and assistant are fully scrubbed and gowned. The skin around the eye is cleaned with povidone iodine 5% which is also used to wet and subsequently flush the conjunctiva with normal saline; adhesive drapes are placed leaving the globe area exposed. A wire speculum is used to part the lids, the superior rectus muscle is picked with toothed forceps and 4/0 silk suture is passed under it. A conjuctival flap is then raised. This can either be fornix or limbal based. Limbal-based flap reduces risk of fibrosis over the filtration drainage site though some believe it allows a freer connection of the surgical site with external conjuctiva and may in theory increase infection risk. Proponents of fornix flap believe it offers greater wound closure and lower infection risk. A caliper is used to demarcate proposed area to raise the outer sclera flap of 5 by 5 mm size. The area is cleared of tenons and haemostasis secured with bipolar wet field cautery. Ideally a separate trolley is used for administration of antimetabolite. A 5% dilution of mytomycin C or 5- fluorouracil is employed. A piece of cotton wool is soaked with the agent and applied over the sclera flap site for five minutes and then washed with 50 millilitres of normal saline. The trolley is subsequently taken away and the surgeons change gloves. The outline of the outer sclera flap is demarcated gently with a scalpel. The proximal part is gently elevated to form the lip of the partial thickness scleral flap. A chooks knife is then used to bluntly dissect the flap from the base of the cornea. A smaller inner sclera flap of 3 by 3 mm is then raised and excised. This is followed by a peripheral iridectomy. The outer flap is sutured at the two proximal edges. Some clinicians prefer to suture all the 4 edges with 10/0 silk sutures. The knots are buried in the sclera. The anterior chamber (A/C) is reformed with saline via a cannula. Conjunctiva is sutured at the edges in fornix-based flap. A running suture with a knot at the two ends can be used to close the conjunctiva in cases that had a limbal-based flap using absorbable 6/0 vicryl. Subconjuctival dexamethasone 4 mg injection is given and tropicamide eye drops applied before the eye is padded. First-day assessment includes measuring visual acuity, IOP, wound site, bleb size and function. Slit lamp bio microscopy is essential in determining state of the eye, such as cornea clarity, depth of A/C, in addition to fundoscopy. Post-operative medications include steroid/antibiotic combination eye drops, a mydriatic and systemic antibiotic such as amoxicillin. Initial follow-up visit is after one week.

5. Complications of trabeculectomy

Intraoperative complication includes hemorrhage, which can be arrested and bleeding vessels cauterized. Shallow A/C on the table usually reforms; in the event of delayed reformation, saline can be injected after the outer sclera flap is sutured.

Post-operative complications include the following:

- Shallow A/C. This is of varied etiology. In case of excessive filtration, the bleb is formed; there is no aqueous leakage as confirmed by a negative Seidel's test and the IOP is not raised. This can be managed by firm pressure padding and observation. In rare instances an additional transconjuctival suture is applied. Wound leakage results in shallow A/C with hypotony and positive Seidel's test detected by dilution of instilled flourescein from the bleb site on inspection with cobalt blue light on the slit lamp. This can be managed conservatively by pressure padding and tends to improve. Failure to improve is addressed by applying one or two additional sutures. Pupil block glaucoma arises from a non-functioning peripheral iridectomy. There is shallow A/C, negative Seidel's test, with raised IOP and iris bombe. Laser iridotomy may be required to relieve the pressure. Malignant glaucoma arises from aqueous back tracking behind the vitreous resulting in hypertony with markedly elevated IOP, corneal edema and shallow A/C with flattened bleb. Management involves administration of systemic osmotic agents such as mannitol, or urea and intravenous carbonic anhydrase inhibitors. In some instances Yag Laser is used to disrupt the anterior vitreous face thus allowing the trapped aqueous to pass through the normal channel.

- Post-operative endophthalmitis. Early manifestation is within 24 to 48 hours. Patient has pain and reduced vision with redness. This requires standard protocol of endophthalmitis management such as aqueous/vitreous aspiration for microscopy culture and sensitivity. Common pathogens are staphylococcus species. Relevant antibiotics are commenced immediately topically, systemically and intra-cameral/intravitreal. Antibiotic can be modified based on culture results.

- Other bleb-related complications include bleb failure which could arise from fibrosis or formation of tenon cyst. Management includes ocular compression, suture manipulation needling and, in some instances, injection of diluted 5-fluorouracil within the first two weeks of surgery. Blebitis is characterized by inflammation and debris (exudates). Without intraocular extension, the vision is normal. Treatment involves taking swab for microscopy, culture and sensitivity. Topical ofloxacin and ciprofloxacin can be used. Large cystic acellular bleb can leak. Mild to moderate leakage can be managed conservatively by pressure padding and antibiotic prophylaxis. Persistent or large area of leakage may require bleb revision such as advancing a conjuctival hood over it.

- Trabeculectomy can accelerate cataract formation. Cataract surgery should be through an approach that does not tamper with bleb function.

6. Conclusion

POAG is a common cause of avoidable blindness in SSA. Due to socio-demographic reasons, patients have poor access to eye care and often present late. Trabeculectomy with antimetabolite is an acceptable procedure that offers good IOP control. Proper education of the patient and caregiver particularly on the goal of treatment is an essential component of management.

Author details

Lawan Abdu

Address all correspondence to: lawal1966@yahoo.com

Department of Ophthalmology, Faculty of Clinical Sciences, College of Health Sciences, Bayero University Kano, Nigeria

References

[1] Cook C, Foster P. Epidemiology of glaucoma: what's new? Can J Ophthalmol 2012 Jun; 47 (3): 223-6

[2] Abdu L. Prevalence and causes of blindness and low vision in Dambatta local government area, Kano state, Nigeria. Niger J Med 2001 Jul-Sep; 11 (3): 108-12

[3] Murdoch IE, Cousens SN, Babalola OE, et al. Afri J Med Med Sci 2001 Dec; 30 (4): 337-9

[4] Adeoye A. Survey of blindness in rural communities of south-western Nigeria. Trop Med Int Health 1996 Oct; 1 (5): 672-6

[5] Agbeja-Baiyeroju AM, Bekibele CO, Bamgboye EA, et al. The Ibadan glaucoma study. Afr J Med Med Sci 2003 Dec; 32 (4): 371-6

[6] Omoti AE, Osahon AL, Waziri-Erameh MJ. Pattern of presentation of primary open angle glaucoma in Benin City, Nigeria. Trop Doct 2006 Apr; 36 (2): 97-100

[7] Dawodu OA, Osahon AI, Emifoniye E. Prevalence and causes of blindness in Otibhor Okhae Teaching Hospital, Irrua, Edo State, Nigeria. Ophthalmic Epidemiol 2003 Dec; 10 (5); 323-30

[8] Mohammed MA, Selvaraj S, Gudlavalleti VS, et al. Causes of blindness and visual impairment in Nigeria: The Nigerian National Blindness and Visual Impairment Survey. Invest Ophthalmol Vis Sci 2009 Sep; 50 (9): 4114-20

[9] Ntim-Amponsah CT, Amoaku WM, Ofosu-Amaah S, et al. Prevalence of glaucoma in an African country. Eye 2004 May; 18 (5): 491-7

[10] Nigerian population report. www.nationmaster.com/country/ni-nigeria/peo-people accessed on 18/10/2014

[11] Osahon AL. Consequences of traditional eye medicine in U.B.T.H Benin City. Nig J Ophthalmol 1995; 3: 51-54

[12] Awoyesuku EA, Ejimadu CS. Visual disability in newly diagnosed primary open angle glaucoma (POAG) in a tertiary hospital in Nigeria. Niger J Med 2012 Jan-March; 21 (1): 78-80

[13] Womald R, Foster A. Clinical and pathological features of chronic glaucoma in north-east Ghana. Eye (Lond) 1990; 4 (Pt 1): 107-14

[14] Mafwiri M, Bowman RJ, Wood M, et al. Primary open angle glaucoma presentation at a tertiary unit in Africa: intra ocular pressure levels and visual status. Ophthalmic Epidemiol 2005 Oct; 12 (5):299-302

[15] Ayena KD, Agbo AD, Attaya AB, et al. [Characteristics of cup/disc ratios in a population of northern Togo aged 20-40 years]. J Fr Ophthalmol 2010 Jun; 33 (6): 408-13

[16] Kovin N, Stephen G, Maria-Gloria B, et al. Prevalence and causes of loss of vision in sub- Saharan Africa 1990-2010. Br J Ophthalmol 2014; 98: 612-8

[17] Sonouvou I, Tchabi S, Monteiro S, et al. Therapeutic of primary open angle glaucoma in Cotonou: a series of 224 cases. J Fr Ophthalmol 2012 Feb; 35 (2): 100-5

[18] Abdu L. Epidemiological properties of primary open angle glaucoma in Nigeria. J Ophthalmol 2013; 2013: 402739.doi:10.1155/2013/402739

[19] Lawan A. Pattern of presentation and outcome of surgical management of primary open angle glaucoma in Kan, Northern Nigeria. Ann Afr Med 2001 Dec; 6 (4): 180-5

[20] Adegbehingbe B, Majengbasan T. A review of trabeculectomies at a Nigerian teaching hospital. Ghana Med J 2007 Dec; 41 (4): 176-80

[21] Kim HY, Egbert PR, Singh K. Long- term comparison of primary Trabeculectomy with 5-fluoracil versus mytomycin C in West Africa. J Glaucoma 2008 Oct-Nov; 17 (7): 578-83

[22] Anand N, Mielke C, Dawda VK. Trabeculectomy outcomes in advanced glaucoma in Nigeria. Eye (Lond) 2001 Jun; 15 (Pt): 274-8

[23] Komolafe OO, Ashaye AO, Bekibele CO, et al. Outcome of Trabeculectomy with 5-fluorouracil using releasable suture technique in a Nigerian Tertiary Hospital. West Afr J Med 2011 May-Jun; 30 (3): 173-7

2

The Risk of Infection in Dry Eye Syndrome Accompanying Primary Sjögren's Syndrome

Maria Maślińska and Brygida Kwiatkowska

Abstract

Primary Sjögren's syndrome (pSS) is an autoimmune disease, which dominates the symptoms resulting from inflammatory infiltrates in exocrine glands. Frequently, patients complain of a feeling of sand under the eyelids, eye irritation, and red eye caused by a decrease in tear secretion. The ophthalmic examination beyond lowering the secretion of tears in Schirmer's test evaluation in cases with a significant intensification of dry eye disease (DED) can be visualized by measuring ocular staining score (OSS) using lissamine green and fluorescein staining. OSS can demonstrate the degree of damage to the corneal surface. It is known that keratoconjunctivitis sicca (KCS) in pSS is not only limited to the complaints of unpleasant feeling of sand under the eyelids but also can lead to serious corneal damage and decreased vision even to blindness. And between the others, complications of KCS in pSS must be replaced with an increased susceptibility to infection. We should also pay attention to possible co-infection with Epstein-Barr virus (EBV) virus and bacterial co-infections, e.g., *Chlamydia pneumoniae, Staphylococcus aureus,* or latent conjunctival infections *Chlamydia trachomatis, Mycoplasma hominis,* and *Ureaplasma urealyticum* in group of patients with DED, not only in pSS group. Another issue is simultaneous with hepatitis C virus (HCV) infection coexistance of clinical and laboratory features of Sjogrens syndrome and accompanying this situation clinical signs of KCS. To sum up symptoms of KCS in primary Sjögren's syndrome and in all patients with DED should be evaluated individually and should take into account the increased risk of infection among these patients.

Keywords: dry eye, infection, Sjögren's syndrome

1. Introduction

Primary Sjögren's syndrome (pSS) is an autoimmune disease in which the symptoms resulting from inflammatory infiltrates in exocrine glands dominate. Frequently, patients complain of a feeling of sand under the eyelids, eye irritation, and red eye caused by a decrease in tear secretion. In pSS, other exocrine glands could be affected—among them: salivary glands, pancreas, vaginal mucous membranes, and glands of gastrointestinal tract or situated in bronchial tree. The patient may complain of dry mouth, dry vagina, and inflammation of the gastric and esophageal reflux. Dry cough may also occur. In the course of pSS interstitial changes in the lungs may occur with a progressive reduction of lung function and a failure of cardiovascular system (in conjunction with the development of right ventricular failure and pulmonary hypertension). Autoimmune inflammatory process may also involve peripheral and central nervous system, including cranial nerves, with symptoms of mixed sensory and motor neuropathy or multiple sclerosis (MS)-like symptoms. In pSS, B lymphocytes (B-cells) play a key role, with their hyperreactivity, leading to the overproduction of autoantibodies. Through the interaction between the cells, stimulation reaches T lymphocytes (T-cells), which are the first to form infiltrates in exocrine glands. The gradual destruction of the exocrine glands by the inflammation and by the autoimmune process causes the above- described symptoms [1].

2. Epidemiology

The epidemiology data of dry eye symptom (DES) reveal that it affects from 5 to 35% of the population. Such discrepancy in the assessment of the frequency of the DES occurrence might be the effect of using different dry eye definitions in each of the studies, as well as the research being performed on different ethnic populations. The data given by the Women's Health Study indicate that Hispanics and Asians display greater predisposition to more severe symptoms of dry eye than Caucasians [2]. The incidence of Sjögren's syndrome, in which DES is a dominant symptom, may also be underestimated. There are no accurate records on the prevalence of this disease, with its milder course prone to be undiagnosed [3,4]. It is estimated that pSS occurs in 0.1–3.0% of the general population. The disease is more common for women (female/male ratio 9:1), affecting mainly individuals between the age of 40 and 60, with the disease most frequently occurring around 50 years of age [5].

3. Outline pathogenesis

The pathogenesis of the disease is not entirely clear and factors responsible for its development are still being sought. It is recognized that environmental or endogenous antigens trigger an inflammatory response in susceptible individuals. Among the environmental factors, several viral infections are considered as primary pSS cause: Epstein-Barr virus (EBV), human T-cell lymphotrophic virus type-1 (HTLV-1), cytomegalovirus (CMV), and hepatitis C virus (HCV) [5–7]. These infections may result in the epithelial barrier damage and the release of autoantigens from the affected epithelial cells. In the case of individual genetic predisposition to pSS, the autoimmune process may develop, involving both mechanisms of innate and adaptive immunity. Genetic factors responsible for the predisposition to pSS development include the presence of HLA-B8, HLA-DW3, HLA-DR3, and DRw52 genes; polymorphism of interferon regulatory factor 5 (IRF 5) gene may also play similar role [1,8]. The release of autoantigens triggers innate immunity through the activation of epithelial (EC) and dendritic cells (DC). DC stimulation promotes interferon I and II pathways; DCs also produce IL-12, which activates natural killer cells (NKCs) and stimulates Th1 cells. Both NKC and Th1 cells secrete interferon gamma (INF-γ), responsible for the tissue damage and stimulating the secretion of B cell activation factor (BAFF). BAFF is produced by T and B cells—both activated by DC; BAFF production is also strongly stimulated by interferon (IFN)-α, released by pDC (plasmocytoid dendritic cells). Moreover, the activation of innate response by Toll-like receptors (TLR-9, TLR-7) additionally increases the secretion of BAFF. This overproduction of BAFF can cause constant stimulation of B cells through different pathways and causes the loss of self-tolerance by T and B cells, overproduction of immunoglobulins, of autoantibodies (predominantly SS-A, SS-B) in particular, and the formation of germinal centres (GC) in the target organs. The affected tissues (especially the salivary glands) display the overexpression of cytokines such as tumor necrosis factor (TNF), lymphotoxin, CXC, and chemokines (ligand 13, 9, 21). This process can lead to the development of lymphoma. The occurrence of primarily marginal zone B-cell lymphoma (MZBCL) has been observed in about 8% of pSS patients—40-fold frequency of the MZBCL in the healthy population [9,10]. The scheme of pathogenesis of pSS is shown on figure1.

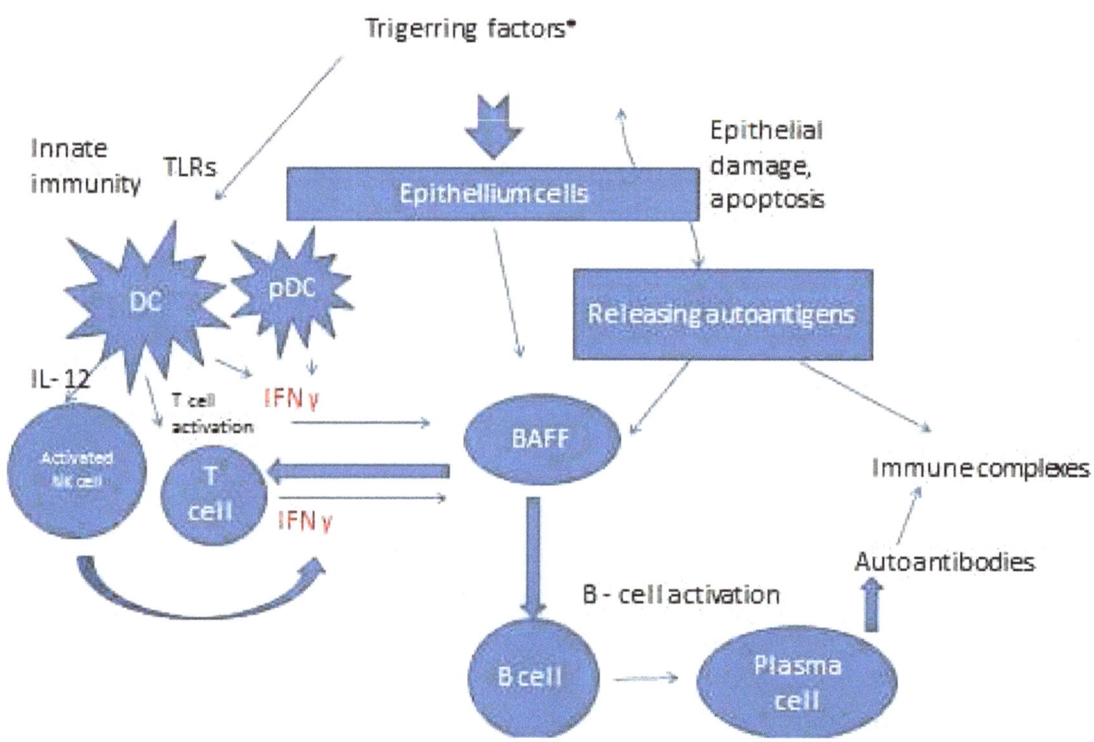

*Triggering factors as viral and bacterial infections, UVA (ultraviolet-A radiation), hormones, genetic predisposition DC-dendritic cell, pDC plasmocytoid DC cell, IFN-γ- interferon gamma, TLRs- Toll-like receptors, IL-12- interleukine 12, TH1-type1 helper cell, BAFF- B cell activating factor, NK-cell natural killer cell

Figure 1. Scheme of pathogenesis [1, 5]

The symptoms of primary Sjögren's syndrome are not homogenous. The autoimmune process involving the epithelium affects many systems and organs, so its manifestations can be very diverse. Symptoms can be divided into two primary groups: common ones, such as dry eyes and mouth, and less frequent symptoms, such as peripheral neuropathy with legs numbness and weakness—with reduced or without reflexes, dysesthesia, feeling of temperature, and vibration. Neurological symptoms may also indicate the seizure of the autonomic nervous system with cardiac arrhythmias or gastrointestinal motility disorder. In the pSS, trigeminal neuralgia and seizure of various nerves ("multiple mononeuropathy") may also occur. The central nervous system can also be involved in pSS therefore myelitis with weakness of limbs and disturbances of urination may occur. Neurological symptoms can also suggest MS, which leads to misdiagnosis. The types of symptoms in pSS are presented in Table 1.

Common symptoms	Less common symptoms/organ involvement
xerophtalmia	intestinal like disease (ILD)
xerostomia	bronchitis
troubles with swallowing	dysphagia, gastrointestinal reflux
dental caries	chronic gastritis
artralgia	symptoms of PBC (primary billary cirrhosis) and AIH
arthritis (non-erosive)	(autoimmune hepatitis)
myalgia	pericarditis
fatigue	pulmonary hypertension
general weakness	celiac-like diseas
weight loss	distal renal tubular acidosis (RTA type 1)
fever	nepritis/glomerulonephritis
Reynaud's phenomenon	chronic renal insufficiency
depression	vasculitis
anxiety	peripheral polyneuropathy,
	cranial neuropathy,
	mononeuritis multiplex
	sensorineural hearing loss
	SM-like syndrome

Table 1. Symptoms of pSS

Keratoconjunctivitis sicca (KCS) is the most frequent cause of complaints from the organ of sight of patients with Sjogren's syndrome, although it can be present in a number of other diseases [11]. KCS is caused by a decreased tear production or increased tear film evaporation. It manifests itself with a feeling of dryness— described as a sandy-gritty eye irritation—burning, stinging, and feeling of tired eyes. In severe cases, the patients suffer from pain, redness, or even decreased vision. The decreased tear production affects the overall reduction of tear secretin as well as limits the aqueous phase of the tears. The causes of DES and complications associated with KCS are presented in Tables 2 and 3.

Primary Sjogren's syndrome may be associated with other autoimmune diseases. Their simultaneous presence can influence both the course and the prognosis of the disease. The most common coexisting diseases are presented in Table 4.

The initial symptoms of an infection in dry eye syndrome—the eye pain, burning, eye redness—can be associated with symptoms of dryness and aseptic KCS, as well as with an incipient infection. However, when the pain and red eye are accompanied by a purulent excretion—a bacterial infection should be suspected. Viral infections primarily cause an eye pain and intense redness. These symptoms may also be associated with general symptoms of infections such as muscle pain, fever, and fatigue. The diagnosis and treatment are determined by the result of the ophthalmological examination.

Keratoconjunctivitis sicca symptoms – conditions and diseases	
Environmental factors as dust, smoke, dry air, aircondition,	Allergic conjunctivitis
Behavior : working at the computer, watching television	Sarcoidosis
long - causing less frequent blinking	Lymphoma
Contact lenses	Graft versus host disease (GvHD)
Age - related dry eye (ARDE)	Autoimmune deficiency (AIDS)
Menopause (low level of estrogens)	Diabetes
Using drugs : antihistamines, β-blockers, diuretics,	Trachoma (cause chlamydia trachomatis)
antispasmodics,	VII cranial nerve damage
diuretics, psychotropic	Meibomian gland dysfunction
Vitami A deficiency	Reflex motor block (central demage of VII cranial nerve)
	Reflex sensory block (trigeminal nerve denervation)
Refractive surgery : laser assisted keratomileusis (LASIK); photorefractive keratoplasty (PRK)	

Table 2. Keratoconjunctivitis sicca —not only symptom of pSS

Eye problems in primary Sjögren's syndrome
discomfort
pain
red eye
conjunctivitis
corneal erosions,
filamentary keratitis,
corneal ulcers
decreased vision

Table 3. Eye complications associated with KCS

The diseases coexisting with p SS
Autoimmune Thyroid Disease (AITD) - Haschimoto disease
Intestinal Lung Disease (ILD)
Primary Billary Cirrhosis (PBC)
Autoimmune hepatitis (AIH)
Cryoglobulinemia
Autoimmune pancreatitis (AIP)
Distal renal tubular acidosis (RTA)
Sclerosis-multiplex like syndrome

Table 4. The diseases coexisting with p SS

4. Risk of eye infections in KCS

The conjunctivitis and changes in the cornea in the pSS are aseptic, yet coexisting infections that may play a part in the development and course of the pSS, KCS in particular. Due to the large differences in estimating the incidence and prevalence of dry eye syndrome (from 5 to 35%) and due to differences in the frequency of recognition of Sjögren's syndrome, it is difficult to accurately estimate the rate of incidence of sicca syndrome associated with eye infections. However, impaired humidification of the eye and related development of KCS undoubtedly significantly increase the risk of bacterial contamination, compared with the normal population.

Among viral infections, EBV plays an important role, which is not limited to the above-mentioned impact on the immune system and lymphocytes. The EBV may be a separate, independent cause of the dry eye syndrome because the infection affects mucosal surfaces and lymphoid tissues. The EBV presence persists in ocular surface epithelia, following primary infection and may cause dacryoadenitis, which leads to abnormal tear secretion [12,13]. Although no direct link between the occurrence of KCS and EBV infection has been established, the influence of EBV on patient's immune status could cause the development of symptoms of dryness. Apart from EBV, other viral infections, which may contribute to the occurrence of KCS and clinical picture of Sjogren's disease, include in particular HCV, human T-cell lymphotropic virus (HTLV), Human (HSV-1), and HIV [7,14]. HCV infection may be responsible for the incidence of ocular symptoms in the course of pSS, such as KCS retinopathy, scleritis, and keratitis. In HSV-1 infection, besides KCS, keratitis, blepharitis, conjunctivitis, uveitis, and retinitis may develop [15]. Viral agents involved in pathogenesis of pSS, EBV in particular, can be simultaneously responsible for causing KCS, conjunctivitis, and reducing resistance of the corneal epithelium.

Although viruses play a significant role in the pathogenesis of pSS, the importance of bacterial co-infections, e.g., *Chlamydia pneumonia* in the course of pSS should not be underestimated [16]. It is known that a tear film has antimicrobial properties, whereas the normal ocular surface contains bacterial flora, including *Staphylococcus epidermidis*, *S. aureus*, and diphteroides (e.g.,

Corynebacterium diphtheriae and *Propionibacterium acnes*). However, in patients with DESs and treated with immunosuppressants, such therapy, along with dryness and cornea damage, results in increased susceptibility to common bacterial infections. In the diagnosis of ocular symptoms, bacterial keratitis should come under consideration. This may more likely be caused by *S. aureus*, *Haemophilus influenzae*, *Streptococcus pneumoniae* and, in the case of use of contact lenses, more often *Pseudomonas aeruginosa*. Hori et al. [17] showed that infections with bacteria resistant to fluoroquinolones (*Staph.* sp. *Staph. aureus*) are more common in patients with dry eye syndrome, although among dry eye patients, regardless of use of punctual plugs or topical steroids, there were no differences in bacteria isolated from conjunctiva.

In the diagnosis of pSS, it must also be considered that some of the commonly known infections, such as HIV, tuberculosis, leprosy, spirochetes, hepatitis A, B, or C, parvovirus B19, Dengue fever, malaria, subacute bacterial endocarditis, and HIV can mimic Sjögren's syndrome with symptoms of eye dryness. Prognosis for the infection occurring in the course of a dry eye in Sjögren's syndrome is more serious compared to the infection cases with no additional risk factors present. This results from the, pre-existing in Sjögren's syndrome, surface damage and use of immunosuppressive therapy in this disease. Therefore, patients with Sjögren's syndrome and a coexisting bacterial infection of the eye belong to a group in which immediate antibiotic therapy should be considered.

5. Cicatrizing conjunctivitis as complication of dry eye disorders

In course of pSS, a slow progressive cicatrizing conjunctivitis (PCC) may also develop with complications such as an impairment of vision (and even blindness), pain, and corneal damage. Cicatrizing is a type of scarring, which can occur as a complication of dry eye accompanied by autoimmune diseases like Sjögren's syndrome or ocular cicatrical pemphigoid. Chronic conjunctival cicatrization (CCC) can also occur as an effect of thermal and chemical burns, postinfectious conjunctivitis, ocular rosacea, atopic keratitis, graft versus host disease, and Stevens-Johnson syndrome (in the latter case prognosis being particularly poor) [18,19]. The presence of cicatrizing conjunctivitis predisposes to microbial keratitis, especially in Sjögren's syndrome. Ormerod et al. [20] described that almost 50% of studied Sjögren's syndrome patients had microbial keratitis as a complication of sterile ulcerations and were subject to recurrent infections. Most common infection in that group was Gram-positive bacteria such as *S. aureus*. It was also noted that patients with conjunctival cicatrization (CC) in the course of Sjögren's syndrome had higher complication rate compared to those in which CC was caused by other factors; such complications included corneal perforation, endophthalmitis, and descementocele. Interestingly, the authors also point out that a long-term therapy with topical corticosteroids and application of bandage contact lenses used in refractive surgery enhanced a risk of microbial keratitis.

Treatment strategies in CC depend on the cause of the underlying disease. In case of microbial keratitis, topical antibiotic use is recommended.

6. Diagnosis criteria of Sjogren's syndrome

Over the years (since 2002), pSS recognition has been based on the criteria set by American-European Consensus Group (AECG) in which both Schirmer's test and tear break-up time (BUT) results are assessed. According to former pSS criteria, the examination of salivary secretory function was assessed by measuring minute salivation and evaluation in sialography. From 2012, the American College of Rheumatology (ACR) has proposed new diagnostic criteria that are presented in Table 5 [21–23].

Sjögren's Syndrome criteria ACR 2012
1. Positive serum anti-SSA/Ro and/or anti-SSB/La or positive rheumatoid factor and ANA titer 1:320
2. Labial salivary gland biopsy exhibiting focal lymphocytic sialadenitis with a focus score 1 focus/4 mm^2
3. Ocular staining score 3 proving keratoconjunctivitis sicca *
Exclusions: Head and neck radiation treatment Active Hepatitis C infection Acquired immunodeficiency syndrome Sarcoidosis Amyloidosis Graft versus host disease (GVHD) IgG4-related disease (IgG4-RD)
*Excluding the patients using daily eye drops for glaucoma and who has had corneal surgery or cosmetic eyelid surgery in the last 5 years

Table 5. Diagnostic criteria of Sjögren's syndrome

It was found that most changes associated with KCS can be demonstrated using the Lissamine green and fluorescein stainings. Both stainings are used for establishing ocular staining score (OSS), determined for each eye separately and used to identify the degree of change in the conjunctiva (Lissamine green) as well as the damage to the cornea (fluorescein) [21]. The slit lamp examination reveals damage to the cornea, but using staining allows for a quantitative and qualitative assessment of these changes. Another test which can be useful in the evaluation of dry eye is a tear osmolality test. However, this test is not included in the criteria for pSS diagnosis [24,25].

The newly proposed criteria also apply to the early stage of diagnosis, when no evidence of the presence of autoantibodies for ribonucleoproteins anti-Ro (SS-A) and anti-La (SS-B) is available. In such a case, the mutual presence of rheumatoid factor (RF) and of antinuclear antibody (ANA, the latter in titer of no less than 1: 320) proves the diagnosis [25].

The important part of establishing pSS diagnosis is confirming the presence of typical changes in histopathology material from minor salivary gland biopsy (MSGB)— mononuclear inflammatory cells form focal infiltrates of more than 50 cells in 4 mm^2 of glandular section. The so-called focus score (FS) is based on the assessment of number of such changes in the tested material. The presence of one or more foci is considered as a positive result. Primary Sjogren's syndrome may be accompanied by other than SS-A, SS-B, or RF autoantibodies [26,27]. Most common pSS-specific antibodies, also associated with other autoimmune diseases, are presented in Table 6.

Autoantibodies in pSS
diagnostic hallmark:
Anti SS-A (Ro)
Anti-SS-B (La)
Autoantibodies in pSS and other autoimmune diseases:
Antinuclear antibodies (ANAs)
Rheumatoid factors (RF)
Anti-centromere antibodies (ACA) (systemic sclerosis)
Anti-mitochondrial antibodies (AMA) - Primary biliary cirrhosis
Anti-cyclic citrullinated peptide antibodies (anti-CCP)
anti-smooth muscle antibodies (ASMA) Autoimmune hepatitis
dsDNA (systemic lupus erythematosus)
Anti- thyreoglobulin (anti TG) – autoimmune thyroiditis
Anti-thyroid peroxidase (anti-TPO)- autoimmune thyroiditis
Novel autoantibodies:
Anti-M3R antibodies
Anti- β fodrin
Anti - protein 1 (SP-1),
Anti - carbonic anhydrase 6 (CA6)
Anti-parotid secretory protein (PSP)

Table 6. Autoantibodies in pSS

Several laboratory tests prove helpful in the diagnosis of pSS, although they do not constitute a part of the present diagnostic pSS criteria. In particular, the deviations in the composition of blood cells and proteins occur and the increased erythrocyte sedimentation rate (ESR) with normal or low concentrations of CRP (a similar situation may exist in multiple myeloma) may be present. Laboratory findings in pSS are presented in Table 7.

Laboratory findings in pSS
Elevated erythrocyte sedimentation rate (ESR),
leucopenia,
anemia
low platelet count
Hypergammaglobulinemia (polyclonal),
ANAs, RF, anti-Ro/SS-A, anti-B/SSB,
decreased level of complement component C4

Table 7. Laboratory findings in pSS

Llissamine green (conjunctiva)		Fluoresceine (cornea)	
grade	dots	grade	dots
0	0-9	0	0
1	10-32	1	1-5
2	33- 100	2	6- 30
3	> 100	3	> 30

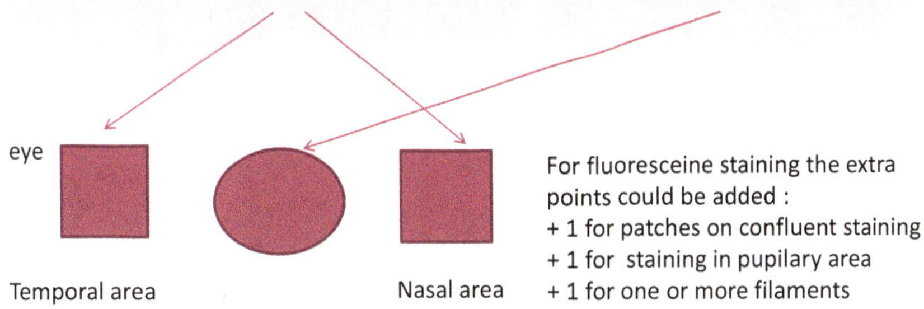

Figure 2. Sicca ocular staining score [25]

7. Prognosis

The emergence of pSS carries an increased risk (by 40 times – comparing to the normal population) of lymphoma development. This imposes necessity of regular monitoring and assessment in pSS of factors/markers determining patient's total capacity for developing lymphoma, including the emergence of cryoglobulins, rheumatoid factor (if previously not present) or of monoclonal proteins, chronic enlargement of the salivary glands, or persistent presence of general symptoms, such as weight loss, fever, and lymphadenopathy.

7.1. Eye examinations for the diagnosis of KCS and pSS

The ophthalmic examination includes first of all a well-known Schirmer's test used to evaluate the extent of decrease in the tear secretion.

In the case of significant intensity of dry eye syndrome, the damage to the cornea can be visualized by applying lissamine green and fluorescein staining [28]. This scoring system has been proposed for the evaluation of KCS in Sjögren's syndrome, but applies in general to the changes in the course of dry eye.

The scoring rules are illustrated in Figure 2, and photographs of eye examination in Figures 3 and 4.

The maximum score for each eye is 12. Scoring more than 3 and higher indicates KCS.

The previous AECG pSS diagnosis criteria consisted, in addition to the Schirmer's test, in other tests confirming the presence of KCS and lacrimation disorder, with Bengal rose staining among the most frequently used. This test allows for the assessment of scaly, dead cells of the corneal epithelium, and conjunctiva as well as mucus particles (filaments) fixed to the corneal

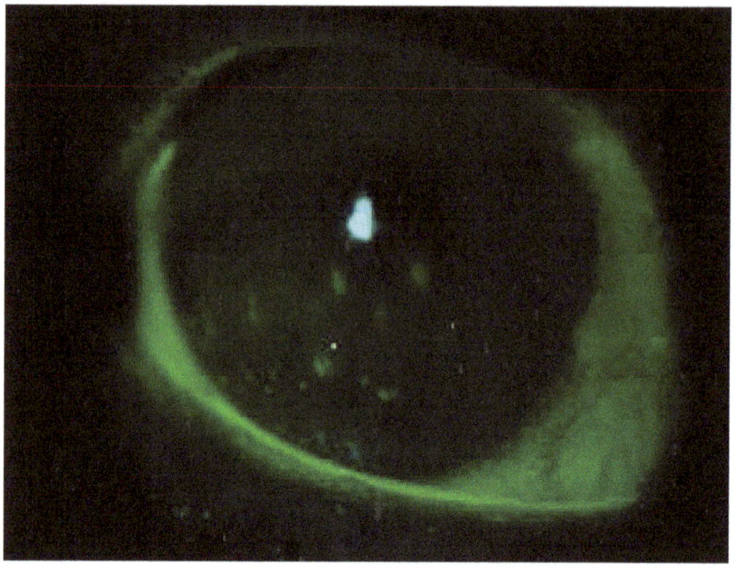

Figure 3. Fluorescein staining

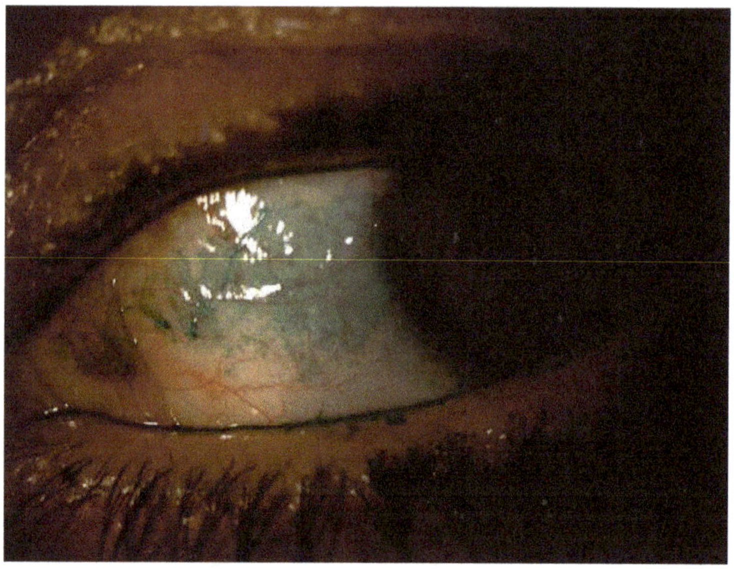

Figure 4. Lissamine green staining

surface, associated with the dry eye syndrome. The results of rose Bengal staining, however, are dose-dependent and cause phototoxicity. The lissamine green dye is less irritating and thus considered better for such use. The quality and quantity of the tear film can be evaluated using tear film break up time (T-BUT)—assessing the time interval between the last complete blink and the first appearance of a dry spot or of disruption of the tear film, observed in the slit lamp. The extension of this test uses fluorescein (F-BUT) staining. The diagnosis of DES is established with BUT result ≤5 seconds. The limitations of this test are eye irritation and increased blink after fluorescein application as well as difficulty in meeting the condition that the patient can blink freely [28].

7.2. Own research

In our study, 30 patients—22 females (73%), 8 males (27%) in mean age of 52 years (from 22 to 85)—diagnosed with pSS revealed stronger correlation of the Schirmer's test results with FS than with OSS. The correlation coefficient of OSS with ANA, anti–SS-A, RF was higher than that of Schirmer's test with anti–SS-A and RF. OSS correlated negatively with Schirmer's test results (r= −0.54; p=0.007). There were no differences between female and male subjects in the Schirmer's test, a group of male patients presented more pronounced symptoms of ocular dryness in the evaluation of staining scores. Our results suggest that the Schirmer's test reflects the intensity of ocular gland infiltration by inflammatory cells, whereas immunostaining proposed in the new Sjögren's syndrome criteria is more closely associated with the immunoactivity and autoantibodies production. It is obvious that the observed correlation requires further support and analysis of research performed on a more numerous group of patients.

7.2.1. Statistical analysis

Correlation analyses were performed with the Spearman correlation coefficient (because of the non-normal distribution of variables). The study was approved by the Bioethics Commission of the Institute of Rheumatology; the subjects have signed written informed consent statements. The study was supported by National Science Center (Narodowe Centrum Nauki) —grant no. 2012/05/N/NZ5/02838. The correlations are shown in Table 8.

Correlations	Correlation coefficient (Spearman test) N=30
OSS mean– SS-A	0,17
OSS mean– SS- B	0,00
OSS mean – FS	0,13
OSS mean – RF	0,04
OSS mean – ANA	-0,16
Schirmer's test mean – SS-A	-0,10
Schirmer's test mean – SS-B	0,14
Schirmer's test mean – FS	0,07
Schirmer's test mean – RF	0,20
test Schirmera średnia – ppj	-0,01
SA-A – SS-B	0,56
OSS mean – Schirmer's test mean	-0,54
Ro – FS	0,04
Ro – RF	0,20
Ro – ppj	0,25
La – FS	0,07
La – RF	0,20
La – ppj	0,27

Table 8. Correlations in patients group with pSS

The data were presented at the 3rd International Congress on Controversies in Rheumatology and Autoimmunity in 2014 [29]. Toker et al. [30] also studied the presence of anti–SS/A and anti–SS/B antibodies in tears and serum as well as assessed the correlations between subjective and objective clinical score of dry eye (then performed Schirmer's test, TBUT test, and rose Bengal staining). This study demonstrated that serum titer of anti-Ro/SSA and anti-La/SSB correlated positively with DESs and negatively with tear production.

7.3. Treatment of pSS

1. Systemic treatment of Sjogren's syndrome

The therapy of autoimmune diseases, such as pSS, is based on the elimination of inflammation and inhibition of stimulation of the immune system. Initially, immunosuppressant drugs, such as corticosteroids, methotrexate, cyclosporine A, and azathioprine are applied. For years, the effectiveness and relevance of applying antimalaria drugs for the treatment of pSS have been debated [31–33]. A number of studies confirm beneficial effects of this drug on the symptoms of dryness and the reduction of BAFF in patients with pSS without significant internal organ involvement [32–34]. In severe cases with life threatening organ involvement, the use of cyclophosphamide, infusions of immunoglobulins, and plasmapheresis are considered necessary.

In the case of renal tubular acidosis, sodium and/or potassium are administered. Considering the role of B cells in pSS, monoclonal anti-CD20 (rituximab RTX) antibodies seem to be a favorable option for therapy. RTX has already shown efficacy in the treatment of rheumatoid arthritis, SLE, and vasculitis [35–37]. The full effectiveness of other biologic drugs causing the depletion of B cells—such as Belimumab (BLyS/BAFF inhibitor) and epratuzumab (humanized anti-CD22 monoclonal antibody)—has not yet been confirmed in pSS treatment [38]. The purpose of the therapy could also be the inhibition of interferon alpha and gamma (IFN-α and IFN-γ) involved in the stimulation of B cells, but this course of therapy requires further study.

Currently, the use of mesenchymal stem cell (MSC) transplantation as a method of treatment of various autoimmune diseases, including Sjogren's syndrome, is also being contemplated [39].

2. Topical treatment—the fight against dryness

Apart from the systemic treatment, no less important for pSS patients is local treatment and alleviation of dryness symptoms. Firstly, in the case of dry eye, the influence of exacerbating factors, such as dryness, dust, long hours of working with computer, and smoking, should be limited. It is recommended to use artificial tears during the day and lubricant ointment at night. Agents used as preservatives in medical drops, even those in moisturizers- among them: benzalkonium chloride (BAK) and disodium (EDTA) pose another problem [40]. The use of over-the-counter (OTC) drops with a higher dose of preservatives increases the symptoms of dryness [41].

The wide array of medications is being used in topical treatment: eye lubricants and moisturizers, such as drops, gels, ointments containing tear substitutes, oils and petrolatum, acrylic acid, hyaluronic acid, glycerin, erythritol, levocarnitine, hydroxymethylcellose, carboxymethylcelulose, or glycol. The preparations without preservatives that replace tears include, e.g., Refresh (Allergan), TheraTears, Soothe (Bausch + Lomb), and System (Alcon) [41].

Ocular lubricants and moisturizers are designed to supplement the shortage of tears, osmolarity, and to improve tear film stability and act protectively. A patient with severe DES both in the course of PSS and from other causes, however, should consult the use of these substances with an ophthalmologist. Increasing the amount of tears can be achieved by permanent occluding of nasolacrimal channel and by the use of biological tear substitutes, namely a drop of the patient's own serum. The inflammatory process in the course KCS also requires anti-inflammatory therapy with cyclosporine drops and topical glucocorticoids. Research is being conducted on the use of pimecrolimus and tacrolimus as immunomodulatory drugs in drops. Also drugs stimulating tear secretion with cholinergic agonists are being used and two of them, namely pilocarpine and cevimeline, are used widely. Currently, studies are being carried out on other stimulants, among others diquafosol (P2Y2 receptor agonist) and rebamipide [42,43].

Tetracyclines (minocycline, tetracycline) might also be considered as important drugs for pSS therapy, showing both antibacterial and immunomodulating effect. They have greater than just antimicrobial effect on inflammation by inhibiting the proinflammatory cytokines as TNF or interleukin-1 (IL-1) and also inhibiting angiogenesis. They have been applied to treat eye infections, ocular and skin manifestations of acne rosacea and are used in the case of meibomian gland dysfunction [44]. In the case of complications of bacterial infection in the course of KCS, typical antibiotics covering the activities of most common pathogens are being used. These include aminoglycosides (e.g., Tobramycin), macrolides, fluoroquinolones, sodium sulfacetamide, or trimethoprim/polymyxin. While wearing contact lenses is as a possible cause of dry eye, in the treatment of DES contact lenses made of special materials such as silicone rubber and highly oxygen permeable materials may protect the eye from drying [45,46].

The surgical treatment, including placement of punctual plugs (collagen or silicone) and cauterization of the puncta, is used in cases of severe corneal injuries and at a risk of a loss of vision. The transplantation of minor salivary glands is an interesting and promising method, but so far with limited use as a therapeutic option [47]. The salivary glands are transplanted as a complex graft to the posterior lamella of the eyelids to increase an ocular surface lubrication and reduce a discomfort in dry eyes.

Frequent blinking is also important for the prophylaxis and complementary action treatment for symptoms of dry eye; avoiding situations that increase the evaporation of the tear film (e.g. wind, air conditioning, and smoking) is recommended as well. The patients with pSS and symptoms of dry eye should be controlled both by a rheumatologist and an ophthalmologist. Routine check of a dry eye should take place at least once every 3 months. However ophthalmologic monitoring frequency will depend on the severity of DESs and the presence of dry eye complications, such as infections. In the latter case, the control should be performed every few days until the infection is cured. The aim of the topical therapy is to eliminate symptoms of dryness and to directly protect mucous membranes. The systemic treatment is directed at achieving a remission—the inhibition of the disease progress, changes in internal organs, and inflammation and infiltration of exocrine glands.

8. Summary

The Sjögren's syndrome is one of the most common rheumatic diseases with predominant symptoms of dryness, particularly of the eye. Therefore, the knowledge on dry eye disease or KCS symptoms is essential not only for ophthalmologic but also for rheumatologic practice. The above section certainly does not exhaust the problem of Sjögren's syndrome, its intricate and still uncertain pathogenesis and a differentiated clinical picture. The author's intention was primarily to draw attention to the problem of DESs and associated complications, including infections.

Author details

Maria Maślińska* and Brygida Kwiatkowska

*Address all correspondence to: maslinskam@gmail.com

Early Arthritis Clinic, National Institute of Geriatrics, Rheumatology and Rehabilitation the name of Prof. Eleonora Reicher, Warsaw, Poland

References

[1] Youinou P, Pers JO. Disturbance of cytokine networks in Sjögren's syndrome. Arthritis Res Ther. 2011;13:227.

[2] McCarty CA, Bansal AK, Livingston PM, Stanislavsky YL, Taylor HR. The epidemiology of dry eye in Melbourne, Australia. Ophthalmology. 1998;105(6):1114–9.

[3] Viso E, Rodriguez-Ares MT, Gude F. Prevalence of and associated factors for dry eye in a Spanish adult population (the Salnes Eye Study). Ophthalmic Epidemiol. 2009;16(1):15–21. doi: 10.1080/09286580802228509.

[4] Lee AJ, Lee J, Saw SM, Gazzard G, Koh D, Widjaja D, Tan DT. Prevalence and risk factors associated with dry eye symptoms: a population based study in Indonesia. Br J Ophthalmol. 2002;86(12):1347–51.

[5] Maślińska M, Przygodzka M, Kwiatkowska B, Sikorska-Siudek K Sjögren's syndrome: still not fully understood disease Rheumatol Int. 2015 ;35:233–41 DOI 10.1007/s00296-014-3072-5

[6] Slobod KS, Sandlund JT, Spiegel PH et al. Molecular evidence of ocular Epstein-Barr virus infection. Clin Infect Dis. 2000;31(1):184–8.

[7] Pinheiro SR, Martins-Filho OA, Ribas JG, Catalan-Soares BC, Proietti FA, Namen-Lopes S, et al. Immunologic markers, uveitis, and keratoconjunctivitis sicca associated with human T-cell lymphotropic virus type 1. Am J Ophthalmol. 2006;142(5):811–5.

[8] Miceli-Richard C, Comets E, Loiseau P, Puechal X, Hachulla E, Mariette X. Association of an IRF5 gene functional polymorphism with Sjögren's syndrome. Arthritis Rheum. 2007;56(12):3989–94.

[9] Huang YF, Cheng Q, Jiang CM, et al. The immune factors involved in the pathogenesis, diagnosis, and treatment of Sjogren's syndrome. Clin Dev Immunol. Vol. 2013(2013). Article ID 160491. doi: 10.1155/2013/160491

[10] Baimpa E, Dahabreh IJ, Voulgarelis M, Moutsopoulos HM. Hematologic manifestations and predictors of lymphoma development in primary Sjögren syndrome: clinical and pathophysiologic aspects. Medicine (Baltimore) 2009; 88(5):284–293.

[11] Lemp MA. Report of the National Eye Institute/Industry Workshop on Clinical Trials in Dry Eyes. CLAO J. 1995;21(4):221–32.

[12] Merayo-Lloves J, Baltatzis S, Foster CS. Epstein-Barr virus dacryoadenitis resulting in keratoconjunctivitis sicca in a child. Am J Ophthalmol. 2001;132(6):922–3.

[13] Rhem MN, Wilhelmus KR, Jones DB. Epstein-Barr virus dacryoadenitis. Am J Ophthalmol. 2000;129(3):372–5.

[14] Bekele S, Gelaw Y, Tessema F. Ocular manifestation of HIV/AIDS and correlation with CD4+ cells count among adult HIV/AIDS patients in Jimma town, Ethiopia: a cross sectional study. BMC Ophthalmol. 2013;27;13:20. doi: 10.1186/1471-2415-13-20.

[15] Alves M, Angerami RN, Rocha EM. Dry eye disease caused by viral infection: review. Arq Bras Oftalmol. 2013;76(2):129–32.

[16] Krásny J, Hrubá D, Netuková M. The role of Chlamydia pneumoniae in the etiology of keratoconjunctivitis sicca (KCS). Recent Pat Inflamm Allergy Drug Discov. 2014;8(3):216–22.

[17] Hori Y1, Maeda N, Sakamoto M, Koh S, Inoue T, Tano Y. Bacteriologic profile of the conjunctiva in the patients with dry eye. Am J Ophthalmol. 2008 Nov;146(5):729-34. doi: 10.1016/j.ajo.2008.06.003. Epub 2008 Jul 30.

[18] Faraj HG, Hoang-Xuan T. Chronic cicatrizing conjunctivitis. Curr Opin Ophthalmol. 2001;12(4):250–7.

[19] Rashida S, Danaa M. Cicatrizing and autoimmune diseases. Chem Immunol Allergy. Basel, Karger, 2007 (92):195–202.

[20] Ormerod LD, Fong LP, Foster CS. Corneal infection in mucosal Scarring Disorders and Sjogren's syndrome. Am J Ophthalmology 1988;105:512–18.

[21] Shiboski SC, Shiboski CH, Criswell L, et al. American College of Rheumatology classification criteria for Sjögren's syndrome: a data-driven, expert consensus approach

in the Sjögren's International Collaborative Clinical Alliance cohort. Arthritis Care Res (Hoboken) 2012;64(4):475–87.

[22] Vitali C, Bootsma H, Bowman SJ, et al. Classification criteria for Sjögren's syndrome: we actually need to definitively resolve the long debate on the issue. Ann Rheum Dis. 2013;72:476–78.

[23] Rasmussen A, Ice JA, Li H, et al. Comparison of the American-European Consensus Group Sjögren's syndrome classification criteria to newly proposed American College of Rheumatology criteria in a large, carefully characterized sicca cohort. Ann Rheum Dis 2014;73(1): 31- 8. doi:10.1136/annrheumdis-2013-203845

[24] Tomlinson A. 2007. DEWS Report, Ocular Surface April 2007 Vol 5 No 2.

[25] Rose-Nussbaumer J, Lietman TM, Shiboski CH, et al. Sjögren's International Collaborative Clinical Alliance Research Groups. Inter-grader Agreement of the Ocular Staining Score in the Sjögren's International Clinical Collaborative Alliance (SICCA) registry. Am J Ophthalmol. 2015 ; 21. pii: S0002-9394(15)00515-2. doi: 10.1016/j.ajo. 2015.08.021. [Epub ahead of print].

[26] Kyriakidis NC, Kapsogeorgou EK, Tzioufas AG. A comprehensive review of autoantibodies in primary Sjogren's syndrome: clinical phenotypes and regulatory mechanisms. J Autoimmun 2003; 51C:67–74.

[27] Shen L, Suresh L, Lindemann M, et al. Novel autoantibodies in Sjogren's syndrome. Clin Immunol 2012;145(3):251–255.

[28] Whitcher JP, Shiboski CH, Shiboski SC, et al. Sjögren's International Collaborative Clinical Alliance Research Groups. A simplified quantitative method for assessing keratoconjunctivitis sicca from the Sjögren's syndrome International Registry. Am J Ophthalmol. 2010;149(3):405–15. doi: 10.1016/j.ajo.2009.09.013. Epub 2009 Dec 29.

[29] Maślińska M. Szymczak – Mikołowska. The degree of correlation between ocular tests, autoantibodies presence and salivary gland inflammatory infiltration in primary Sjögren's syndrome. Index No.260 3rd International Congress on Controversies in Rheumatology and Autoimmunity in 2014.

[30] Toker E, Yavuz S, Direskeneli H.Anti-Ro/SSA and anti-La/SSB autoantibodies in the tear fluid of patients with Sjögren's syndrome. Br J Ophthalmol. 2004;88:384–87.

[31] Bron JB, Abelson BM, Ousler G, et al. Methodologies to diagnose and monitor dry eye disease: Report of the Diagnostic Methodology Subcommittee of the International Dry Eye Workshop. Ocul Surf. 2007;5(2):108–52.

[32] Mumcu G, Biçakçigil M, Yilmaz N, Ozay H, Karaçayli U, Cimilli H, Yavuz S. Salivary and serum B-cell activating factor (BAFF) levels after hydroxychloroquine treatment in primary Sjögren's syndrome. Oral Health Prev Dent. 2013;11(3):229–34. doi: 10.3290/j.ohpd.a30172.

[33] Yavuz S1, Asfuroğlu E, Bicakcigil M, Toker E. Hydroxychloroquine improves dry eye symptoms of patients with primary Sjogren's syndrome. Rheumatol Int. 2011;31(8):1045–9. doi: 10.1007/s00296-010-1415-4. Epub 2010 Mar 23.

[34] Rihl M1, Ulbricht K, Schmidt RE, Witte T. Treatment of sicca symptoms with hydroxychloroquine in patients with Sjogren's syndrome. Rheumatology (Oxford). 2009;48(7):796–9. doi: 10.1093/rheumatology/kep104. Epub 2009 May 11.

[35] Chen S, Liu Y, Shi G. Anti-CD20 antibody in primary Sjögren's syndrome management. Curr Pharm Biotechnol. 2014;15(6):535–41.

[36] St Clair EW, Levesque MC, Prak ET, Vivino FB, Alappatt CJ, Spychala ME, Wedgwood J, McNamara J, Moser Sivils KL, Fisher L, Cohen P. Autoimmunity Centers of Excellence. Rituximab therapy for primary Sjögren's syndrome: an open-label clinical trial and mechanistic analysis. Arthritis Rheum. 2013;65(4):1097–106. doi: 10.1002/art.37850.

[37] Vossenkämper A, Lutalo PM, Spencer J Translational Mini-Review Series on B cell subsets in disease. Transitional B cells in systemic lupus erythematosus and Sjögren's syndrome: clinical implications and effects of B cell-targeted therapies. Clin Exp Immunol. 2012; 167(1):7–14.

[38] Steinfeld SD, Tant L, Burmester GR et al. Epratuzumab (humanised anti-CD22 antibody) in primary Sjögren's syndrome: an open-label phase I/II study. Arthritis Res Ther. 2006;8(4):R129.

[39] Xu J, Wang D, Liu D, Fan Z, et al. Allogeneic mesenchymal stem cell treatment alleviates experimental and clinical Sjögren syndrome. Blood 2012;120(15):3142–51.

[40] Sarkar J, Chaudhary, Namavari A, et al. Corneal neurotoxicity due to topical benzalkonium chloride. Invest Ophthalmol Vis Sci. 2012;53(4):1792–802.

[41] Stephenson M. OTC Drops: Telling the Tears Apart. When choosing an over-the-counter artificial tear for your dry-eye patient, consider severity of disease and form of dry eye. Rev Ophtalmol. 2012; 19 (10):31-37. www.reviewofophthalmology.com/content/i/2133/c/36940/

[42] Keating GM. Diquafosol ophthalmic solution 3 %: a review of its use in dry eye. Drugs. 2015;75(8):911–22. doi: 10.1007/s40265-015-0409-7.

[43] Ueda K, Matsumiya W, Otsuka K, Maeda Y, Nagai T, Nakamura M. Effectiveness and relevant factors of 2% rebamipide ophthalmic suspension treatment in dry eye. BMC Ophthalmol. 2015;15:58. doi: 10.1186/s12886-015-0040-0.

[44] Kwiatkowska B, Maslinska M, Przygodzka M, Dmowska-Chalaba J, Dabrowska J, Sikorska-Siudek K. Immune system as a new therapeutic target for antibiotics. Adv Biosci Biotechnol. 2013;4:91–101.

[45] Bacon AS, Astin C, Dart JK. Silicone rubber contact lenses for the compromised cornea. Cornea. 1994;13(5):422–8.

[46] Romero-Rangel T, Stavrou P, Cotter J, Rosenthal P, Baltatzis S, Foster CS. Gas-permeable scleral contact lens therapy in ocular surface disease. Am J Ophthalmol. 2000;130(1):25–32.

[47] Geerling G, Raus P, Murube J. Minor salivary gland transplantation. Dev Ophthalmol. 2008;41:243–54. doi: 10.1159/000131093.

3

Analysis of the Disturbances Caused by Intraocular Forced Convection Mechanism Failure

Humberto D. Silva, Eduardo D. Silva,
Maria Tamires D. Silva, Cristiana P. Dória and
Cristiane P. Dória

Abstract

In this chapter, we show the refractive error treatment result of a patient, the first author, who restarted in 2000, after a 4-year break, at the study start. According to previous publications, the treatment consists of rehydration and elimination of agglutinated, dehydrated and deposited metabolic residues in the cornea, the trabecular meshwork, the crystalline lens and the retina, as a consequence of the failure in the mechanism of intraocular mass transfer by forced convection. However, the forced movement of the metabolic mass to rehydrate one region can cause dehydration in another region. Therefore, the patient developed posterior and capsular cataract in their respective eyes, right and left. This dehydration, during the treatment, increases the difficulties for the success of the treatment. The first part is a chronological record of the most important components of the treatment. Then, the research method and the material used are discussed. The main symptoms and signs are analyzed and correlated with the failure of the mass transfer process and the accumulation of metabolic residues. The anatomy of binocular vision is analyzed as a part of the forced convection mechanism, and in conclusion, the report shows the main oculomotor functions, topographic mapping of corneas over an interval of 17 months.

Keywords: cataract, glaucoma, saccadic movement, torsional movement, refractive error, uveitis, floaters

1. Introduction

The research began in 1996 when the first author (will be called the patient) realized that after 4 h of working on a computer, his vision was blurred and, after performing other activities, the view was retrieved. Then, the patient realized the possibility of regaining his vision, which was showing the beginning of the symptoms of presbyopia. The patient presented visual acuity OD 6/10 and OS 9/10 and corrective lenses NV, OD +0.25 and OS +0.75. Work interruption occurred in the same year due to anterior recurrent uveitis of unknown cause in the left eye, which increased the intraocular pressure to 40 mmHg in the first crisis. Two years before the start on this study, the patient had his first two cases of uveitis, but the most important crisis occurred after the study began and the patient took a few days to get medical help. To control intraocular pressure, the patient received three intraocular injection on alternate days. Even with the patient's narrative that he did not feel well, the doctor reduced the dosage of medications. The patient still felt pain when pressing the left eye in the superior nasal position through the superior eyelid. The patient returned to the doctor after 2 days, having noticed the blurred image in the left eye. The physician diagnosed the recurrence of uveitis and intraocular pressure at 40 mmHg. At the end of treatment, the pain in the sclera did not exist. Many other painful inflammations had occurred in the left eye, but at this early stage, physicians consulted in Brazil and France did not prescribe any treatment. Treatment was started the next day after uveitis was diagnosed. At that time when the pain symptom occurred in the sclera, the patient used a medication eye-drop prescribed for the treatment of uveitis to impede damage progression. A single drop once was sufficient to eliminate the symptom and avoid uveitis, but when the symptom did not go away, the patient used another dose the next day. On June 15, 1998, the patient had visual acuity 8/10, with corrective lenses. The research for vision recovery was restarted in the year 2000 after an oculomotor relaxation procedure, advised by the patient's brother, who had read in a self-help book on eyesight.

After 2009, the same ophthalmologist periodically examines the patient, but sometimes the patient looks for another professional in order to obtain information from the doctor when he first examines the patient. A posterior cataract had developed in the right eye and capsular in the left eye. **Table 1** shows the lenses prescribed by doctors. The prescribed lenses do not change the direction of the elimination treatment of the intraocular metabolic residues. In 2012, ophthalmologists informed the patient that, without surgical intervention in the left eye, the patient would have great difficulty in passing the eye examination to renew his driver's license, scheduled for 2014. So, 15 days before the date of renewal, the patient underwent 12 sessions of 30-min exercise on different days with occlusion of the right eye and added 2 days without exercises. The patient was approved in the exam.

Although the patient perceived changes in visual perception during treatment progress, however, it was not possible to establish treatment phases through these changes. The changes in visual perception depend on the element being observed. The observed element can be an object, a light source or an image, with or without letters, that is near or far, in a certain environment. The environment can be dark, or light, with or without diffused light, under the influence of various luminous intensities. In addition to the environment, visual perception is severely influenced by dehydration, agglutination and the amount of metabolic residues accumulated.

The physical characteristics of the residue disposed orally vary with the progress of the treatment of recovery of sight. Eliminated residue is the one with the least resistance to movement. The movement resistance depends on the location of the accumulation region and the

Calendar date	Rx		Spherical	Cylindrical	Axis
1975	D.V.	O.D.	–	–	–
		O.S.	–	–	–
	N.V.	O.D.	+0.25	–	–
		O.S.	+0.25	–	–
1994	D.V.	O.D.	–	–	–
		O.S.	–	–	–
	N.V.	O.D.	+2.50	0.50	35°
		O.S.	+2.50	0.50	155°
December 02, 1996	D.V.	O.D.	–	–	–
		O.S.	–	–	–
	N.V.	O.D.	+0.50	–	–
		O.S.	+0.75	–	–
1997	D.V.	O.D.	+1.50	0.50	30°
		O.S.	+1.50	0.25	140°
	N.V.	O.D.	+2.50	0.50	30°
		O.S.	+2.50	0.25	140°
1999	D.V.	O.D.	+1.50	0.50	35°
		O.S.	+1.50	0.50	140°
	N.V.	O.D.	+3.50	0.50	35°
		O.S.	+3.50	0.50	140°
July 18, 2003	D.V.	O.D.	+1.50	0.50	180°
		O.S.	1.25	–	–
	N.V.	O.D.	+2.50	0.50	180°
		O.S.	+2.50	–	–
June 20, 2006	D.V.	O.D.	+1.25	0.50	65°
		O.S.	+1.00	0.50	125°
	N.V.	O.D.	+2.75	0.50	65°
		O.S.	+2.75	0.50	125°
June 30, 2006	D.V.	O.D.	+1.25	–0.50	30°
		O.S.	+1.00	–0.50	155°
	N.V.	O.D.	+2.75	–0.50	30°
		O.S.	+2.75	–0.50	155°
March 19, 2007	D.V.	O.D.	+1.00	–0.50	35°
		O.S.	+1.00	–0.50	120°
	N.V.	O.D.	+2.25	–	–
		O.S.	–2.25	–	–

Calendar date	Rx		Spherical	Cylindrical	Axis
October 01, 2012	D.V.	O.D.	—	−0.50	100°
		O.S.	−0.50	−1.50	100°
	N.V.	O.D.	+2.50	add	—
		O.S.	+2.50	add	—
November 12, 2012	D.V.	O.D.	+0.50	−0.75	90°
		O.S.	−1.00	−0.75	105°
	N.V.	O.D.	+3.25	−0.75	90°
		O.S.	+1.75	−0.75	105°
February 07, 2013	D.V.	O.D.	−0.75	—	—
		O.S.	−2.00	—	—
	N.V.	O.D.	+2.25	add	—
		O.S.	+2.25	add	—
July 22, 2013	D.V.	O.D.	+0.50	−1.25	85°
		O.S.	−1.50	−1.00	105°
	N.V.	O.D.	+2.75	add	—
		O.S.	+2.75	add	—

Table 1. Lenses prescribed by doctors.

physical and biochemical characteristics. These characteristics are mainly associated with the compositions of their components, viscosity, dehydration, color, transparency and acidity. Some of these characteristics can be observed in oral elimination.

At the beginning of treatment, it was very easy to perceive the negative afterimage, but it has not been observed for a long time. This pathology was solved. Initially, the appearance of new floaters was observed. Then, there were floaters that changed their appearance, one divided into two, maintaining a discreet connection. The oldest floater had already added new expansion, but kept its round, black core. Sometimes after the beginning of treatment, the oldest floater changes in appearance and returns to the initial appearance.

When the light source, in a dark environment, is refracted in light rays projected on the retina, it may suggest the beginning of the residue elimination phase; the perception of the colored arc, around the light source, indicates residues with a high index of refraction, very dehydrated, with great viscosity; blurry sight can indicate residues available on the cornea for disposal.

The intraocular process of accumulation of metabolic residues, as well as its intraocular process of elimination of metabolic residues, occurs essentially through the involuntary oculomotor movement that acts with the objective of producing the best projection in the temporal retina. In the process of eliminating the accumulated metabolic residue, the patient voluntarily interferes in the oculomotor movement so that the metabolic residue interferes in the projected image in the temporal retina, and then, the involuntary movement rehydrates the accumulated residues in the region, reduces its viscosity, and produces the best projection in the temporal retina. Much attention, just as there is anterior ocular torsional movement, due to the difficulty of adaptation of the cornea, a posterior ocular torsional movement can occur, cause physical tension in the optic nerve and cause normal tension glaucoma.

2. Method

Teamwork was used to interview professionals and patients. Team studies, based on the interpretation of symptoms, among others, corneal burning, tear production and resistance to visual adaptation to a fixed target, performed through the horizontal periodic movement of the head (the duration of the exercise is within the range of 5-30 min). Studies of anatomy and biophysics of the eyes as a system of dynamic action are made. Simulation of a physical model to reproduce the studies of Scheiner, apud [1], was used to associate the main refractive errors and the patient's symptomatology. Simulation of a hypothetical mathematical model was made to study the daily intraocular pressure variation. As the main form of treatment progress evaluation, a light source, at the same distance, was initially used to measure the diameter of its dispersion, evaluated in the number of adjacent diameters of the source. At the present, a traffic light is used as the light source for measurement. Visual acuity and corrective lens parameters are not used to evaluate the reduction of intraocular metabolic residue.

3. Eyesight regeneration and analysis of symptoms and signs

3.1. Materials

In this section, the main materials used for vision recovery are listed in alphabetical order, together with a brief description of the use.

Corrective lenses, +19 D, +10 D, +5 D, +2.5 D, −5D: Negative lenses were abandoned shortly after starting treatment because they did not present difficulties during exercises. Corrective lenses have been included in vision recovery exercises because anyone, without accumulation of intraocular metabolic residue, can read a text with any corrective lens.

Cotton-polyester fabric, nylon mesh: Light obstruction acts as a load for oculomotor movement. The mesh with thicker wire requires more oculomotor effort. By having a greater aperture in its mesh, the nylon mesh interferes in the elimination of the metabolic residues that are sheltered by the shadow of the light obstructed by its wires. The cotton-polyester fabric, by having a smaller opening in its mesh, can eliminate the residuals left by the nylon mesh.

Eyewear (temporal): Occlusion of temporal visual fields to increase the power of the rectus and ciliary muscles without the help of the oblique muscles.

Eyewear (nasal): Occlusion of the nasal visual fields to stimulate the movements related to the projection of the image in the nasal retina (needed but with little use).

Pinhole glasses: Used only at the beginning of treatment as a test. The use of these glasses can cause patient well-being because it eliminates a small volume of metabolic residue, but the volume eliminated is insufficient to solve the problems of refraction error. In addition, its use is not recommended during activities involving patient control or movement, such as driving a vehicle or walking. The holes in the lenses select the visual axis direction, and Scheiner's experiment apud [1] shows that the selection of the visual direction presents to the patient's target at different distances, making it impossible to evaluate the distance of the target and cause an accident.

Sun: Treatment using sunlight has been used several times because it is a source of light with greater intraocular penetration power. It is because of its power that, when looking at the Sun, one or more regions become dark. This strong light causes movements in the dehydrated and viscous metabolic residue that becomes opaque for some time, the accumulation region. Opacity ends due to involuntary intraocular movement. It is the involuntary movement of adaptation to the dark.

Compact fluorescent lamp: Used as fixation point.

Treadmill equipment: Ocular exercise performed on a treadmill does not cause sleep. Six is a great speed for the exercises. It is necessary that there is ample front and lateral visual space.

3.2. Symptoms and signs

During the exercises, there may be, in one or both eyes, fiery sensation along with bloodshot eye. After, there may be itching. Sweat can be severe on one side of the head or on both sides. Exercises can stimulate bruxism, pain in the jaw joint, tongue, and marks on the face. Although there is no direct relationship in many cases, this takes a lot of time and effort to perform the image fusion in a certain direction, or to maintain the fusion of images during the movement of the fixation point. By carrying out the exertion for a long time, it can divert the attention of the patient and it passes on to transmit force to these other parts of the body. After the exercises, sight may become blurry or there may be some other painless modification. For a short time, there may be a foreign body sensation in the cornea or intraocular. There may be acute pain of short duration.

Auditory perception: In 2003, on routine examination, the patient became aware of the absence of 6 kHz frequency perception and the presence of permanent noise, only in the left ear. In the analysis performed by an otorhinolaryngologist, no other pathology was found. In subsequent years, the patient was evaluated to verify the evolution of auditory perception. The patient began to perceive small hearing in the frequency of 6 kHz and reduced the perception in the adjacent frequencies, including in the right ear. Currently, the patient has noticed some relationship between the exercises for recovery of sight and the perceived noise, because the noise in the right ear stops and the amplitude of the remaining noise varies with the direction of the exercise. Then, among the criteria of choice of exercises are the direction of greater variation in the amplitude of the noise and displacement of fixed images. Thus, the variation in noise should be considered, in the choice of the exercise for the eyesight recovery.

Dizziness: Exercising may cause dizziness, and in this way, the patient should hold onto the equipment support during the exercises.

Imbalance: May be perceptible or imperceptible. The imperceptible can cause the patient to knock down nearby objects, can in certain situations move one or more steps, as if drunk, for a short time, can cause pain in the sciatic nerve, and can produce dry callus on the bottom of the feet (**Figure 1**). Sometime later, they suffered fatigue in the right leg. Tiredness settled in the upper posterior region of the knee and then settled in the upper posterior region of the thigh, and the same symptom started in the left leg. This caused a great deal of suffering. It was not thought to be due to muscle strain. The hypothesis was that there was a problem of balance, since the dry callus had already been treated, and balance requires many activities of the lower limbs. Early in the morning, when the patient was seated, he began the eye exercise with eyewear (temporal), to strengthen and straighten the muscles, the symptoms immediately disappeared. The patient worked all day with the symptom of one who had walked for a long time. Two days later, the patient spent a lot of time with the symptom of muscle relaxation in both legs.

Torticollis: The most common signs are the sensation of contraction and pain on one side of the neck that can radiate to the back. It can be caused by stimuli of recurring displacement of the projected image on the retina.

3.3. Analysis of some ocular pathologies

The analysis was based on the progress of the recovery of the patient's vision, in addition to the conclusions reached in our other publications. The ocular refractive error has its origin in the accumulation, dehydration and agglutination of the intraocular metabolic residue [2] caused by the defect in the mechanical system of mass transfer in the cornea (between the corneal layers) [2–4], trabecular meshwork [5], lens [6] and retina [7, 8]. Congenital and acquired pathologies increased the mass transfer deficiency.

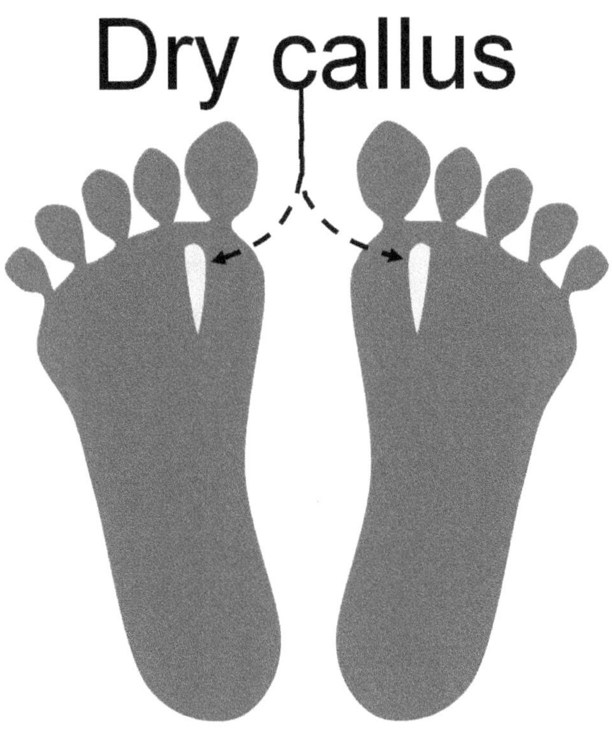

Figure 1. Diagram showing the dry callus location.

Cataract: It is the accumulation of dehydrated metabolic residue in the lens. As the residue is translucent, its dehydration is opaque.

Because it is an accumulation, it is natural to increase the volume and rigidity of the lens, as well as to associate the age of the person with its consequences, among them visual acuity. During the exercises, there may be an intraocular foreign body sensation as well as a small, rapid and uncomfortable intraocular pain because of cataracts.

Dark adaptation: The eye takes longer than 20 min to fully adapt from bright sunlight to dark [9].

The eyes are organs of the visual system. The eye transmits the luminous image to the retina that, through electrochemical impulses, transmits to the brain. The image interpretation can trigger a physical protection action, that is, the person through the image can move the hand or foot to perform a body protection action. The hand and foot take well less than 20 min to make the maximum displacement. So "the eye is a radar that spends 20 minutes to identify an attack, and in defence, it can trigger a missile attacking the target in a minute, so this radar is not for this operation." This means a serious visual impairment. A person without accumulated intraocular metabolic residue can look at the sun and then read a text written in black ink on white paper. In the appendix, it is shown that the adaptation time to the dark is not greater than 0.24 s (Eq. 7).

Glaucoma:

- **Open-angle:** It is caused by slow obstruction of the trabecular meshwork, resulting in increased eye pressure.

In Ref. [5], *it shows how the metabolic residues coming from the cornea can slowly obstruct the trabecular meshwork, increasing the resistance of the aqueous humor and, consequently, increasing the intraocular pressure.*

- **Angle-closure:** It is the result of the closing of the angle between the iris and the cornea.

The accumulation of dehydrated metabolic residue causes formation of a large refractive error and may cause defective coordination between the movement of the lens and the movement of the oculomotor muscles. See in keratoconus analysis.

- **Normal-tension:** The optic nerve is damaged without the eye pressure being too high [5].

The accumulation of intraocular metabolic residue modifies the shape, volume and mass of the eye, and as a result, the oculomotor muscles move out of their ergonomic movement and change the position of the eye in the ocular cavity. These changes can strain the optic nerve.

Eye movements [10]:

- **Conjugate:** They are those that preserve the angular relationship between the right and left eyes.
- **Saccadic:** They are very fast jumps from one eye position to another.

Saccadic and vergence movements are acquired pathologies associated with agglutinated metabolic residues. These clusters form intraocular lenses, which project images into the retina, in different places.

In 1619, Scheiner described these images apud [1]. *Then, when the visual axis changes agglutination, the image of interest jumps from the fovea to another location. This jump causes a rapid movement of the eye in the opposite direction (saccadic movement) to transfer the image to fovea. If the jump of the eye causes the return of the visual axis to the anterior agglutination in order to cause recurrent periodic movement, then it can cause photosensitive epilepsy* [2].

- **Vergence:** Eye movement for fusion of retinal images and obtaining binocular vision.

Floaters: These are deposits of metabolic residue, in the cornea or lens, with various sizes, shape, consistency and refractive index and can be transparent, translucent or opaque.

During treatment, the oldest floater is opaque, but on many days, it presents itself in different forms and opacity. Another floater was divided in two and maintained connection between both.

Headache: This is a warning symptom of a greater problem that is occurring in the body.

You should not take medicine and you should do exercises. If you delay in taking action, the treatment is much longer. Precisely, on the day that the writing of this work is being finalized, the right eyeball of the patient presented a pain sensation, similar to the occurrence, shortly after the injection in the left eye of the same patient. It is probable that the right eye has performed movements that cause mechanical tension in the optic nerve. If immediate corrective action is not provided, it can cause glaucoma with normal pressure. In both cases, the treatment is the same given in relation to the imperceptible imbalance of the body, motor coordination and increase of the power of the rectus muscles.

Keratoconus: Changes of the cornea to a cone-like shape and its thickness reduction.

The torsional accommodation of the cornea is a movement of variation of the radius of its curvature. This may be caused by personal habits and ocular structure, which can progressively increase the radius of curvature, causing keratoconus, or by modifying its cylindrical periphery to the conical shape, blocking the drainage of the aqueous humor, causing angle-closure glaucoma. **Figure 2** *shows the two possibilities.*

Ocular dominance: This is the fixation of the eye with less movement (called the dominant eye) on the target and the adjustment of the contralateral one.

In Ref. [4], *it is treated as visual impairment.*

Phosphene: This can be directly induced by retina mechanical stimulation. It is easy to check when rubbing or applying pressure to closed eyes.

In Ref. [7], *it is written without naming the acquired pathology. "The metabolic secretions are accumulated in the retina forming clusters without any regularity therefore when the eyes are pressed on*

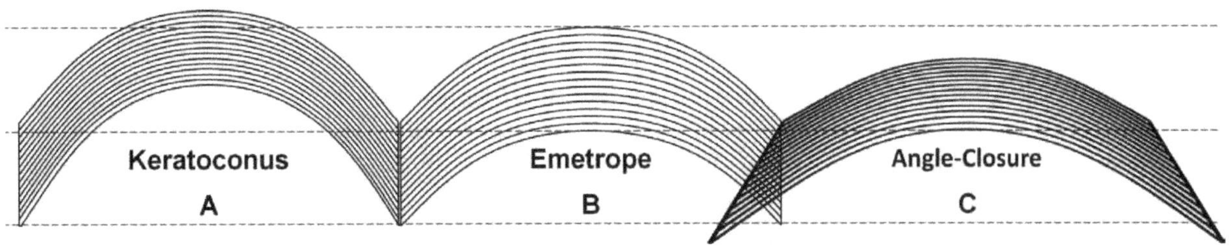

Figure 2. Scheme of the formation of keratoconus, and the angular closure.

by the hands, the photoreceptors are also pressed, and the process affects its biochemical transduction that produces an electrical signal to the brain which interprets it as a light signal." At the present, only, some blue dots are still perceived.

Photophobia: It is a symptom of abnormal light sensitivity.

When the iris fails to reduce interference from the brightness of the incident light to improve the sharpness of the temporal retinal projection. This is one of the effects of accumulation of intraocular metabolic residue. If the physician needs to use different corrective lenses between the exams with and without dilated pupils, it is necessary to verify the need to eliminate the stagnant metabolic residues in regions that are not usually used to design images in the retina.

Refractive error

- **Myopia:** When there is a need for the use of concave lens, to correct the convergence of light rays.
- **Hyperopia:** When there is a need for the use of convective lens, to correct the convergence of light rays.
- **Presbyopia:** When there is a need for the use of bifocal or progressive lens, to correct the convergence of light rays.
- **Astigmatism:** When there is a need for the use of cylindrical lens, to correct the convergence of light rays.

In Ref. [2], *it is shown that refractive error causing myopia, hyperopia, presbyopia and astigmatism has the same origin: dehydration and agglutination, intraocular, of accumulated metabolic residues.*

4. Binocular vision anatomy

Binocular eyesight uses the image fusion for greater visual accuracy. **Figure 3** shows, schematically, the main elements to explain the oculomotor control mechanism, obtained from the images projected on the retina.

Binocular vision of the fixation point on a screen (F in **Figure 3**) occurs when the visual axes of the eyes converge at this point. The F-point protrudes into the central fovea at points F_R and F_L (**Figure 3**), respectively, in the right and left eyes. The two visual axes define the visual plane. The visual plane intercepts the retina in both eyes on two anatomical horizontal meridians, in the right and left eyes. Each anatomical horizontal meridian has two sides, the temporal and the nasal. The nasal anatomical horizontal meridian includes a segment, corresponding to the optic disc, which does not send an image to the brain.

The nasal anatomical horizontal meridian intercepts the neural communication periphery of the optic nerve, closer to the left fovea, at the P_{LL} point (**Figure 3**). In the right eye, the P_{LR} retinal point is the closest to the fovea, obtained by the interception of the temporal anatomical horizontal meridian with the corresponding neural communication periphery of the

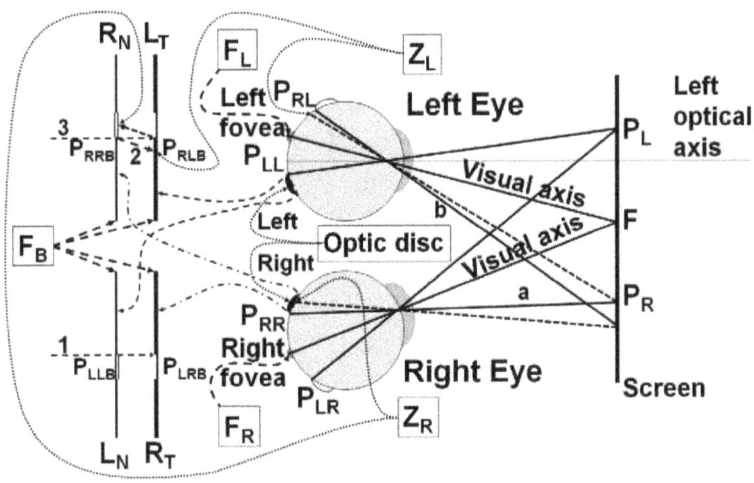

Figure 3. Binocular vision representation scheme.

contralateral optic disc (projection of the contralateral blind spot periphery). If the P_{LL} and P_{LR} retinal points are the neurologically corresponding signals to the P_L screen point retinal projections, the image fusion is perfect. The projection on the right temporal anatomical horizontal meridian, containing the P_{LR} point, sends the visual signals to the ipsilateral cerebral hemisphere in the R_T line (right temporal side), shown in **Figure 3**. The projection on the left nasal anatomical horizontal meridian, containing the P_{LL} point, sends the visual signals to the contralateral cerebral hemisphere, in the L_N line (left nasal side), shown in **Figure 3**. In the L_N line, there is a small segment for the optic disc representation. The arrow "1" locates in the brain at the intersection with the L_N line and the neural point P_{LLB} (left horizontal nasal anatomical meridian) corresponding to the signal received from P_{LL} retinal point and reaches the R_T line at the neural point P_{LRB} (right horizontal temporal anatomical meridian) corresponding to the signal received from P_{LR} retinal point. If the P_{LLB} and P_{LRB} neural points are the neurologically corresponding signals to the P_L screen point retinal projections, the images fusion is perfect, that is, the horizontal diameter of the contralateral blind spot is projected on the R_T line white highlight, indicated by "1" arrow.

The nasal anatomical horizontal meridian intercepts the neural communication periphery of the optic nerve, closer to the right fovea, at the P_{RR} point (**Figure 3**). In the left eye, the P_{RL} retinal point is the closest point of the fovea, obtained by the interception of the temporal anatomical horizontal meridian with the neural corresponding of communication periphery of the contralateral optic disc (projection of the contralateral blind spot periphery). If the P_{RR} and P_{RL} retinal points are the neurologically corresponding signals to the P_R screen point retinal projections, the image fusion is perfect. In this case, retinal points are not the neurologically corresponding signals to the P_R screen point retinal projections; therefore, there is no fusion of images, and there is binocular diplopia. The projection on the left temporal anatomical horizontal meridian, containing the P_{RL} point, sends the visual signals to the ipsilateral cerebral hemisphere in the L_T line (left temporal side) shown in **Figure 3** diagram. The projection on the right nasal anatomical horizontal meridian, containing the P_{RR} point, sends the visual signals to the contralateral cerebral hemisphere in the R_N line (right nasal side) shown in **Figure 3** diagram. In the R_N line, there is a small segment for the optic disc representation. Arrow "2" locates in the brain at the intersection with the R_N line and the neural point P_{RRB} (right horizontal nasal anatomical meridian) corresponding to the signal received from P_{RR} retinal point and reaches the L_T line at the neural point P_{RLB} (left horizontal temporal anatomical meridian) corresponding to the signal received from P_{RL} retinal point. If the P_{RRB} and P_{RLB} neural points are the neurologically corresponding signals to the P_R screen point retinal projections, the image fusion is perfect. The image fusion follows the neural correspondence shown by the "3" arrow, which does not correspond to the respective P_R screen point retinal projections; thus, there is binocular diplopia. The right superior oblique muscle action can accommodate the cornea to perform the angular displacement of "2" arrow until reaching "3" arrow (make the Z_L point coincide with P_{RL} point corresponding to P_{RLB} point in brain). That is, intersect "a" line (**Figure 3**) with the "b" line on the screen, or move the Z_R point (**Figure 3**), projected on the optic disc of the right eye, to overlap the P_{RR} point or P_{RRB} in brain. As the control is contralateral, the right superior oblique muscle action moves the Z_L point until it coincides with the P_{RL} point, that is, the horizontal diameter of the contralateral blind spot is projected on the LT line white highlight, indicated by "3" arrow.

5. Conclusion

As is well known, the brain is "cross-wired" with body movement control and superior oblique muscle but is ipsilateral to the other oculomotor muscles. For the reception of visual signals, the brain is ipsilateral to the projection in the temporal retina and contralateral to the projection in the nasal retina. In the binocular limit of lateral vision, the nose contralateral shadow is the contralateral temporal projection, so that the ipsilateral nasal projection is the only contralateral control signal of the third and sixth cranial nerve functions. Therefore, contralateral ocular movement occurs only under the influence of the projections in the ipsilateral eye. The image fusion influences only the contralateral movement of the superior oblique muscle to avoid binocular diplopia. In summary, the ipsilateral and contralateral nasal projections form the contralateral oculomotor control signals, and the ipsilateral temporal projection transmits, for the brain, the reference signal in motor control of the contralateral superior oblique muscle. In addition, the inferior oblique muscle can correct some angular deviation of ipsilateral temporal projection, without any influence of control of the superior oblique ipsilateral muscle (it does not have a reference image for motor control). In this way, it is easy to understand the contralateral influence resulting from a monocular stimulus.

Rectus muscles: Its main function is to maintain the designed fixation point in the fovea centralis. The superior and inferior rectus muscles avoid and stabilize the vertical displacement of the ipsilateral retinal projection, and the lateral and medial rectus muscles avoid and stabilize the horizontal displacement of the ipsilateral retinal projection. Maintaining eyesight at a fixation point is extremely important for proper accommodation of the crystalline lens and cornea. The fixation point can be a light source or not, and it can be fixed or movable and can be in an ambience with or without changing the lighting level. Vision may be with or without ocular occlusion, may be with or without corrective lenses and may or may not be through a mesh. The head may have a rotating, extension and flexing motion, or it may remain motionless. These are possible combinations that depend on the goal to be achieved. Exercise can cause itching in the sclera nasal region.

Ciliary muscle: It has the main function of maintaining and stabilizing the projection in the ipsilateral temporal fovea and giving it the same dimension as in the contralateral nasal fovea image. These muscles also have the ability to correct the distance from the fixation point, which may be invisible to the eye and act as a mass transfer mechanism by forced convection in the lens.

Superior oblique muscle: It has the main function of enlarging or reducing the projection in the horizontal nasal anatomical meridian, so that the same projected image in the periphery of the optical disc is the same projected image in the corresponding neural region of the periphery of this optic disc, in the contralateral temporal retina. The deviation in the ipsilateral temporal projection causes a force antagonistic to the superior obliquus muscle movement.

Inferior oblique muscle: It has the main function of correcting the angular deviation of the projection in the temporal retina in relation to the projected image in the contralateral nasal retina. The torsional accommodation of the cornea is a joint action of the oculomotor muscles to obtain fusion of the temporal and contralateral nasal images, in addition to varying the intraocular pressure. This accommodation is the mechanism of forced convective mass transfer on the cornea and retina, and it may be inferior, cylindrical or superior, but the difficulty in twisting the cornea may cause twisting of the eyes. Because of the cornea torsional accommodation, a circle in the binocular view can project with the same radius in the retinas of the eyes, with duplication of the monocular vision information, adjustable, and able to obtain a much greater mathematical precision than the accuracy of monocular vision, in accordance with human perception.

Iris: It is a thin circular structure with the main function of reducing incident light when this brightness interferes with the sharpness of the temporal retinal projection as well as diaphragmatic action, to avoid the aqueous humor return, when the pressure in the anterior chamber is greater than the pressure in the posterior chamber due to corneal accommodation.

Eyelid movement: It has the main function of mechanical transport of nutrients and metabolic residues, in addition to being able to reduce the ocular opening voluntarily or involuntarily, when the iris reaches the minimum limit of its opening. The eyelid, on a regular basis, spreads tears, for rehydration and entrainment of the metabolic residue throughout the anterior ocular surface. Tears and metabolic residues are drawn into the puncta (an opening near the nasal bridge) by capillary action and conducted to lacrimal sac through the lacrimal canaliculi and then to the nasal cavity through the nasolacrimal duct. In the nasal cavity, the tear goes out through the nose or the metabolic residue can dehydrate; the resulting mucus accumulates in the nasal cavity; or the viscous residue passes through the throat and is eliminated orally or through the digestive tract. Elimination of the metabolic residue during sleep can cause a very inflamed throat, which may be accompanied by hoarseness for a few days. Cough and sneezing may occur with the expulsion of metabolic residue. Shedding of tears (or eye discharge) of one or both eyes may occur in response to the elimination of metabolic residue from the corneal epithelium, and it can last more than a day. The elimination of metabolic residue in the cornea can be accompanied by the sensation of foreign body in the eye.

Because of the personal habits, the mobile intraocular mass may remain stagnant for a long time, so the metabolic secretions of this medium can dehydrate by decantation, increasing its viscosity and, consequently, increasing the absorption and refraction of light penetrating the eyes. This is the process of accumulation of metabolic residues in the cornea, the trabecular meshwork, the lens and the retina, causing the most known intraocular problems such as refractive errors, keratoconus, glaucoma, cataract, retinal detachment, retinitis pigmentosa and macular degeneration among other problems, which may be added with other factors. Involuntary oculomotor movement exists to reduce the refractive error of the projected image in the temporal retina. However, this involuntary movement can add other problems such as change in the volume and shape of the eyeball, cornea and lens. However, this same involuntary movement can be used to rehydrate and remove the intraocular metabolic residue, in the form of solution or suspension.

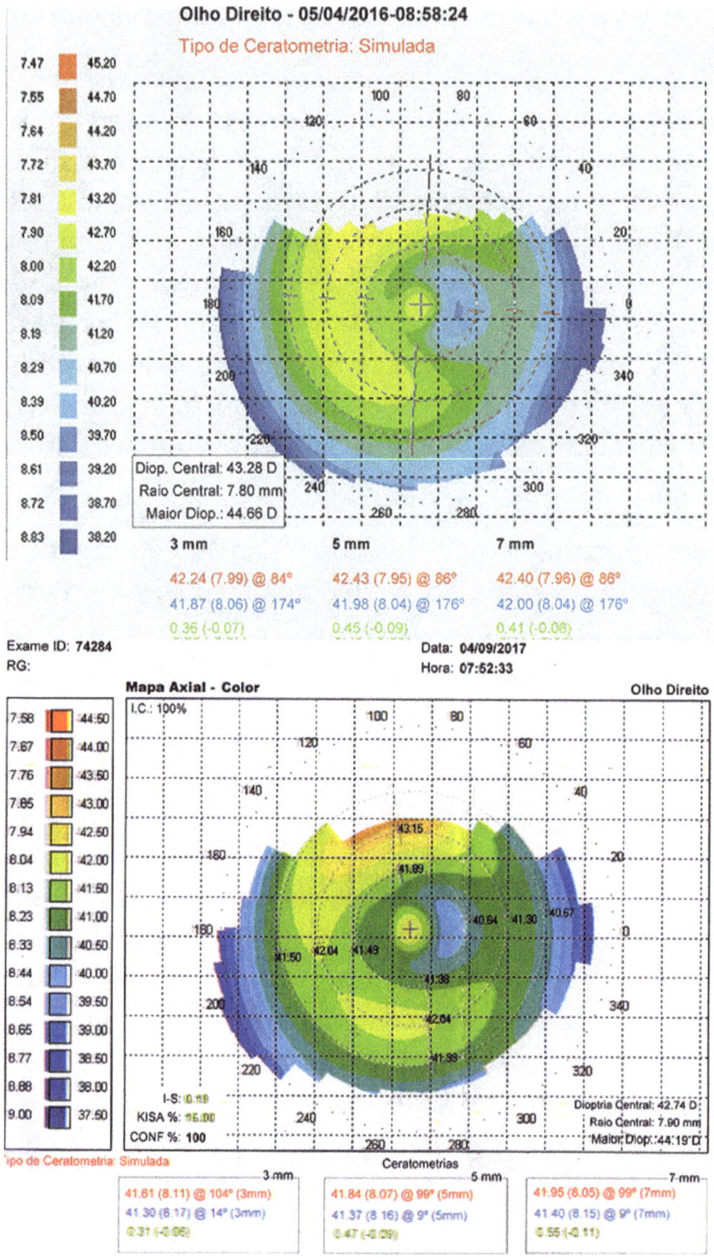

Figure 4. Corneal topography of the right eye performed on April 04, 2016, and September 05, 2017.

From the examinations performed on the patient, only a computerized corneal topography could provide some information to evaluate the progress of the treatment. For each eye and in both, it was necessary to add, on examination, the complementary volume, surplus volume and volume to be distributed, to obtain a uniform corneal lens. At the end of the work, these volumes will be null. **Figure 4** shows the corneal topography of the right eye performed on April 04, 2016, and September 05, 2017, and **Figure 5** shows the result of the same exam for the left eye. Visually, it is possible to verify the progress of the work performed, but there is no measure that can evaluate the volume of metabolic mass moved in the cornea, during 17 months. The region of the left cornea, with the most dehydrated metabolic mass, is indicated in the last examination, shown in **Figure 5**. This region has lower diopter and higher viscosity. Its rehydration causes a foreign body sensation in the cornea, but because of cataract, it can cause foreign body sensation intraocular.

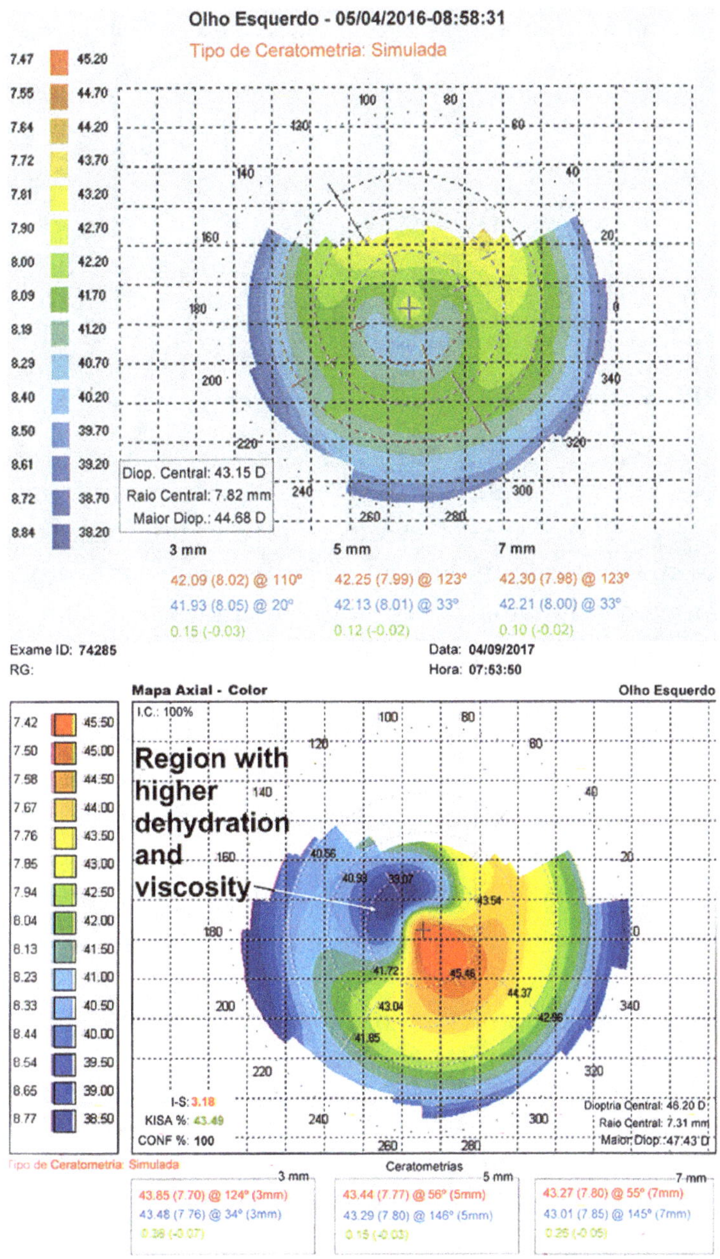

Figure 5. Corneal topography of the left eye performed on April 04, 2016, and September 05, 2017.

Acknowledgements

To God for having helped the first author, in troubles during many years of suffering that led him to become an analytical observer of events in his own body, because of his mother, under the doctor's permission, 15 days before the birth of the first author, traveled by plane. In addition, by helping us to coexist, long ago, with the harms of internal political and economic decisions. For Marcos, brother of the first two authors, who showed in 1999, in a self-help book, the importance of oculomotor relaxation for the eyesight treatment. To colleagues, of the first two authors, ANDES-SN Sindicato Nacional members, and its Seção Sindicato ADUFEPE members, who, during the intervals of some of the societies' meetings, provided with important scientific information for the study. To those who were interviewed to friends, colleagues and family members who directly or indirectly have contributed to this work. There was no public or private financial participation for publication of this work. The authors agree with the individual mentions.

A. Appendix

A.1. Dynamic comparison of the agility of change of state among different activities of the body, eyesight adaptation to dark and movements of the limbs and superior eyelids

In Ref. [5], it was shown that in a first-order system, the percentage change of the final state from an initial state is given by Eq. (1) (see the graphic in **Figure 6**), where $e = 2.71828$, t is the time and τ is the time constant. In the human body, the eye movement has less constant time than the arm movement, that is, the eye movement is faster than the arm movement.

$$f(t) = 100 \cdot (1 - e^{-t/\tau}) \tag{1}$$

In this appendix, a first-order linear mathematical model is used to determine the time constant (numerical value of agility evaluation of a system) to find the maximum displacement time of the upper limbs in personal defense, considering concepts exposed and the maximum time with eyes closed, due to the movement of the eyelid with 287 winks per minute [5]. The result is compared to the value obtained, considering the adaptation to dark with 20 min. With the data obtained, it is verified that the time of 20 min for the adaptation to the dark is unacceptable, because it would have to admit the agility of the superior members much greater than the one of the vision.

The verification of the speed between two systems is performed through the percentage execution of the activity for multiple values of the time constant. If two systems named "A" and "B" with τ_A and τ_B their respective time constants and have the relation $\tau_A = 2\tau_B$, then, when time is equal to τ_A, "A" system performed 63.2% of its final state; however, "B" system has

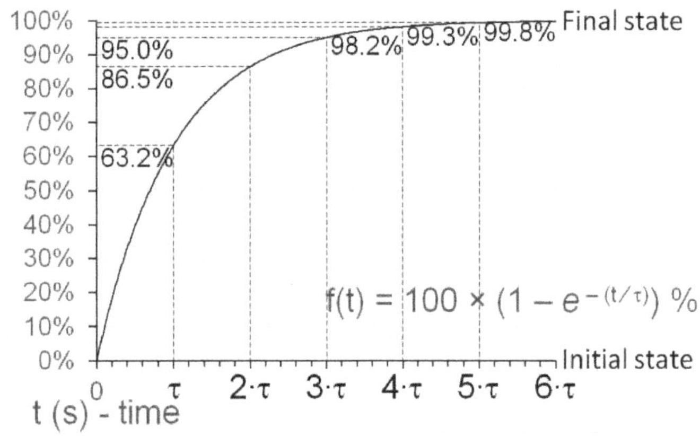

Figure 6. Graph of the function $f(t) = 100 \cdot (1 - e{-t/\tau})$.

already achieved 86.5%. Therefore, the system with the shortest time constant is the fastest, in this case the "B" system.

a. **Eyelid**—287 flashes per min [5]

To simulate the movement of the eyelid, you should consider the maximum distance traveled by the eyelid should be considered as 100%. In the initial state, the eyelid is closed (or open) when the instantaneous time is equal to zero and, in the final state, the eyelid is open (or closed) when the instantaneous time is equal to τ_e, $2\tau_e$, $3\tau_e$, $4\tau_e$, $5\tau_e$, $6\tau_e$ or more, depending on the accuracy.

When t is equal to τ, the system executes 63% of the activity. When t is equal to 2τ, the system executes 86% of the activity. When t is equal to 3τ, 4τ or 5τ, the system executes 95, 98 or 99% of the activity, respectively.

Eq. (2) gives the time t_{oc} that the eyelid passes to open or close the eye, in seconds.

$$t_{oc} = 60/(2 \cdot 287) = 0.10453 \text{ s} \tag{2}$$

If **0.10453** represents 99% of the opened or closed eyelid, then the minimum time constant is $\tau_i = 0.10453/5 = 0.02091$ s and, if 95% of the maximum time constant is $\tau_a = 0.10453/3 = 0.03484$ s, then the eyelid time constant τ_e is in the range $0.02091 \text{ s} \leq \tau_e \leq 0.03484$ s. Eq. (3) gives the eyelid mean time constant τ_{em}.

$$\tau_{em} = (0.02091 + 0.03484)/2 = 0.02788 \text{ s} \tag{3}$$

Thus, the eyelid system completes its activity between $3\tau_{em}$ and $5\tau_{em}$, so its average time is $4\tau_{em}$, and the eyelid opens or closes the eye with time t_e given by Eq. (4), which is considered the transition time for the state change (from opened or closed eye to closed or opened eye or from light to dark).

$$t_e = 4 \cdot 0.02788 = 0.1115 \text{ s} \tag{4}$$

The neural system of reception and comprehension of the retinal image spends the same eyelid time t_e, to complete the whole process, after the conclusion of the eyelid movement, so that the total processing time t_{na} is given by Eq. (5), for the situation **a** (eyelid—287 flashes per minute).

$$t_{na} = (1+1) \cdot t_e = 2 \cdot 0.1115 = 0.223\text{ s} \tag{5}$$

If the neural system has the completion time t_{na}, its time constant varies between $\tau_{nia} = 0.223/5 = 0.0446$ s and $\tau_{naa} = 0.223/3 = 0.07433$ s and then the neural time constant τ_{na} is in the range $0.0446\text{ s} \le \tau_{na} \le 0.07433\text{ s}$. Eq. (6) gives the neural mean time constant τ_{nma}, for the situation **a** (eyelid—287 flashes per minute).

$$\tau_{nma} = (0.0446 + 0.07433)/2 = 0.05947\text{ s} \tag{6}$$

The neural system completes its activity between $3\tau_{nma}$ and $5\tau_{nma}$, so its average time is $4\tau_{nma}$, and the image interpretation occurs with time t_{na} given by Eq. (7), which is considered the transition time for the state change (the time of interpretation of the retinal image).

$$t_{na} = 4 \cdot 0.05947 = 0.23786\text{ s} \tag{7}$$

The superior limb movement system, to reach the maximum displacement, takes twice the time t_{na} of the reception and comprehension of the retinal image process, after its completion, so that Eq. 8 gives the total processing time t_{sa}, that is, slightly less than one second for superior limb maximal displacement.

$$t_{sa} = (2+1) \cdot t_{na} = 3 \cdot 0.23786 = 0.71359\text{ s} \tag{8}$$

b. Dark adaptation—30 min [9]

If the neural system has the completion time $t_{nb} = 20.0$ min (in Ref. [9] cites 30 min), its time constant varies between $\tau_{nib} = 20/5 = 4.0$ min and $\tau_{nab} = 20/3 = 6.66667$ min, that is, $4.0\text{ min} \le \tau_{nb} \le 6.66667$ min. Eq. 9 gives the neural mean time constant τ_{nmb}, for the situation **b** (dark adaptation—30 min [9]).

$$\tau_{nmb} = (4.0 + 6.666)/2 = 5.33333\text{ min} \tag{9}$$

The neural system completes its activity between $3\tau_{nmb}$ and $5\tau_{nmb}$, so its average time is $4\tau_{nmb}$, and the image interpretation occurs with time Eq. (10), which is considered the transition time for the state change (the time of interpretation of the retinal image).

$$t_{nb} = 4 \cdot 5.33333 = 21.33333\text{ min} \tag{10}$$

The movement system of the superior limbs takes twice the time, t_{nb}, to reach the maximum displacement of the reception and comprehension of the retinal image process, after its completion, so that Eq. 11 gives the total processing time t_{sb}, that is, slightly more than an hour for superior limb maximal displacement.

$$t_{sb} = (2+1) \cdot t_{nb} = 3 \cdot 21.33333 = 64.0 \text{ min} \tag{11}$$

Thus, the mathematical model and its parameters have shown that if the measured eyelid movement, 287 flashes per minute [5], is considered as a reference, it obtains, for the displacement of the upper limbs, the time $t_{sa} = 0.71359$ s, compatible with the reality. However, if the time of 20 min (30 min [9]) is considered as a reference for adaptation to the dark, it obtains, for the displacement of the upper limbs, the time $t_{sb} = 64$ min, incompatible with reality.

The exposed model does not consider dead time (the time lag between the beginning of stimulus given to a system and the beginning of resulting response); however, it is possible to adopt $t_{na} = 0.23786$ s and $t_{nb} = 21.33333$ min as the dead time in the respective simulations. In this case, the dead time, considering the eyelid movement, is compatible with reality and confirms the simplified representation of the event, whereas for the second case, the waiting time is incompatible for the defense of the body, therefore, or the parameter adopted is incompatible or the model chosen is not applicable. This work adopted the first alternative.

Author details

Humberto D. Silva[1]*, Eduardo D. Silva[1], Maria Tamires D. Silva[2], Cristiana P. Dória[2] and Cristiane P. Dória[2]

*Address all correspondence to: hdoria@ufpe.br

1 Universidade Federal de Pernambuco, Recife, Brazil

2 Independent Professional, Recife, Brazil

References

[1] Werner L, Trindade F, Pereira F, Werner L. Physiology of accommodation and presbyopia. Arquivos Brasileiros de Oftalmologia. 2000;**63**:503-509. DOI: 10.1590/S0004

[2] Silva HD, Dória LCP, Dória CP, Dória CP, Silva MCTD, Silva HD Jr, MTD S. Simulation of the Errors of Refraction in the Human Eye. In: Öchsner A, da Silva LFM, Altenbach H, editors. Analysis and Design of Biological Materials and Structures. Berlin, Heidelberg: Springer Berlin Heidelberg; 2012. pp. 187-200. DOI: https://doi.org/10.1007/978-3-642-22131-6_15

[3] Silva HD, Dória LCP, Dória CP, Dória CP, Silva Md CTD, Júnior HDS, Silva MTD. Nutrients and metabolic secretions transfer in cornea. Defect and Diffusion Forum. 2011;**312-315**:737-742. DOI: 10.4028/www.scientific.net/DDF.312-315.737

[4] Silva HD, Dória LCP, Dória CP, Dória CP, do Carmo M, Silva TD, Silva HD Jr, Silva MTD. Analysis of failure mechanism of forced convection in the cornea of the human eye. In: Öchsner A, da Silva LFM, Altenbach H, editors. Characterization and Development of Biosystems and Biomaterials. Berlin, Heidelberg: Springer-Berlin-Heidelberg; 2013. pp. 217-226. DOI: http://www.springer.com/materials/biomaterials/book/978-3-642-31469-8

[5] Silva HD, Dória LCP, Dória CP, Dória CP, Carmo M, Silva TD, Silva HD Jr, Silva MTD. Simulation of variation of intraocular pressure. In: Öchsner A, da Silva LFM, Altenbach H, editors. Characterization and Development of Biosystems and Biomaterials. Berlin, Heidelberg: Springer-Berlin-Heidelberg; 2013. pp. 235-253. DOI: http://www.springer.com/materials/biomaterials/book/978-3-642-31469-8

[6] Silva HD, Dória Silva E, Dória LCP, Dória CP, Dória CP, Silva Md CTD, Júnior HDS, Silva MTD. Forced convection mechanism failure in the eye can cause cataract. Defect and Diffusion Forum. 2013;**334-335**:225-229. DOI: 10.4028/www.scientific.net/DDF.334-335.225

[7] Silva HD, Dória LCP, Dória CP, Dória CP, Silva Md CTD, Júnior HDS, Silva MTD. Mass transport mechanism in the retina of the human eye. Defect and Diffusion Forum. 2012;**326-328**:18-23. DOI: 10.4028/www.scientific.net/DDF.326-328.18

[8] Agarwal M, Ulmer JL, Chandra T, Klein AP, Mark LP, Mohan S. Imaging correlates of neural control of ocular movements. European Radiology. 2016;**26**:2193-2205. DOI: 10.1007/s00330-015-4004-9

[9] Bye LA, Modi NC, Stanford M, editors. Basic Sciences for Ophthalmology. 1st ed. United Kingdom: Oxford University Press; 2013. 288 pp. 0191004073, 9780191004070

[10] Silva HD, Dória Silva E, Dória LCP, Dória CP, Dória CP, Silva Md CTD, Júnior HDS, Silva MTD. Forced convection mechanism failure in the eye can cause macular degeneration. Defect and Diffusion Forum. 2013;**334-335**:230-234. DOI: 10.4028/www.scientific.net/DDF.334-335.230

4

Bacterial Endophthalmitis

S. Malhotra, S. Sharma, N. J. K. Bhatia, C. Hans and P. Kumar

Abstract

Endophthalmitis is an ocular inflammation involving vitreous cavity along with the retinal and uveal components of the eye mostly due to infectious agent. The source of infection could be exogenous or endogenous. Exogenous endophthalmitis results from direct inoculation as a complication of ocular surgery, foreign bodies or penetrating ocular trauma, while endogenous endophthalmitis results from haematogenous spread of organisms from a distant source of infection. Endophthalmitis often results in partial or complete loss of vision despite aggressive therapeutic and surgical intervention and hence it is considered as a medical emergency. Diagnosis of infectious agent is critical in the management of these agents. Intravitreal antimicrobial therapy along with anti-inflammatory agents is the key ingredient for successful management of endophthalmitis, while surgical procedures like vitrectomy become necessary in severe endophthalmitis cases. This is a brief review regarding classification, etiological agents causing endophthalmitis, diagnosis and therapeutic challenges of endophthalmitis that will help in improving the visual outcome.

Keywords: Bacterial endophthalmitis, diagnosis, therapeutic challenge

1. Introduction

Endophthalmitis is an ocular inflammation into the posterior segment of the eye usually involving vitreous cavity along with the retinal and uveal components of the eye [1] due to infectious agent, usually bacterial or fungal or non-infectious causes. Normally, the blood–ocular barrier prevents invasion from infective organisms, but if this is breached (directly through trauma or indirectly due to a change in its permeability secondary to inflammation), infection can occur. Endophthalmitis often results in partial or complete loss of vision despite aggressive therapeutic and surgical intervention and hence it is considered as a medical emergency [2, 3]. When inflammation spreads throughout the globe involving all the layers including the Tenon's capsule with or without involvement of the peri-ocular tissues, the condition is known as panophthalmitis. Hence, in endophthalmitis there is involvement of all ocular tissues except the sclera while in panophthalmitis there is involvement of all ocular tissues including the sclera. Panophthalmitis is a devastating fulminant condition associated with complete loss of vision and with very poor prognosis [3].

Features	Infectious endophthalmitis	Non-infectious endophthalmitis
Symptoms	Severe vision loss with moderate to severe pain.	Vision loss is mild to moderate with mild pain.
Signs	Conjunctival congestion is seen along with hypopyon and fibrin deposits. Also vitreous opacity is prominent.	Conjunctival congestion, hypopyon and fibrin deposits are usually not seen. Vitreous opacity is usually mild.
Slit lamp examination	Retinal infiltrates and intra-retinal haemorrhages are common.	Retinal infiltrates and intra-retinal haemorrhages are very rarely seen.
Clinical course	Rapidly progressive.	Slow improvement.
Treatment	Antibiotics and surgery.	Topical and/or systemic corticosteroids.

Table 1. Difference between infectious and non-infectious endophthalmitis [4]

2. Sterile/non-infectious endophthalmitis

Sterile endophthalmitis is an acute intra-ocular inflammation of the vitreous cavity that resolves without the need of intra-vitreal antibiotics and/or vitreo-retinal surgery. In these cases if vitreous microbiological study is done, it needs to be culture negative. This condition has diverse etiologies and includes systemic auto-immune diseases, local ocular inflammations of unknown cause, endophthalmitis related to lens material and endophthalmitis attributable to intra-ocular foreign bodies.

Phacoanaphylactic endophthalmitis (lens-induced granulomatous inflammation) is a type of non-infectious endophthalmitis which represents an auto-immune response to lens protein. This is a rare consequence of lens injury which may occur after trauma causing rupturing of the lens capsule, or post surgery such as following extracapsular cataract extraction when residual lens cortex is present. There is a mixed neutrophilic and granulomatous response seen around the lens in histology [5].

Phacotoxic endophthalmitis is a condition which was previously used to cover a mixed group of conditions related to cataract surgery and intra-ocular lens implant surgery. However, since inflammation is seen mostly in the anterior segment, the term was changed to toxic anterior segment syndrome (TASS). TASS is caused due to reactions to chemicals (irrigationsolutions, preservatives, drugs, denatured viscoelastics), IOL (intra-ocular lens) materials, instrument sterilization and preparation-related compounds [6,7]. TASS presents with marked decrease in vision and diffuse corneal oedema within 12–24 h of anterior segment surgery, most commonly cataract surgery and, more recently, it has been reported after phakic intra-ocular lens implantation [6,8].

Sterile endophthalmitis has also been noted following intra-ocular injection, post vitrectomy and after glaucoma drainage device implantation surgery. Intra-vitreal triamcinolone acetonide has also been associated with sterile endophthalmitis when triamcinolone crystals migrate into the anterior chamber [9]. Clinically, sterile endophthalmitis presents within 24 h of surgery, Gram stain and culture negative, involving the anterior segment in the case of TASS, and showing no response to antibiotics but improvement is seen with topical and/or oral steroids. However, it is difficult to rule out infectious etiology because some infectious cases mayhave rapid onset and have initial negative cultures [6].

3. Classification of bacterial endopthalmitis

Endophthalmitis can be categorized as exogenous and endogenous endophthalmitis. Exogenous endophthalmitis results from direct inoculation as a complication of any intra-ocular surgery (**post-operative endophthalmitis**) and/or blunt or penetrating ocular trauma (**post-traumatic endophthalmitis**). Destruction of intra-ocular tissues may be due to direct invasion by the organism and/or inflammatory mediators of the immune response. **Endogenous endophthalmitis** results from the haematogenous spread of organisms from a distant source of infection [10]. Rarely, keratitis (infection of the cornea), if left untreated, can result in corneal perforation and intra-ocular seeding of organisms leading to endophthalmitis [11]. According to British report, 59% of endophthalmitis were exogenous while 41% were endogenous in origin [12]. In comparison, another study from India suggested that 92.6% were exogenous endophthalmitis and only 7.4% were endogenous endophthalmitis [13]. There are multiple factors responsible for variation in incidence, namely, number of patients included in the study, duration of study, urban versus rural population, pre-disposing factors present, inpatient versus outpatient population and geographical areas of study.

3.1. Post-operative endophthalmitis

Post-operative endophthalmitis is the most common form of endopthalmitis and it occurs most frequently following cataract surgeries like phacoemulsification and intra-ocular lens implantation. However, other procedures namely corneal surgeries (penetrating keratoplasty, keratoprosthesis insertion, refractive corneal surgeries), vitreous procedures (intra-vitreal injections, vitrectomies), glaucoma surgical treatments (blebs, glaucoma valve placements), procedures to correct retinal detachment including scleral buckling, and strabismus correction are also associated with varying risks of endophthalmitis. The organisms are generally acquired from eyelid margin and pre-ocular tear film [2,3]. Contributing factors for development of endophthalmitis include dry eye, corneal perforation, systemic immune dysfunction, previous presence of infection like bacterial conjunctivitis, cicatricial disorders (e.g. ocular cicatricial pemphigoid and Steven-Johnson), chronic use of topical antibiotics and both topical and oral corticosteroid use [11]. In various vitrectomies (Pars plana vitrectomy or 25 gauge vitrectomy), diabetes mellitus is recognized as an important risk factor for exogenous endophthalmitis [14]. Sometimes, cases of clustering of the endophthalmitis are seen, suggesting contaminated materials/solutions or problems with instrument sterilization as responsible [15,

16]. Bacterial infections are the most common cause of post-operative endophthalmitis, and Gram-positive isolates account for the majority of these cases [2]. Coagulase negative *Staphylococcus* accounts for majority of cases followed by *enterococci* and *streptococci* of viridans group. Among Gram-negative isolates, *Pseudomonas aeruginosa* endophthalmitis is identified [17, 18]. Fungal infections are less common and occur particularly in association with the use of contaminated ocular irrigation fluids [19]. *Candida* spp. (especially *C. parapsilosis*), *Aspergillus* spp. and *Fusarium* spp. are common fungal pathogens responsible for post-operative endophthalmitis [20]. *E. faecalis* is the causative agent in 4% to 8% of post-operative endophthalmitis cases and is isolated most frequently from infected filtering blebs following glaucoma surgery [10]. The visual outcome is poor and has become a key public health concern because of the emergence of antibiotic resistance to useful antibiotics including vancomycin [21].

Delayed onset infection (> 6 weeks post-operative) may occur due to sequesteration of low-virulence organisms introduced at the time of surgery or to delayed inoculation of organisms [22, 23]. *S. epidermidis, Propionibacterium acnes,* filamentous bacteria (including *Actinomyces* and *Nocardia* sp.), *Hemophilus influenzae,* non-tuberculous mycobacteria (*M. abscessus, M. chelonae* etc.) and *candida* spp. are responsible for chronic or delayed endophthalmitis [24, 25]. In cases with delayed onset infection, organisms gain access to the eye through either wound abnormalities, suture tracks or filtering blebs. It is more common with glaucoma filtering surgery [26].

3.2. Post-traumatic endophthalmitis

Penetrating injuries are accompanied by higher infection rate of 1–17% compared to post-surgery cases [10]. The broad prevalence range is due to factors such as frequency of intra-ocular foreign bodies, distribution of trauma causes, and management strategies. Onset may be acute or delayed, but the most virulent organisms can destroy an eye within hours. Important risk factors for post-traumatic endophthalmitis are the presence of an intra-ocular foreign body (IOFB), the length of time between injury and foreign body removal, delay in closure of the globe, poorer visual acuity at presentation, virulence of organisms and the immune system of the affected individual [27]. Post-traumatic-endophthalmitis-associated isolates are mostly derived from the environment, and hence includes greater variety of organisms than those following ocular surgery. *Staphylococcus* and *Streptococcus* sp. are the most frequent pathogens, followed by *Bacillus cereus and P. aeruginosa* [28]. Filamentous fungi, especially *Aspergillus* sp. and *Fusarium* sp., are also responsible for post-traumatic endophthalmitis [29]. Bacillus infection is noteworthy as it causes rapid destruction of eye leading to decline in retinal function and vision loss within 24 to 48 h post-infection, despite aggressive treatment and/or surgical intervention. This suggests that even if the infected eye is rendered sterile by antibiotics, ocular damage continues to occur due to the bacterial toxins produced – haemolysins, lipases, enterotoxins and proteases – acting together [30].

3.3. Endogenous endophthalmitis

Endogenous endophthalmitis is relatively rare accounting for 2% to 8% of all endophthalmitis cases [31]. It results from the introduction of organisms into the eye as a result of haematogenous spread from a remote primary site of infection [31]. Populations at greatest risk include immunocompromised patients like diabetes, HIV, organ transplant, cardiac disease and malignancy or those on immunosuppressive therapy, patients with prolonged indwelling devices and intra-venous drug abusers [32]. Endogenous endophthalmitis is more common with fungal isolates than with bacterial isolates. Most common fungal pathogens include *Candida* spp., *Aspergillus* sp. and *Fusarium* spp. *Candida albicans* remains the most important although others such as *C. glabrata, C. tropicalis, C. dubliniensis* and *C. krusei* are being increasingly detected [33]. *Aspergillus* sp. (*A. fumigatus* followed by *A. flavus*) have been reported less frequently than *Candida* sp., but Aspergillus endophthalmitis cause rapidly progressive retinal damage and is more visually devastating compared to Candida endophthalmitis [34]. Common causes of endogenous bacterial endophthalmitis include *S. aureus, B. cereus* and Gram-negative organisms, including *Escherichia coli, Neisseria meningitidis* and *Klebsiella* spp. [10]. *Bacillus* spp. is a primary cause of endogenous endophthalmitis in intra-venous drug abusers due to contaminated injections and drug solutions [10]. Rarely, protozoa like Microsporidia and Amoebae may be the pathogens for endogenous endophthalmitis [35]. It is seen that visual outcomes are poorer with endogenous fungal endophthalmitis compared to endogenous bacterial endophthalmitis. The common foci of infection may be urinary tract infection, septic arthritis, pneumonia and endocarditis [35]. Seriously ill patients may neglect eye symptoms until vision is permanently compromised. Hence, it has been recommended that ophthalmic screening should be routine in high-risk situations such as intra-venous drug use, long-term antibiotics, immunosuppressive therapy, primary or secondary immunodeficiency, prolonged central line use, debilitated patients and pre-mature infants [36].

3.3.1. Endophthalmitis associated with microbial keratitis

Cornea gets infected in situations like contact lens wearer, any pre-existing corneal disease and rarely due to dry cornea (as seen in chronic blepharoconjunctivitis or dacrocystitis, tear film deficiency or topical steroid therapy). If corneal infection is severe enough to cause progressive ulceration of cornea, then it can lead to bacterial endophthalmitis [11].

The incidence rates [37, 38] and etiologial agents of different types of endophthalmitis have been enumerated in Tables 2 and 3, respectively.

Source of infection	**Causes**	**Incidence rate**
Exogenous endophthalmitis		
1. Post-operative	Overall	0.05–0.3%
	Post-cataract surgery	0.02–0.11%
	Post-intravitreal injection	0.03–0.87%
	Post-penetrating keratoplasty	0.1–0.5%
	Post-keratoprostheses	0–12.5%
	Glaucoma valve surgery	1.7–1.9%
	Filtering blebs	0.2–9.6%

Source of infection	Causes	Incidence rate
	Vitrectomy	0.05–0.14%
	Episcleral surgery	0.01%
	Strabismus surgery	Very rare (1 in 30,000)
1. Post-traumatic		1–17%
Endogenous endophthalmitis		2–8%

Table 2. Incidence rates of different types of endophthalmitis

Source of infection	**Classification**	Causative agents
Exogenous	**1. Post-operative endophthalmitis**	
	Acute (within 6 weeks of surgery)	Coagulase-negative staphylococci (Most common "/>60%), *Staphylococcus aureus,* viridans group streptococci, and enterococci. Gram-negative organisms like *Pseudomonas aeruginosa* [2]. Fungi like *Candida* spp. (especially *C. parapsilosis*), *Aspergillus* spp. and *Fusarium* spp.
	Delayed or chronic (after 6 weeks of surgery)	*Propionibacterium acne* (most common), *Streptococcus* spp., coagulase negative staphylococci (*S. epidermidis*), filamentous bacteria (including *Actinomyces and Nocardia* sp.), *Hemophilus influenzae,* non-tuberculous mycobacteria (*M. abscessus, M. chelonae,* etc.) and *candida* spp. (*Candida parapsilosis*).
	2. Post-traumatic endophthalmitis	Staphylococci (most common), *Bacillus cereus, Streptococci, P. aeruginosa* and polymicrobial infections. Filamentous fungi, especially *Aspergillus* sp. and *Fusarium* sp.
Endogenous	**Endogenous endophthalmitis**	Fungi like *Candida spp. (Candida albicans, C. glabrata, C. tropicalis, C. dubliniensis, C. krusei), Aspergillus* sp. (*A. fumigatus, A. flavus*) and *Fusarium* spp. Gram-positive bacteria include *S. aureus, B. cereus* and Gram-negative organisms, including *Escherichia coli, Neisseria meningitidis* and *Klebsiella* spp. Rarely, protozoa like Microsporidia and Amoebae.

Table 3. Etiological agents of different types of endophthalmitis

4. Clinical presentation

Clinical presentation of the disease depends on the virulence and toxin production of the infecting pathogen, the mechanism of introduction into the eye, how quickly treatment is initiated and the patient's age [10]. Symptoms of endophthalmitis range from a relatively painless anterior chamber inflammation, such as that typically caused by *Staphylococcus epidermidis* to an indolent and protracted intra-ocular infection caused by *P. acnes*, to an explosive ocular and periorbital infection caused by *B. cereus* [10]. The clinical presentations of various endophthalmitis are depicted in Table 4.

Types	Symptoms	Signs
Acute post-operative endophthalmitis	• Sudden decrease of vision and increasing eye pain • Red eye, ocular discharge and blurring of vision [38, 39].	• Lid oedema, intense conjunctival injection and chemosis, corneal oedema, papillary fibrin membrane and hypopyon [Figures 1 and 2]. • Severe inflammation in the anterior chamber and the vitreous [38, 39].
Delayed post-operative endophthalmitis	• Insidious decrease of vision and gradually increasing redness with minimal pain [40].	• Conjunctival injection, hypopyon, corneal oedema and clumps of exudates on the iris or around the pupillary margin.
Bleb associated endophthalmitis	• Rapidly worsening pain and vision • Red eye	• Marked conjunctival injection and hypopyon. • Bleb appears milky white with area of necrosis in the sclera (Figure 3).
Post-traumatic endophthalmitis	Same as acute post-operative endophthalmitis, but more severe and early onset in *Bacillus cereus* infection (Figure 4).	Same as acute post-operative endophthalmitis • Fever, proptosis and corneal oedema [38, 39].
Endogenous endophthalmitis	• Acutely ill immunocompromised patient presenting with decreased vision	• Lid and conjunctival oedema • Flame-shaped retinal haemorrhages. • Hypopyon, vitreous inflammatory reaction and microabscesses on the iris [39].
Candida endogenous endophthalmitis	• Decreased vision, floaters and pain • Usually bilateral and follow an indolent course	• Fluffy yellow white retinal lesions and retinal haemorrhages. • Hypopyon and widespread inflammation.

Table 4. Clinical presentation of various endophthalmitis

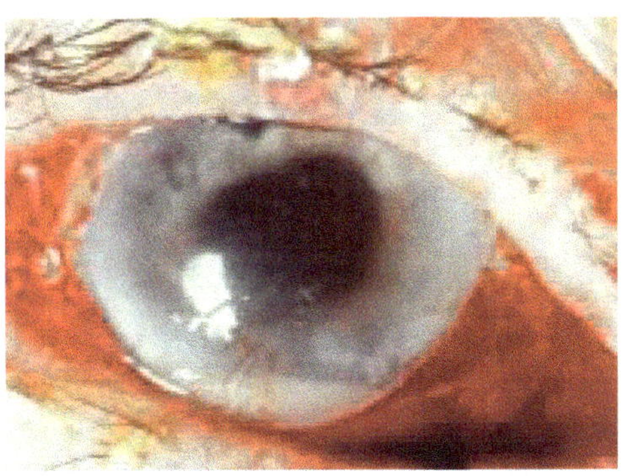

Figure 1. Intense conjunctival congestion with corneal edema and hypopyon

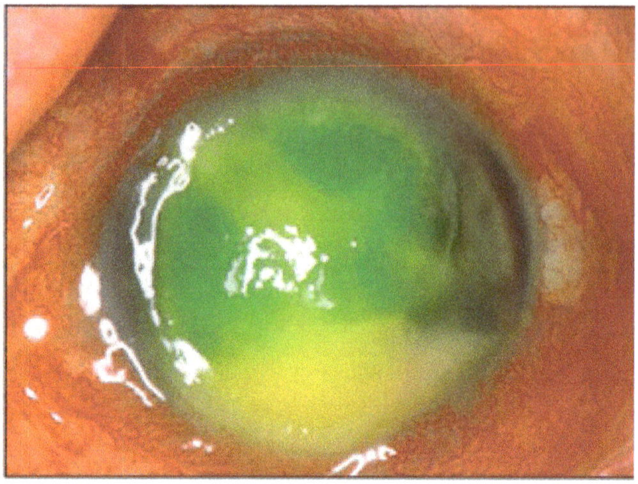

Figure 2. Endophthalmitis affecting the cornea

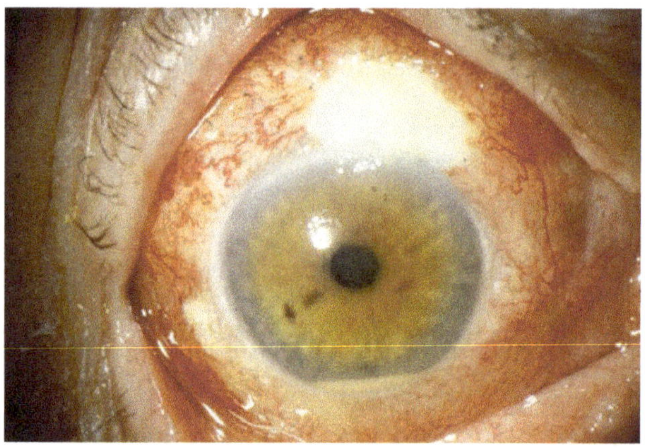

Figure 3. White bleb with intense conjunctival injection suggestive of bleb-associated endophthalmitis

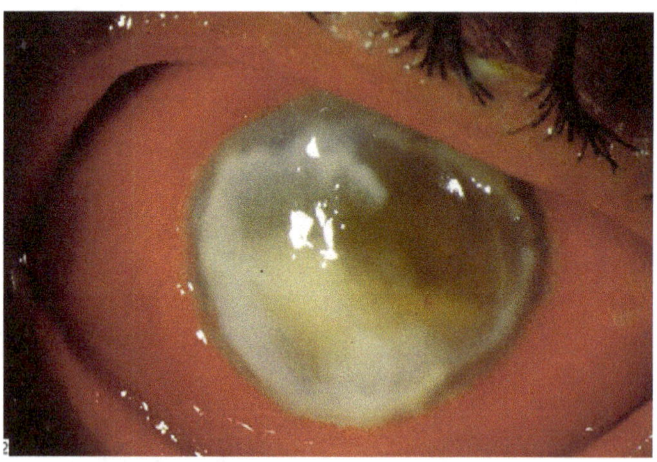

Figure 4. Post-traumatic endophthalmitis caused by *Bacillus cereus* showing prominent conjunctival congestion, corneal ring infiltrate and dense hypopyon

5. Pathogenesis of bacterial endophthalmitis

5.1. Protective mechanisms in eye

5.1.1. Blood–ocular fluid barrier

Under normal circumstances, the blood–ocular barrier provides a natural resistance against invading organisms and it ensures proper functioning of intra-ocular tissues and is essential for immune privilege [10]. The blood–ocular fluid barrier consists of inner and outer blood–retina barriers and the blood–aqueous humour barrier. The inner blood–retina barrier is formed by tight junctions between the endothelial cells and basement membrane of retinal capillaries and retinal pericytes, which control the blood supply for the inner retinal layers, preventing leakage of plasma constituents into the vitreous. The tight junctions between retinal pigment epithelial cells constitute the outer blood–retina barrier and control the blood supply to retinal photoreceptor cells and the choriocapillaris. The blood aqueous humour barrier is formed by the iris and ciliary epithelium and thus divides the highly perfused iris from its neighbouring compartments, the anterior chamber and the anterior vitreous [41]. Certain cytokines, such as transforming growth factor β, α-melanocyte stimulating hormone and vasoactive intestinal peptide, are known to have immunosuppressive property and have been detected in healthy aqueous humour [10].

5.1.2. Anterior Chamber-Associated Immune Deviation (ACAID)

Ocular antigen presenting cells, namely macrophages and dendritic cells, are found in the iris and the choriocapillaris [42]. In most cases of post-operative endophthalmitis, bacteria enter the eye via the anterior chamber, where antigen presentation initially occurs and hence antigen presenting cells residing in the iris are the most likely to first encounter these pathogens. This process may be facilitated by the mild inflammatory reaction in the anterior segment, resulting from tissue manipulation of surgery. Retinal and uveal antigen presenting cells may not have access to antigen under physiological conditions but can activate during the later stages of infection, if the microbes have gained access to the posterior segment. When the defense mechanisms of immune privilege are overwhelmed, then only fulminant inflammation occurs [10].

5.1.3. Invading mechanisms of organisms

Organisms causing endophthalmitis are mostly part of conjunctival flora. They adhere to IOLs and create microcolonies through biofilm formation and within biofilms they are protected from host inflammatory responses, both physically and through multiple genetic changes that alter antigenicity. Organisms in the biofilm are thus difficult to eradicate and may persist despite antibiotic treatment, resulting in relapsing endophthalmitis [43].

Various toxins and enzymes are produced and secreted by the invading organisms causing destruction of protective mechanisms in the eye in case of fulminant infection in eye. *B. cereus* produces a number of cytolysins and enzymes that could contribute to the rapid course and severity of endophthalmitis, including haemolysins, lipases, enterotoxins and proteases

[30]. *E. faecalis* strains frequently harbour conjugative plasmids that encode a cytolysin which effectively lyses both eukaryotic and prokaryotic cells [44]. Cytolysin causes destructive changes in retinal architecture and vitreal structures. Adhesin, aggregation substance, produced by enterococci is a virulence-enhancing factor and helps them to attach to membranous vitreous structures. *S. aureus* secretes cell wall-associated products and adhesions (e.g. clumping factor, fibronectin-binding protein and protein A) and extracellular virulence factors (e.g. toxins such as alpha-toxin, beta-toxin, gamma-toxin and leukocidin, proteases and lipases) which are responsible for high virulence of this organism in endophthalmitis. These virulence factors are controlled by quorum-sensing systems namely, *agr* (accessory gene regulator) and *sar* (staphylococcal accessory regulator) [45]. Hence, therapeutics designed to inactivate global regulation of *S. aureus* during the early stages of infection may be more effective in arresting tissue damage than targeting individual toxins.

6. Role of complement and proinflammatory cytokines in endophthalmitis

IL-1 initially mediates the acute-phase response, inducing other inflammatory mediators such as prostaglandins, phospholipase A2, collagenases and other proinflammatory cytokines (IL-6 and tumour necrosis factor alpha [TNF-α]). IL-1 induces the breakdown of the blood–retina barrier and leukocyte recruitment into the intra-ocular tissue [10]. IL-6 induces production of acute phase proteins such as C-reactive protein and fibrinogen by the liver and promotes B- and T-cell differentiation [46]. In the eye, IL-6 plays a local role in negative feedback on IL-1 and TNF-α production. TNF-α also provokes an intra-ocular inflammatory reaction and acts synergistically with IL-1. IL-8 promotes the recruitment of neutrophils, and because dense neutrophil infiltration is a characteristic feature of endophthalmitis, its involvement in intra-ocular infection is probable but has not yet been determined [10].

7. Brief overview of pathogenesis

During bacterial growth, toxin production by virulent organisms results in loss of retinal function. Cell envelopes, fragments of peptidoglycan, and teichoic acid or lipopolysaccharides are released in intra-ocular spaces during intra-ocular growth or antibiotic killing. These components may come in contact with resident immune cells and stimulate them to produce pro-inflammatory cytokines or other immune mediators which initiate a cascade of inflammatory events, including increased permeability of the blood–ocular fluid barrier, with influx of additional soluble mediators and recruitment of phagocytic inflammatory cells to the site of infection. Inflammatory cells may in turn produce more inflammatory cytokines, in addition to toxic enzymes and reactive oxygen species. During the later stages of protracted endophthalmitis, lymphocytes migrate into inflamed intra-ocular tissues, and an immunoglobulin response results as shown in Figure 5. The ultimate result is the disruption of retinal architecture and death of non-regenerating retinal photoreceptor cells and a significant intra-ocular inflammatory response which can exacerbate the harmful effects of bacterial growth and toxin production by causing bystander damage [10].

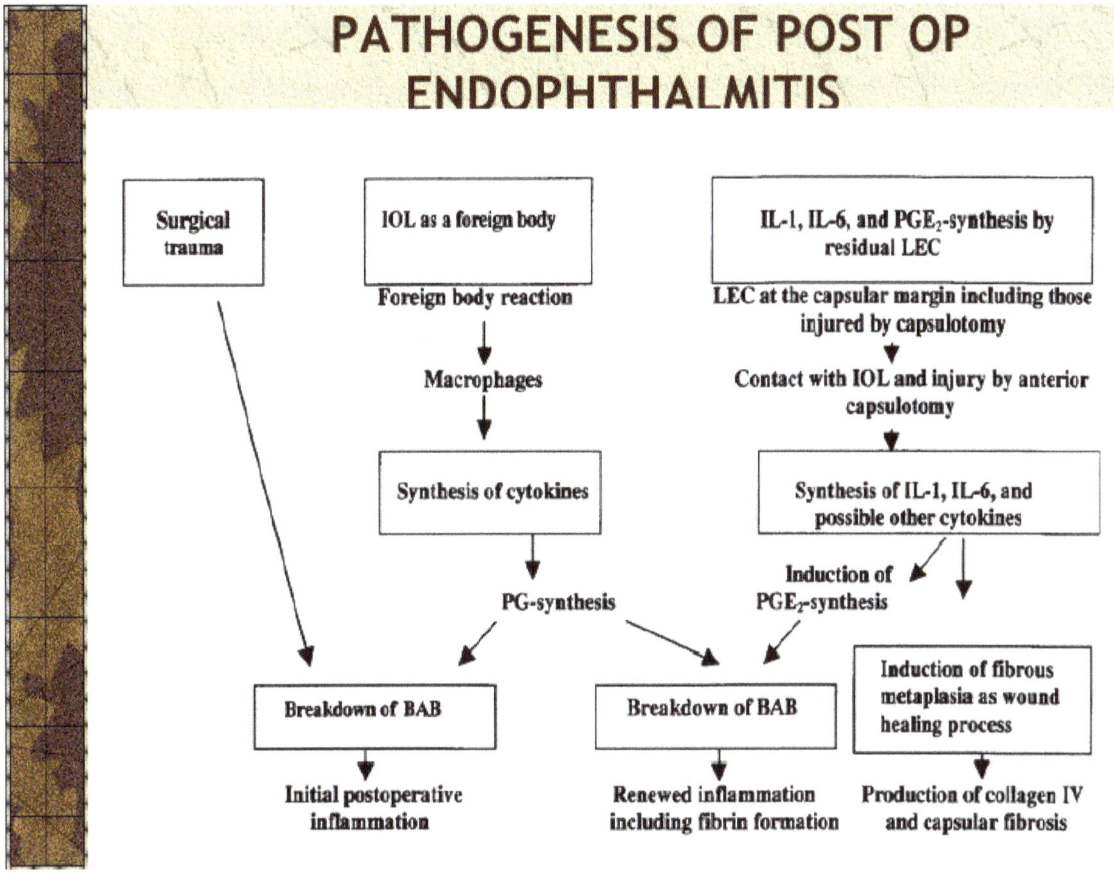

Figure 5. Brief overview of pathogenesis of bacterial endophthalmitis

7.1. Diagnosis of bacterial endophthalmitis

7.1.1. Laboratory diagnosis

The clinical diagnosis of endophthalmitis is confirmed by obtaining intra-ocular specimens like aqueous and vitreous specimen [47]. The possibility of isolating a microorganism from the vitreous specimen is 56–70%, whereas it is 36–40% from the anterior chamber (AC) humour [48]. Culture and sensitivity studies on aqueous and vitreous samples are necessary to determine the type of organism and antibiotic sensitivity.[9, 10] If endogenous bacterial endophthalmitis is suspected, a systemic workup for the source of infection is required, with cultures of blood, sputum and urine. Anterior chamber tap can be done by introducing 30-gauge needle on a tuberculin syringe to anterior chamber through limbus to obtain a 0.1 ml sample under topical anesthesia. The vitreous specimen can be obtained either by vitreous tap, vitreous biopsy or by using an automated vitrectomy instrument. In vitreous tap, a 21-gauge needle on a tuberculin syringe is used to obtain 0.1–0.2 ml of vitreous sample under sub-Tenon block. Vitreous biopsy can be taken using a 23-gauge vitrectomy cutter. Direct inoculation of the intra-ocular fluid specimen onto specific culture media is especially important when limited specimens are obtained. Specimens obtained with automated vitrectomy instruments can be processed by two methods. Vitrectomy specimen is either passed through 0.45 mm filter paper that concentrates the microorganisms and particulate matter and filter paper is sectioned and distributed on the appropriate media or vitrectomy specimen is directly inoculated into standard blood culture bottle [49]. Specimens can be inoculated on 5% sheep blood agar for recovery of the most common bacterial and fungal isolates. Sabouraud dextrose agar is also inoculated for recovery of fungal isolates. Chocolate agar: can be used for the recovery of fastidious organisms (i.e. *Neisseria gonorrhoeae* and *Hemophilus influenzae*). Thioglycollate broth and anaerobic blood agar are useful for recovery of small numbers of aerobic or anaerobic (including *Propionibacterium acnes*) organisms from ocular fluids and tissues. Blood culture bottles contain specially prepared medium for the recovery of both aerobic and anaerobic bacteria and fungi and it can be directly inoculated by intra-ocular fluids. Immunologic and molecular genetic technologies enable rapid and specific identification of infectious agents. In culture negative cases, the additional use of polymerase chain reaction was reported to aid in the identification of the organism [49]. These real-time techniques have been used in both clinical and experimental settings, and their future use in this area appears promising [50, 51].

In the Endophthalmitis Vitrectomy Study (EVS), Gram stain result did not reveal any sub-groups in which vitrectomy had a beneficial value and therefore is not useful in making initial therapeutic decisions [26]. Also in EVS, there was no difference in the culture positivity rate and operative complications between samples obtained by tap and those obtained by vitrectomy [52].

7.1.2. Imaging studies

In B-scan ultrasound of the posterior pole, choroidal thickening and ultrasound echoes in the vitreous support the diagnosis of endophthalmitis. Retained lens material and associated retinal detachment are also visible. The ultrasound also provides a baseline prior to intra-ocular intervention and allows assessment of the posterior vitreous face and areas of possible traction [53]. In traumatic cases, a CT scan can be performed, which may show thickening of the sclera and uveal tissues associated with various degrees of increased density in the vitreous and peri-ocular soft tissue structures. In endogenous cases, imaging modalities like two-dimensional echocardiography and chest x-ray can be done to rule out potential sources of infection.

8. Prevention of endophthalmitis

The most effective therapy for endophthalmitis is prevention. Sterile technique during any type of ocular surgery is important. All instruments for surgery should be thoroughly sterilized with autoclaving; tubing is preferably sterilized with ethylene oxide gas sterilizer. BSS (balanced salt solution) bottles should never be kept or used for more than one operating session. Proper preparation before any intra-ocular surgery including peri-ocular and ocular surface (cul-de-sac) sterilization with povidone iodine 5% applied for 3 min is the best means for prevention of endophthalmitis (superior to topical antibiotics) [54]. In allergic patients, 0.05% chlorhexidine can be used. Large bottles of diluted povidone iodine or chlorhexidine should be avoided and single-use vials be used as they get contaminated with *P. aeruginosa*. A prophylactic antibiotic like topical 0.5% levofloxacin or ofloxacin one drop 1 h and one drop 30 min before surgery and three drops at 5 min intervals immediately following surgery is effective in reducing the rate of post-operative endophthalmitis according to the European Society of Cataract and Refractive Surgery (ESCRS) study [55]. Topical antibiotic should be continued four times a day for two weeks post-operatively. The use of antibiotics in the irrigation and infusion fluid is also an option. In addition, washing the surgical gloves whether containing talc or not, after wearing them in sterile saline and washing any surgical instrument before introducing it into the eye and avoiding touching any non-sterile place including the body surface with anything. Biodegradable scleral plugs impregnated with antibiotics, antiviral and anti-inflammatory drugs have been tested for drug release *in vitro*. Scleral plugs containing vancomycin, amikacin and dexamethasone have been used for slow delivery of drugs in the vitreal cavity at a concentration well above MIC (minimum inhibitory concentration) for a period of time needed to treat bacterial endophthalmitis in place of repeated vitreal injections [56, 57]. All patients with ocular penetration injuries should be treated with IV broad-spectrum antibiotics for 3 days. The common regimen is cefazolin 1 g tds and gentamycin 80 mg BD. If injury is through contaminated object, vancomycin 1 g bd (in slow infusion to prevent "red man" syndrome) should substitute cefazolin. In patients allergic to penicillins or cephalosporins, moxifloxacin 400 mg once a day may be used.

8.1. Treatment strategy for endophthalmitis

Endophthalmitis is an ocular emergency, and urgent treatment is required to reduce the potential of significant visual loss. Microbial endophthalmitis is a therapeutic challenge due to delicate anatomy and physiology of ocular tissues. Retina has a rich blood supply, but the vitreous and anterior chambers are avascular and are isolated from systemic circulation via blood–ocular fluid barrier [4]. These features represent a barrier for the delivery of cellular and humoral mediators of host immunity and also antimicrobial or anti-inflammatory agents administered systemically. This leaves clinicians with few treatment options like injecting drug directly into intra-ocular space, but there is a risk of vitreous or sub-retinal haemorrhaging, retinal toxicity, corneal abrasions, central artery occlusion, uveitis or lens opacification [58]. Also, retinal photoreceptor cells are highly sensitive not only to the offending pathogen and the resulting inflammatory response but also to antimicrobial agents administered locally to treat the infection [59].

8.2. Antimicrobial agents and anti-inflammatory agents

Outcome of endophthalmitis management depends on several factors, including the responsible pathogen, the patient's age, the duration between injury and treatment, the therapy chosen and the condition of the eye upon presentation [60]. Delay in therapy results in poor visual outcome, especially in severe cases of endophthalmitis. Bacterial endophthalmitis is treated with repeated injection of antibiotics into the vitreous concurrently with systemic antibiotics, although some potentially effective antibiotics like vancomycin and aminoglycosides do not penetrate readily into the vitreous, due to the protective effect of the blood–ocular fluid barrier; however, intra-ocular inflammation increases the permeability of the blood–

ocular fluid barrier, enhancing penetration of systemic antibiotics into the vitreous cavity [61]. Another reason for poor systemic antibiotic effect in endophthalmitis is poor penetration through the blood flow because of the inflammation and necrosis of blood vessels. Because of variable penetration into the vitreous cavity of aminoglycosides, vancomycin and cephalosporins, the EVS evaluated their clinical efficacy in a post-cataract surgery endophthalmitis controlled trial and found that systemic antibiotics did not enhance visual outcomes in these patients. However, this recommendation does not hold true following other types of ocular surgery, trauma or suspected endogenous endophthalmitis [62]. Systemic antibiotics are important for therapeutic management of endogenous endophthalmitis where there is concomitant bacteremia, while intravitreal antibiotic is a key component for clinical management of exogenous bacterial endophthalmitis. Fluoroquinolones are currently used by many clinicians in combination with intravitreal antibiotics like vancomycin, amikacin and ceftazidime for severe endophthalmitis cases. The two drug regimens commonly used by clinicians include vancomycin (1 mg/0.1 ml) to cover Gram-positive organisms and a third-generation cephalosporin (ceftazidime 2 mg /0.1 ml) or amikacin (0.4 mg/0.1 ml) to cover Gram-negative organisms [63]. Repeated intravitreal injections of antibiotics may be necessary if there is no response to the initial therapy.

Fungal endophthalmitis carries a poor prognosis and there is no standard management available for treating this condition. In fungal endophthalmitis cases, systemic antifungal agents namely amphotericin with or without flucytosine or fluconazole are used. In fluconazole-resistant strains voriconazole may be helpful; however, information on new antifungal agents for endophthalmitis is limited. It is seen that chorioretinitis infections can be more readily cured with systemic antifungal agents, whereas more aggressive treatment including pars plana vitrectomy with intravitreal amphotericin (5–10mg/0.1mL) or voriconazole and systemic antifungal is required for patients with vitritis. Topical antifungal agents (natamycin 5%) are also included, especially in cases of corneal involvement [64].

The use of corticosteroids is controversial. In endophthalmitis, ocular inflammation is induced by growing bacteria and also due to breakdown of cell wall or other components due to use of antibiotics. This overt inflammatory response can damage sensitive neurologic tissues. They should not be administered without proper coverage of all infective microorganisms and when the infection is not controlled. Intravitreal dexamethosone in the concentration of 400 microgram in 0.1 ml has been used, but is contraindicated in fungal endophthalmitis [65].

8.3. Pars plana vitrectomy

Although intravitreal antibiotic therapy can provide effective bacterial killing during endophthalmitis, vitrectomy is an appealing adjunct to management. Vitrectomy (surgical cutting and aspiration of vitreous contents and replacement with balanced salt solution) (Figure 6) debrides the vitreous cavity of bacteria, inflammatory cells and other toxic debris; promotes better diffusion of antibiotics; helps in obtaining adequate sampling for microanalysis and helps in speedy recovery of vision [66, 67]. Timing of vitrectomy is controversial, and investigators advocate aggressive early treatment with early vitrectomy in suspected bacterial metastatic endophthalmitis, and more conservative approach in suspected fungal cases. Also,

3 port pars plana 23 or 25 gauge complete vitrectomy is preferred over core vitrectomy. However, in an inflamed eye certain complications like retinal detachment, hypotony and pthisis bulbi can occur. The definite indications for vitrectomy include worsening of signs and symptoms, rapid progression, infections uncontrolled by systemic and /or intravitreal antibiotics, retinal necrosis, extensive subretinal abscess, retinal detachment and intra-ocular foreign body [65].

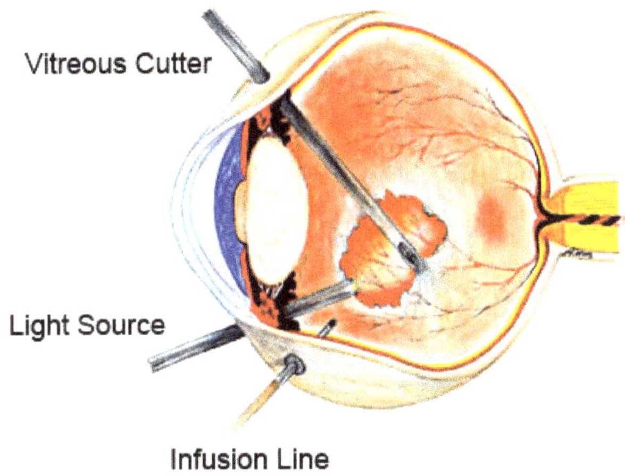

Figure 6. showing Cutting and aspiration of vitreous contents in pars plana vitrectomy

9. Conclusion

Endophthalmitis may cause severe visual loss and detailed understanding of the offending organisms and the intra-ocular host response and its early recognition is necessary for effective treatment of endophthalmitis and improving visual outcome. The key to successful therapy for endophthalmitis is rapid sterilization of the posterior segment by antibiotics and arrest of potentially harmful inflammation, while concurrently limiting risks associated with penetration of the eye by injections or surgery.

Author details

S. Malhotra*, S. Sharma, N. J. K. Bhatia, C. Hans and P. Kumar

*Address all correspondence to: drshalinimalhotra@yahoo.com

Department of Microbiology, Dr. Ram Manohar Lohia Hospital and PGIMER, New Delhi, India

References

[1] Peyman G, Lee P, Seal DV. Endophthalmitis: Diagnosis and Management. Taylor & Francis, London & New York: 2004, pp. 1–278.

[2] Kresloff MS, Castellarin AA, Zarbin MA. Endophthalmitis. Surv Ophthalmol 1998;43:193–224.

[3] Kernt M, Kampik A. Endophthalmitis: pathogenesis, clinical presentation, management, and perspective. Clin Ophthalmol 2010;4:121–35.

[4] Moshfeghi A, Rosenfeld PJ, Flynn HW Jr, et al. Endophthalmitis after intravitreal anti-vascular endothelial growth factor antagonists: a six-year experience at a university referral center. Retina 2011;31:662–8.

[5] Marak Jr GE. Phacoanaphylactic endophthalmitis. Erratum in: Surv Ophthalmol 1992;36:454.

[6] Mamalis N, Edelhauser HF, Dawson DG, Chew J, LeBoyer RM, Werner L. Toxic anterior segment syndrome. J Cataract Refract Surg 2006;32:324–33.

[7] Holland SP, Morck DW, Lee TL. Update on toxic anterior segment syndrome. Curr Opin Ophthalmol 2007;18:4–8.

[8] Carolee M, Cutler P, Jacob B, Sue C, Chris D, Henry EE, Nick M. Toxic anterior segment syndrome: Common causes J Cataract Refractive Surg July 2010;36(7):1073–80.

[9] Stepien KE, Eaton AM, Jaffe GJ, Davis JL, Raja J, Feuer W. Increased incidence of sterile endophthalmitis after intravitreal triamcinolone acetonide in Spring 2006. Retina 2009;29:207–13.

[10] Callegan MC, Engelbert M, Parke DW, Jett BD, Gilmore MS. Bacterial endophthalmitis: epidemiology, therapeutics, and bacterium-host interactions. Clin Microbiol Rev 2002;15:111–24.

[11] Scott IU, Flynn HW, Feuer W, Pflugfelder SC, Alfonso EC, Forster RC, Miller D. Endophthalmitis associated with microbial keratitis. Ophthalmology 1996;103:1864–70.

[12] Krause L, Bechrakis N, Heimann H, Kildal D, Foerster M. Incidence and outcome of endophthalmitis over a 13-year period. Can J Ophthalmol 2009;44:88–94.

[13] Ramakrishnan R, Bharathi M, Shivkumar C, et al. Microbiological profile of culture-proven cases of exogenous and endogenous endophthalmitis: a ten-year retrospective study. Eye (Lond) 2009;23:945–56.

[14] Bahrani HM, Fazelat AA, Thomas M, et al. Endophthalmitis in the era of small gauge transconjunctival sutureless vitrectomy – meta analysis and review of the literature. Semi Ophthalmol 2010;25:275–82.

[15] Akçakaya AA, Sargin F, Erbil HH, et al. A cluster of acute-onset postoperative endophthalmitis over a 1-month period: investigation of an outbreak caused by an uncommon species. Br J Ophthalmol 2011;95:481–4.

[16] Korah S, Braganza A, Jacob P, Balaji V. An "epidemic" of post cataract surgery endophthalmitis by a new organism. Indian J Ophthalmol 2007;55:464–6.

[17] Jamulingam M, Parameswaran SK, Lysa S, Selvaraj M, Madhavan HN. A study on the incidence, microbiological analysis and investigations on the source of infection of postoperative infectious endophthalmitis in a tertiary care ophthalmic hospital: an 8-year study. Indian J Ophthalmol 2010;58:297–302.

[18] Anand AR, Therese KL, Madhavan HN. Spectrum of aetiological agents of postoperative endophthalmitis and antibiotic susceptibility of bacterial isolates. Indian J Ophthalmol 2000;48:123–8.

[19] Peponis V, Rosenberg P, Chalkiadakis SE, Insler M, Amariotakis A. Fungal scleral keratitis and endophthalmitis following pterygium excision. Eur J Ophthalmol. 2009;19:478–80.

[20] Narang S, Gupta A, Gupta V, et al. Fungal endophthalmitis following cataract surgery: clinical presentation, microbiological spectrum, and outcome. Am J Ophthalmol 2001;132:609–17.

[21] Huycke MM, Sahm DF, Gilmore MS. Multiple-drug resistant enterococci: the nature of the problem and an agenda for the future. Emerg Infect Dis 1998;4:239–49.

[22] Forster RK. Etiology and diagnosis of bacterial postoperative endophthalmitis. Ophthalmology Apr 1978;85(4):320-6.

[23] Arshinoff SA, Bastianelli PA. Incidence of postoperative endophthalmitis after immediate sequential bilateral cataract surgery. J Cataract Refract Surg Dec 2011;37(12): 2105–14.

[24] Adán A, Casaroli-Marano RP, Gris O, et al. Pathological findings in the lens capsules and intraocular lens in chronic pseudophakic endophthalmitis: an electron microscopy study. Eye (Lond) 2008;22:113–9.

[25] Al-Mezaine HS, Al-Assiri A, Al-Rajhi AA. Incidence, clinical features, causative organisms, and visual outcomes of delayed-onset pseudophakic endophthalmitis. Eur J Ophthalmol 2009;19:804–11.

[26] Soltau JB, Rothman RF, Budenz DL, Greenfield DS, Feuer W, Liebmann JM, Ritch R. Risk factors for glaucoma filtering bleb infections. Arch. Ophthalmol 2000;118:338–42.

[27] Andreoli CM, Andreoli MT, Kloek CE, Ahuero AE, Vavvas D, Durand ML. Low rate of endophthalmitis in a large series of open globe injuries. Am J Ophthalmol 2009;147:601–8.

[28] Vedantham V, Nirmalan PK, Ramasamy K, Prakash K, Namperumalsamy P. Clinico-microbiological profile and visual outcomes of post-traumatic endophthalmitis at a tertiary eye care centre in South India. Indian J Ophthalmol 2006;54:5–10.

[29] Gupta A, Srinivasan R, Kaliaperumal S, Saha I. Post-traumatic fungal endophthalmitis—a prospective study. Eye (Lond) 2008;22:13–7.

[30] Callegan MC, Kane ST, Cochran DC, et al. Bacillus endophthalmitis: roles of bacterial toxins and motility during infection. Invest Ophthalmol Vis Sci 2005;46:3233–8.

[31] Romero CF, Rai MK, Lowder CY, and Adal KA. Endogenous endophthalmitis: case report and brief review. Am Fam Phys 1999;60:510–14.

[32] Binder MI, Chua J, Kaiser PK, et al. Endogenous endophthalmitis: an 18-year review of culture- positive cases at a tertiary care center. Medicine 2003;82:97–105.

[33] Ruhnke M, Rickerts V, Cornely OA, et al. Diagnosis and therapy of candida infections: joint recommendations of the German Speaking Mycological Society and the Paul-Ehrlich-Society for Chemotherapy. Mycoses 2011;54:279–310.

[34] Lamaris GA, Esmaeli B, Chamilos G, et al. Fungal endophthalmitis in a tertiary care cancer center: a review of 23 cases. Eur J Clin Microbial Infect Dis 2008;27:343–7.

[35] Safneck JR. Endophthalmitis: a review of recent trends. Saudi J Ophthalmol 2012;26:181–9.

[36] Khan A, Okhravi N, Lightman S. The eye in systemic sepsis. Clin Med 2002;2:444–8.

[37] Lundstrom M, Wejde G, Stenevi U, et al. Endophthalmitis after cataract surgery: a nationwide prospective study evaluating incidence in relation to incision type and location. Ophthalmology 2007;114:866–70.

[38] Behndig A, Montan P, Stenevi U, et al. One million cataract surgeries: Swedish National Cataract Register 1992–2009, J Cat Refract Surg 2011;37:1539–45.

[39] Al-Mezaine HS, Kangave D, Al-Assiri A, Al-Rajhi AA. Acute-onset nosocomial endophthalmitis after cataract surgery: incidence, clinical features, causative organisms, and visual outcomes. Cataract Refract Surg 2009;35:643–9.

[40] Al-Mezaine HS, Al-Assiri A, Al-Rajhi AA. Incidence, clinical features, causative organisms, and visual outcomes of delayed-onset pseudophakic endophthalmitis. Eur J Ophthalmol 2009;19:804–11.

[41] Chaudhry IA, Shamsi FA, Elzaridi E, Al-Rashed W. Al-Amri AM, Al-Anezi F, Arat YO, Holck DEE. Outcome of treated orbital cellulitis from a tertiary eye care center in the Middle East. Ophthalmology 2007;114:345–54.

[42] Cunha-Vaz JG. The blood-ocular barriers: past, present, and future. Doc Ophthalmol 1997;93:149–57.

[43] Steptoe RJ, Holt PG, McMenamin PG. Functional studies of major histocompatibility class II-positive dendritic cells and resident tissue macrophages isolated from the rat iris. Immunology 1995;85:630–7.

[44] Miller KV, Eisley KM, Shanks RM, et al. Recurrent enterococcal endophthalmitis seeded by an intraocular lens biofilm. J Cataract Refract Surg 2011;37:1355–9.

[45] Gilmore MS, Callegan MC, Jett BD. Enterococcus faecalis cytolysin and Bacillus cereus bi- and tri-component toxins. In: Alouf JE, Freer JH. (Eds.) The Comprehensive Sourcebook of Bacterial Protein Toxins, 2nd edn. Academic Press, London, United Kingdom 1999, pp. 419–434.

[46] Projan SJ, Novick RP. The molecular basis of pathogenicity. In: Crossley KB, Archer GL. (Eds.) The Staphylococci in Human Disease. Churchill Livingstone, New York, NY, 1999, pp. 55–82.

[47] Van Snick J. Interleukin-6: an overview. Annu Rev Immunol 1990;8:252–78.

[48] Donahue SP, Kowalski RP, Jewart BH, et al. Vitreous cultures in suspected endophthalmitis: biopsy or vitrectomy? Ophthalmology 1993;100:452.

[49] Spadea L, Fiasca A. Treatment of post-operative endophthalmitis. Eur Ophthal Rev 2012;6(3):149–56.

[50] Joondeph BC, Flynn HW Jr, Miller D, et al. A new culture method for infectious endophthalmitis. Arch Ophthalmol 1989;107:1334.

[51] Dworkin LL, Gibler TM, Van Gelder RN: Real-time quantitative polymerase chain reaction diagnosis of infectious posterior uveitis. Arch Ophthalmol 2002;120:1534–9.

[52] Wittwer CT, Kusukawa N: Real-time PCR. In: Persing DH. (Ed.) Molecular Microbiology: Diagnostic Principles and Practice. Washington, DC: ASM Press, 2004, pp. 71–84.

[53] Results of the Endophthalmitis Vitrectomy Study. A randomized trial of immediate vitrectomy and of intravenous antibiotics for the treatment of postoperative bacterial endophthalmitis. Endophthalmitis Vitrectomy Study Group, Arch Ophthalmol 1995;113:1479–96.

[54] Chan IM, Jalkh AE, Trempe CL, Tolentino FI. Ultrasonographic findings in endophthalmitis. Ann Ophthalmol Aug 1984;16(8):778–84.

[55] Alp BN, Elibol O, Sargon MF, et al. The effect of povidone iodine on the corneal endothelium. Cornea 2000;19:546–50.

[56] ESCRS Endophthalmitis Study Group: Prophylaxis of postoperative endophthalmitis following cataract surgery: results of the ESCRS multi-centre study and identification of risk factors. J Cataract Refract Surg 2007;33:978–88.

[57] Liu SJ, Kau YC, Liaw CW, Peng YJ. In vitro elution of vancomycin/amikacin/ steroid from solvent-free biodegradable scleral plugs. Int J Pharm 2009;370:75–80.

[58] Peng YJ, Kau YC, Wen CW, Liu SJ. Solvent-free biodegradable scleral plugs providing sustained release of vancomycin, amikacin, and dexamethasone—an *in vivo* study. J Biomed Mater Res Part A 2010;94:426–32.

[59] Nelson ML, Tennant MTS, Sivalingam A, et al. Infectious and presumed noninfectious endophthalmitis after intravitreal triamcinolone acetonide injection. Retina 2003;23:686–91.

[60] Wiechens B, Neumann D, Grammer JB, Pleyer U, Hedderich J, Duncker GI. Retinal toxicity of liposome-incorporated and free ofloxacin after intravitreal injection in rabbit eyes. Int Ophthalmol 1998–1999;22:133–43.

[61] Foster RE, Martinez JA, Murray TG, Rubsamen PE, Flynn HW, Forster RK. Useful visual outcomes after treatment of Bacillus cereus endophthalmitis. Ophthalmology 1996;103:390–7.

[62] Ferencz JR, Assia EI, Diamantstein L, Rubinstein E. Vancomycin concentration in the vitreous after intravenous and intravitreal administration for postoperative endophthalmitis. Arch Ophthalmol 1999;117:1023–7.

[63] Ferencz JR, Assia EI, Diamantstein L, Rubinstein E, Vancomycin concentration in the vitreous after intravenous and intravitreal administration for postoperative endophthalmitis. Arch Ophthalmol 1999;117:1023–7.

[64] Recchia FM, Busbee BG, Pearlman RB, Carvalho-Recchia CA, Ho AC. Changing trends in the microbiologic aspects of postcataract endophthalmitis. Arch Ophthalmol 2005;123:341–6.

[65] Lamaris GA, Esmaeli B, Chamilos G, et al. Fungal endophthalmitis in a tertiary care cancer center: a review of 23 cases. Eur J Clin Microbiol Infect Dis 2008;27:343–7.

[66] Mathews AS, Pillai GS, Natasha R, Shetty M. Endogenous endophthalmitis – a review. Kerala J Ophthalmol 2011;23:25–31.

[67] Fujii GY, De Juan E Jr, Humayun MS, et al. Initial experience using the transconjunctival sutureless vitrectomy system for vitreoretinal surgery. Ophthalmol 2002;109:1814–20.

[68] Fine HF, Iranmanesh R, Iturralde D, Spaid RF. Outcomes of 77 consecutive cases of 23-gauge transconjunctival vitrectomy surgery for posterior segment disease. Ophthalmol 2007; 114:1197–200.

5

Cataract Surgery in Patients with Uveitis: Preoperative and Surgical Considerations

Alejandro Rodriguez-Garcia and C. Stephen Foster

Abstract

Cataract is one of the most frequent visual impairment complications of uveitis, accounting for up to 40% of the visual loss seen in these patients. In general, uveitis patients differ from the general cataract population in that they are younger and have a higher rate of comorbidities, however the rates of inflammatory sequelae vary markedly among uveitic entities. Cataract development may be influenced by the cause and duration of uveitis, the degree of inflammation control, and the use of corticosteroid therapy. Cataract surgery in patients with uveitis represents a serious challenge due to pre-existing ocular comorbidities that may limit the visual outcome and difficult the surgical procedure; the need for preoperative control of inflammation; and the efficacy of postoperative management to avoid immediate and late ocular complications. A detailed ophthalmologic exam prior to surgery is essential to know the status of pre-existing pathologic changes, adjust the medical therapy to achieve absolute control of inflammation, establish a surgical plan, and deliver an objective visual prognosis to the patient or the relatives. The key point to surgical success is the absolute control of inflammation, meaning no cells in the anterior chamber for at least 3 months prior to surgery. Today, minimally invasive phacoemulsification with acrylic foldable intraocular lens implantation is the standard of care for most patients with uveitis. It must be taken into consideration that higher rates of intraoperative and postoperative complications may occur. Vision-limiting pathology related to pre-existing uveitis complications are the major contributing factors for limited postoperative visual outcome.

Keywords: uveitis, cataract, phacoemulsification, intraocular lens, steroids, macular edema, glaucoma

1. Introduction

Cataract represents a significant burden in the management and visual outcome of uveitis patients. Up to 40% of the visual loss seen in these patients is either solely or largely due to cataract [1]. Lens opacification is caused by repeated episodes or sustained intraocular inflammation characterized by the release of free oxygen radicals, lysosomal enzymes, immune complex deposition on the lens capsule, hypoxia, and altered composition of the aqueous humor [2]. The development of cataract depends on the type of uveitis, the degree and duration of the inflammatory process, and on the prolonged and excessive use of corticosteroids [3–5].

Cataract surgery in patients with uveitis represents a serious challenge for the anterior segment surgeon [6, 7]. Nowadays, clear cornea phacoemulsification with intraocular lens (IOL) implantation is the standard of care for most patients with uveitis [8, 9]. However, despite remarkable progress on surgical techniques and IOL materials, certain specific considerations should be taken into account regarding patient selection, preoperative preparation, as well as perioperative and postoperative management for successful long-term results [10, 11]. Nearly one-third of all uveitic eyes have small pupils, which represent a surgical technical difficulty [2]. In such cases, higher rates of additional intraoperative maneuvers are required to obtain proper visualization and phacoemulsification of the cataract [4, 12, 13]. And, while surgery is associated with an improvement in best corrected visual acuity (BCVA), higher rates of both, intraoperative and postoperative complications have been reported [14, 15]. Moreover, it has been shown that the final BCVA in uveitic eyes is worse than in non-uveitic ones [14]. Therefore, identifying the cause of uveitis and pre-existing pathologic changes that affect the visual outcome, achieving absolute control of inflammation before surgery, careful surgical planning, and solving intraoperative and postoperative complications are crucial to obtain a successful result (BCVA ≥ 20/40).

2. Epidemiology

Cataract is the most common ocular complication in children with chronic uveitis with an estimated rate from 35 to 52.0% [16]. In juvenile idiopathic arthritis (JIA)-associated uveitis, the prevalence varies from 40 to 60% and the incidence of new-onset cataract formation has been estimated as 0.04/eye-year [17, 18]. On the other hand, in adult patients it is one of the most frequent complications of uveitis with a prevalence rate as high as 50% as seen in Fuchs uveitis [6, 14, 19, 20]. In HLA-B27-associated anterior uveitis, the most common cause of uveitis in adults, cataract formation is the third most frequent complication with an estimated prevalence of 14%, and an incidence rate of 0.091 during follow-up time (**Table 1**) [21]. Cataract prevalence varies among different causes of uveitis and depends on multiple factors including etiology, localization of the inflammatory process, time elapsed between the onset and diagnosis of uveitis, the degree of inflammation, the clinical course, and the use of corticosteroids [1, 18, 22, 23].

Cause of uveitis	Cataract prevalence range (median)	Successful outcome BCVA ≥ 20/40 (Snellen)	Frequent complications	References
Fuchs uveitis	15–75% (50%)	83%	Intraoperative AC hemorrhage (3.6–76%) Hyphema Ocular hypertension (glaucoma) (3–35%) PCO (14.6%) Progressive vitreous opacification	[20, 27, 48, 49]
Herpetic uveitis	15–75% (24%)	72.2%	Viral reactivation Iris posterior synechiae Secondary glaucoma	[63, 151–153]
Juvenile idiopathic arthritis-associated uveitis	40–60% (50%)	60–70% (67%)	Exuberant postoperative inflammation Iris posterior synechiae Secondary glaucoma (25%) CME Cyclitic membrane Hypotony (Phthisis bulbi)	[4, 17, 18, 25, 26, 81, 95, 97–99, 101, 110]
HLA-B27 associated uveitis	9.2–20.1%	NA	Recurrent uveitis CME Iris synechiae	[21]
Pars planitis	36–42% (40%)	50–83%	Persistent vitritis (haze) CME (50%) Glaucoma (10%) PCO (10%) IOL Cocooning (29%) ERM Optic nerve atrophy	[23, 28, 140, 154]
Adamantiades-Behcet disease	21–26% (38.5%)	72.5% (42.4%)	Exuberant inflammation (12.5%) Iris posterior synechiae (17.5%) CME (12.5%) ERM (7.5%) Papillitis (optic nerve atrophy) (5%) PCO (37.5% most common)	[148, 155, 156]
Vogt-Koyanagi-Harada disease	10–35%	68%	Exuberant inflammation Iris anterior and posterior synechiae Pupillary membrane PCO (76%) Macular scarring	[135, 157]

Cause of uveitis	Cataract prevalence range (median)	Successful outcome BCVA ≥ 20/40 (Snellen)	Frequent complications	References
Sympathetic ophthalmia	31.8%	67.79% (72.2%)	PCO (77.7%) Glaucoma	[158]
Sarcoidosis	21%	61%	PCO (57.1%) Recurrent uveitis CME Glaucoma	[159]

AC = anterior chamber; PCO = posterior capsule opacification; CME = cystoid macular edema; ERM = epiretinal membrane.

Table 1. Prevalence, visual outcome, and complications of cataract surgery in uveitis.

3. Clinical characteristics of diverse forms of uveitis

In general, the uveitic population differs from the general population suffering from cataract in that they are younger and have a higher rate of comorbidities [15]. However, the rates of inflammatory sequelae vary markedly among uveitic entities [7, 24]. For this reason, each uveitis syndrome must be analyzed separately with respect to ocular complications and visual outcome [6, 14] (**Table 1**). While Fuchs uveitis regularly has the best visual prognosis and the least postoperative complications, JIA-associated uveitis has one of the most fear prognosis due to frequent pre-existing pathology, difficulties in reaching absolute control of inflammation, and multiple intraoperative and postoperative complications [4, 25–27].

4. Preoperative evaluation

A correct classification and etiologic diagnosis of the uveitic entity is very helpful to establish the appropriate surgical strategy and to determine the prognosis [8]. Moreover, a complete preoperative ophthalmologic examination is essential since pre-existing pathology will have significant therapeutic and prognostic visual implications [16, 28]. For instance, corneal opacity, vitreous haze, macular edema, and optic nerve atrophy usually result in a poor visual outcome [6, 19]. Therefore, it is very important that the patient and/or their relatives have an objective report on the status of the eye to be operated in order to have a realistic expectation of the final visual result. Ancillary diagnostic tests are always necessary to detect pre-existing pathologic changes that will allow us to render a more accurate visual prognosis. In most cases, it is helpful to perform a macular function test. Several methods are available for this purpose including the potential acuity meter (PAM), the laser interferometer (LI), and the focal electroretinogram (fERG) [29, 30]. The PAM test has proven an accuracy of 84% in patients with poor visual acuity (<20/40) [30]. On the other hand, LI has shown a lower accuracy (65%) and a tendency for over-predicting vision compared to the PAM in these patients [29, 30]. Focal cone ERG is very sensitive for detecting macular pathology, showing 91% accuracy in eyes with poor visual acuity [30].

Linear A-B ultrasound is necessary to identify vitreous hemorrhage and opacity, as well as posterior segment changes like, retinal detachment, optic nerve swelling, and sclerochoroidal thickness [31]. Another very useful device is high-frequency ultrabiomicroscopy (UBM), which generates high-resolution images at an almost histological level. *In vivo* image sections may be obtained up to 3–6 mm in depth, permitting visualization of anterior segment structures [32]. Frequent indications for UBM in uveitis include uveitis-glaucoma-hyphema syndrome (UGH), sclerouveitis, herpetic anterior uveitis, pars planitis, pseudophakic uveitis, hypotony, peripheral toxocariasis, and ciliary body pathology [32, 33].

Retina fluorescein angiography (FA) allows the detection of many different forms of posterior segment inflammatory changes. It is used to evaluate the activity and extent of chorioretinitis and optic nerve involvement; identify macular edema and choroidal neovascularization; diagnose certain posterior uveitic entities with typical features; evaluate retinal vascular involvement and neovascularization; and to monitor the therapeutic response [34]. However, many inflammatory changes occur in the peripheral retina where visualization may be difficult with conventional angiography. Wide field scanning laser ophthalmoscopy performs ultra-wide angle FA allowing clear identification of peripheral lesions and accurate documentation of disease progression [35]. This recently new image technology has replaced conventional angiography for the diagnosis and monitoring of intermediate and many forms of posterior uveitis [35].

Indocyanine green angiography (ICGA) allows the detection of choroidal inflammation. Two patterns of choroidal vasculitis have been described: primary inflammatory choriocapillaropathy and stromal inflammatory vasculopathy [36]. The first pattern is characterized by non-perfusion of the choriocapillaris found in entities like, multiple evanescent white dot syndrome, acute posterior multifocal placoid pigment epitheliopathy, multifocal choroiditis, and serpiginous choroidopathy [36]. The choroidal stromal inflammatory vasculopathy pattern is seen in active Vogt-Koyanagi-Harada disease (VKH), ocular sarcoidosis, tuberculosis, and birdshot chorioretinopathy [37]. In Behcet's disease, as in other forms of uveitis, both ICGA vascular patterns may be seen at different stages of inflammation [38].

Today, the most frequently used imaging technique to detect and monitor macular inflammatory changes is optical coherence tomography (OCT). With an axial resolution in the 5–7 μm range, it provides close to an *in-vivo* histologic view of the retina [39]. There are several types of OCT available for clinical purposes. The spectral-domain OCT is the most used method [40]. It allows high-speed, accurate images of the retina, particularly macular pathology like, cystoid and diffuse macular edema, subretinal fluid accumulation, epiretinal membrane formation, macular holes, and choroidal neovascularization [41]. Longer wavelength OCT systems, including the swept-source technology and en-face imaging, enhance the detection of subtle microstructural changes in chorioretinal disorders by improving imaging of the choroid [42–44]. A technique that produces high-resolution cross-sectional images of the entire choroid called enhanced depth imaging technique (EDI-OCT) has identified increased subfoveal choroidal thickness in patients with active Behcet [45] and VKH disease, as well as loss of focal hyperreflectivity of the inner choroid in the acute and convalescent phases of VKH [46].

Once the preoperative evaluation is completed, a postoperative visual prognosis may be assumed, therapeutic adjustments may be applied, and a surgical plan is prepared based on pre-existing pathologic findings.

5. Preoperative preparation and therapeutic strategies

The key to surgical success in patients with uveitic cataract is the absolute control of inflammation, meaning no cells in the anterior chamber for at least 3 months prior to surgery [7]. This requisite is crucial to obtain an optimal surgical result and to minimize postoperative complications [7, 24]. Active uveitis at the time of cataract surgery has been associated with worse visual outcomes [15, 47]. Moreover, postoperative cystoid macular edema (CME) is more likely to develop in eyes with active inflammation within a 3-month period before surgery (relative risk 6.19) than those under control [41]. However, this general consensus of no cells in the anterior chamber prior to surgery has its exemptions [2]. In Fuchs uveitis, minimal but persistent anterior chamber cells and flare are frequently found despite intensive and sustained treatment with topical corticosteroids [48]. Hence, anti-inflammatory treatment is not indicated for the low-grade anterior chamber reaction seen in Fuchs uveitis and only occasionally, a short-course of corticosteroids is indicated for symptomatic exacerbations [49]. Other exemptions are related to the necessity for prompt surgical intervention in cases like, lens-induced uveitis, cyclitic membrane formation with hypotony, persistent vitreous opacity or hemorrhage, and retinal detachment [50, 51].

Preoperative management depends specifically on the type and etiology of uveitis. For inactive idiopathic anterior non-granulomatous uveitis as for Fuchs uveitis, topical administration of prednisolone acetate 1% four times a day, starting 3–7 days before surgery may be sufficient to avoid an outburst of postoperative inflammation [24]. On the contrary, patients with JIA-associated uveitis, anterior granulomatous uveitis, intermediate, posterior, and panuveitis also require oral prednisone (1.0 mg/kg/day) starting 3 days before surgery and continued for a week after cataract removal and then tapered slowly according to the inflammatory status [52, 53]. Preoperative oral steroids have been shown to be effective in reducing the risk of CME [41]. If patients are on immunosuppressive chemotherapy and/or biologics, they should be continued at current dosage [11]. In case that systemic corticosteroids are contraindicated (e.g., diabetes mellitus, metabolic disease, acid-peptic disease, obesity, or osteoporosis), periocular administration (transseptal or sub-Tenon's) of triamcinolone acetonide (40 mg/ml) should be considered [54, 55]. Alternative immunosuppressive agents like, cyclosporin-A, tacrolimus, or anti-metabolites may be administered to these patients considering that most of these medications require a longer period of time (usually 4–6 weeks) to reach an optimal therapeutic effect [56].

The use of topical non-steroidal anti-inflammatory drugs (NSAIDs) like, ketorolac 0.4%, nepafenac 0.15%, or bromfenac 0.09%, have become a standard of care practice for the perioperative management of inflammation, pain, surgical-induced miosis, and cystoid macular edema in uneventful and also in uveitic cataract surgery [57–59]. A systematic review found high-quality evidence that topical NSAIDs are more effective than topical steroids in preventing the short-term pseudophakic CME in non-uveitic cataract surgery [60]. On the other hand, a recent evidence-based review conducted by the American Academy of Ophthalmology found that the claimed made about the synergistic effect of combined topical steroids and NSAIDs remains unproven [61]. In addition, NSAIDs have only a short-term therapeutic effect on prompt visual recovery and reduction of established CME, but no effect on the long-term visual outcome [57, 58, 61]. There is good collective clinical evidence and rationale that the application of a topical NSAID 3 days before surgery reduces CME and improves vision in the short-term [61]. Because the COX-2 enzyme is inducible and mostly responsible for the inflammatory process, the selective inhibitory effect of nepafenac and bromfenac makes them more suitable for this purpose [62]. Nepafenac has shown the shortest time to reach maximal concentration and the greatest aqueous humor peak concentration compared to ketorolac and bromfenac in eyes having cataract surgery [62]. After the surgical procedure, topical NSAIDs use is usually extended for 4–6 weeks [1, 10].

There are other special conditions in uveitis in which certain specific actions should be taken before cataract extraction is performed. Such is the case of herpetic uveitis in which prophylactic anti-viral therapy with acyclovir or valacyclovir should be administered at least 1 week before surgery in order to avoid recurrent viral infection [63, 64]. Other special consideration is the preoperative management of prominent band keratopathy interfering with cataract visualization which may be treated with EDTA 1–2% calcium chelation, or Excimer laser PTK before cataract surgery [65, 66].

Cataract and glaucoma frequently coexist as uveitis complications, and a combined surgical procedure may be associated with an increased risk of glaucoma surgery failure [67, 68]. In such cases, it may result better to perform a clear cornea small-incision cataract extraction first, followed later on by filtration surgery or a valve implantation with anti-metabolites [69, 70]. One must consider that uveitic glaucoma eyes operated for trabeculectomy with mitomycin-C which had previous cataract surgery or granulomatous uveitis, have a higher risk of surgical failure (RR = 2.957, P = 0.0344, and RR = 3.805, P = 0.0106, respectively) [71]. A higher risk of glaucoma surgical failure has also been associated with idiopathic, intermediate, and Fuchs uveitis; active intraocular inflammation at the time of surgery; and relapse of uveitis [72]. Moreover, the success rate of filtration surgery in uveitic eyes is significantly lower than that of non-uveitic, and many patients with successful intraocular pressure (IOP) control still require anti-glaucoma therapy to maintain adequate IOP levels in the postoperative period [72].

Posterior vitrectomy and cataract extraction may be an alternative for patients with prominent posterior segment pathology including vitreous opacity, hemorrhage, cystoid macular edema, and tractional retinal detachment [73]. There is reasonable evidence that cataract phacoemulsification combined with posterior vitrectomy has a favorable visual outcome for some patients with refractory inflammation, particularly those with significant vitreous opacity and chronic macular edema [13, 74]. In children, this combined surgical approach has been used for JIA-associated uveitis, pars planitis, and other forms of posterior uveitis [75].

However, this technique is not exempt of serious postoperative complications like, glaucoma, macular edema, and exuberant inflammation [75, 76]. For specific cases with various ocular complications, multiple combined surgical strategies have been postulated including phacoemulsification with IOL implantation, posterior vitrectomy, intravitreal sustained-release corticosteroid injection, and glaucoma tube implantation with promising results [77].

6. Surgical technique and intraoperative maneuvers

Nowadays, small clear corneal incision phacoemulsification surgery is preferred over extracapsular cataract extraction (ECCE) and lensectomy for most patients with uveitis [78, 79]. Since cataract surgery in these patients is frequently complicated by corneal opacification, iris synechiae, pupillary and cyclitic membranes, among others, the surgical technique should be minimally invasive with precise and delicate maneuvers [10, 24] (**Figure 1**). Most studies report a higher rate of additional maneuvers, notably iris and pupillary manipulation within a range between 19 and 67% of eyes [4–6, 25].

Dealing with unexpected intraoperative complications like, corneal stromal edema; anterior chamber hemorrhage; pigment dispersion; posterior capsule rupture with vitreous exposure is key to achieve the best surgical outcome possible [6, 19, 75]. The first challenge that the surgeon faces is an adequate exposure and visualization of the cataract. Iris synechiolysis, pupillary membrane removal, and pupil distension with iris hooks or iris stretch devices are frequently required for proper cataract visualization [80, 81]. There is no general consensus on what is the best way to deal with the pathologic changes of the anterior segment encountered in uveitic eyes. However, it is generally agreed that

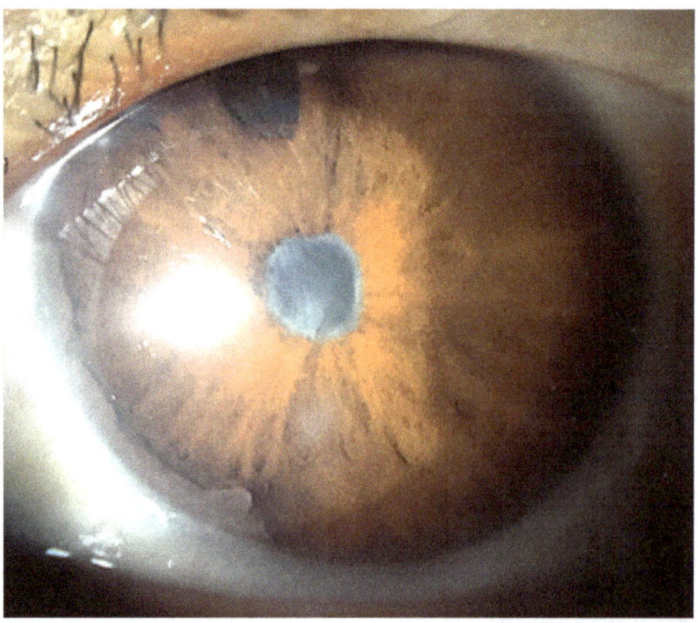

Figure 1. Anterior segment appearance of a patient with Vogt-Koyanagi-Harada disease showing extensive peripheral anterior and posterior synechiae, shallow anterior chamber and a pupillary membrane in front of a secondary cataract.

attempts should be made to minimize surgical maneuvers in order to lessen tissue manipulation and trauma as possible [6, 24, 26].

The capsulorhexis should measure between 5 and 6 mm in diameter because smaller apertures are frequently associated with capsular phimosis and posterior iris synechiae to the anterior capsule remnant [82–84] (**Figure 2**). On the other hand, larger diameter capsulorhexis may affect the IOL centration and stability [83]. The phacoemulsification technique may vary depending on the density and zonular status of the cataract, but an effort should be made to use the less ultrasound power and time possible, to perform vigorous cortical and posterior capsule cleaning, and to avoid posterior capsule rupture [11, 19]. Avoiding the latter is crucial to obtain a good postoperative result, especially in chronic and recurrent uveitis like, herpetic uveitis, pars planitis, VKH disease, toxoplasmosis, among others [6, 24, 85]. In these cases, posterior capsule rupture with vitreous exposure may be a contraindication for IOL implantation due to a high probability of postoperative excessive and persistent inflammation [12, 86]. In uveitic eyes with encapsulated and subluxated IOLs with extensive fibrosis, IOL removal may be necessary at some point of the postoperative period to control severe inflammation and reduce its consequences [87–89]. For eyes with extensive membrane formation in the anterior vitreous, vitrectomy after performing a posterior central capsulorhexis must be considered [90].

Decision making regarding the type of IOL to be used; anterior or posterior chamber IOL implantation; possible IOL sulcus fixation; combined filtration surgery, MIGS, or valve implantation; central posterior capsulorhexis after PC-IOL implantation with anterior vitrectomy; lensectomy, as well as posterior vitrectomy with or without retinal surgery are frequently met during uveitic cataract surgery, and the surgeon must be prepared to make the best decision for the particular case [91–94]. The implantation of a foldable IOL "in the bag" is ideal for most cases of uveitis with certain exceptions [4, 95]. Until now, it is not clear how to proceed in children with uveitic cataract, and randomized controlled trials (RCT) are necessary to elucidate

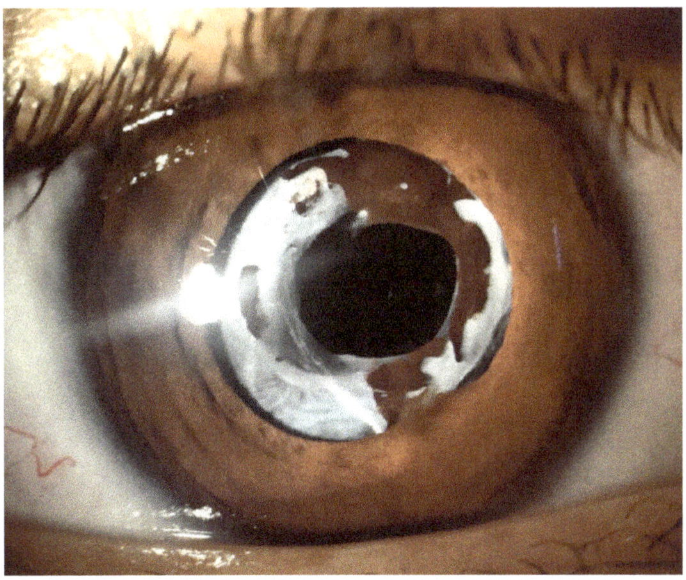

Figure 2. Patient with ankylosing spondylitis and HLA-B27-associated uveitis after cataract surgery showing capsular phimosis and partial adherence of the pigmentary epithelium of the iris to the anterior capsule remnant.

this matter [4, 25, 26, 81]. Historically, uveitic cataract surgery during childhood has been associated with a higher rate of surgical complications, particularly excessive postoperative inflammation [6, 10]. In the past, this situation made that the preferred surgical techniques for cataract extraction in this group including ECCE with posterior pars plana vitrectomy or lensectomy [4, 95]. However, recent evidence favors the implantation of foldable PC-IOLs in children with uveitis, including patients with JIA-associated iridocyclitis [25, 26, 96–101].

Intraocular corticosteroids can be administered during surgery. Intracameral dexamethasone phosphate (400 μg/0.1 ml) or intravitreal triamcinolone (4 mg/0.1 ml) injection (IVTA) may be administered intraoperatively, except in advanced secondary glaucoma or known steroid-responsive patients [4, 102]. A prospective and comparative RCT between oral corticosteroids and preservative-free IVTA injection showed no differences in postoperative anterior chamber reaction, IOP levels, and central macular thickness (CMT) [103]. Another study found a better effect of IVTA versus orbital floor TA on macular edema and postoperative inflammation after cataract surgery in patients with uveitis [55]. However, IVTA injections have a temporary effect therefore, may require repeated injections which are not exempt of serious ocular complications like, elevated IOP (30–43% eyes), bacterial endophthalmitis, vitreous hemorrhage, and retinal detachment [104]. For those eyes at higher risk for intravitreal injection, sub-Tenon's or transseptal TA can be administered at the end of surgery [19].

Intravitreal steroid sustained-release devices containing fluocinolone acetonide 0.59 mg or dexamethasone phosphate 0.7 mg have proven to be beneficial for the control of inflammation, prevention of CME, or reduction of CMT if applied a few days to weeks before or during cataract surgery [105]. Although no general consensus exists on the appropriate surgical time, it seems reasonable to perform the cataract surgery within 4–6 weeks from the last steroid implantation [105–107]. The most fear complication of sustained-release steroid devices is ocular hypertension (OHT). A meta-analysis found that 66% of eyes develop OHT after the implantation of the 0.59 mg fluocinolone acetonide device, compared to 32% following 4 mg IVTA, and only 15% with the 0.7 mg dexamethasone implant [108]. Risk factors for developing OHT include, pre-existing glaucoma, higher baseline IOP, younger age, OHT following previous injection, uveitis, higher steroid dosage, and fluocinolone implant [108]. A new sustained-release implant containing 0.19 mg fluocinolone acetonide has shown promising results improving visual acuity and reducing CMT with a significant reduction of IOP compared to the dexamethasone implant and IVTA [109].

7. Considerations for intraocular lenses

The general consensus regarding cataract surgery in patients with uveitis is that implantation of IOLs may be safely performed when ocular inflammation is completely abolished for a minimum period of 3 months [4, 7]. However, a debate still exists if an IOL should be implanted in specific circumstances like, lens-induced uveitis, JIA-associated iridocyclitis, young children with posterior or panuveitis, and intraoperative rupture of the posterior capsule with vitreous exposure [25, 26, 91, 110]. The implantation of an IOL triggers different intraocular responses including inflammation and foreign body reaction, as well as activation of the complement and coagulation cascades [83, 111–113]. These reactions along with the breakdown of the blood-aqueous barrier induced by surgery may increase cellular adhesion and lens epithelial cell (LEC) proliferation on the anterior surface of the IOL, resulting in anterior capsule phimosis, fibrosis, and posterior capsule opacification (PCO) [114]. With the advent of technologic development, many advances have been made to reduce IOL-induced reactions and to improve their biocompatibility [115]. The inflammatory response induced by IOLs is inversely related to its biocompatibility, so the higher the biocompatibility, the lower the inflammatory response [15, 83, 115]. Even though they were considered biologically inert, the first IOLs made of polymethyl-methacrylate (PMMA) were capable of producing foreign body reaction, as well as activate the complement and coagulation cascades [113, 116].

Different strategies have been used to reduce the host response, including the modification of the IOL surface by making it hydrophilic, like in heparin-coated PMMA IOLs, or hydrophobic such as surface passivated [83]. Heparin surface-modified IOLs have improved biocompatibility compared with unmodified PMMA IOLs in eyes at risk for severe postoperative inflammation, including those with uveitis [117, 118].

Foldable IOLs may be hydrophobic, including silicone IOLs or hydrophilic, and both surfaces have demonstrated to be relatively inert [114, 119]. Hydrophobic surfaces resist cell adhesion while hydrophilic ones reduce electrostatic forces and cellular adhesion, preventing the attraction of inflammatory cells and their activation, as well as adherence of fibroblasts to the IOL surface [120, 121].

Anterior capsule phimosis has been related to the degree of fibrotic reaction produced by pro-inflammatory cytokines released by residual LEC [122, 123]. Careful vacuuming the undersurface of the anterior capsule helps to reduce the number of LEC [82, 124]. Capsular phimosis has been reported more frequently with hydrogel (poly-HEMA) than acrylic, and silicone IOLs [83, 125]. Foreign body giant cell precipitates are less frequently seen in hydrophilic than on hydrophobic IOL surfaces and heparin-coated PMMA IOLs [115, 126]. The frequency of posterior capsule opacification (PCO) is highest with PMMA IOLs, less with silicone and minimal with acrylic IOLs [124, 127].

Few studies have evaluated the visual outcome following cataract surgery in uveitis with silicone IOL implantation. Overall, only 30% of eyes have achieved 20/40 of better vision with silicone IOLs, fewer than any other type of IOL [15]. Silicone was the first material available for foldable IOLs, but its use has declined particularly because it cannot be used for a monobloc open-loop designed, the preferred choice for preloaded injectors that allow implantation through small corneal incisions [128].

With the advent of acrylic foldable IOLs, the biocompatibility issue has become a minor concern, but controversy still exists of which material, hydrophilic or hydrophobic is best suitable for patients with uveitis [120, 126, 129]. Since the lens is surrounded by aqueous humor, it was thought that hydrophilic materials were more biocompatible than hydrophobic for patients with uveitis [89, 92]. However, there is insufficient evidence to determine the effects of different types of IOL materials, including hydrophobic and hydrophilic acrylic IOLs in patients with uveitis [129]. Results from the largest RCT provide only preliminary evidence that acrylic IOLs may perform better than silicone IOLs in terms of improving vision and reducing the chances of postoperative inflammation and complications [129, 130]. A large multicenter RCT with standardized outcome measurements is necessary to properly address the surgical outcome of patients with uveitic cataract.

8. Immediate postoperative management

The postoperative management is as important as the preoperative preparation and the surgical procedure itself. Since the first postoperative moments, intense topical corticosteroids (1% prednisolone acetate hourly), topical NSAIDs (anti-COX-2 selective), topical wide spectrum antibiotics (fourth generation fluoroquinolones), overnight steroid ointment, as well as mydriatic-cycloplegic combinations (e.g., 1% tropicamide + 5% phenylephrine every 6-hours × 5–7 days) should be administered [11, 24, 131]. Topical corticosteroids are wined down according to the grade of anterior chamber inflammatory reaction, the presence of glaucoma, or OHT in steroid-responders [54]. In case the patient was given systemic corticosteroids, they should be maintained at immunosuppressive levels (1 mg/kg/day) for 7–10 days before reducing them slowly to a minimum dose of 7.5 mg/day [56]. In case the patient is on immunosuppressive chemotherapy or biologic therapy, it should be continued at maintenance dose [19, 131]. Systemic anti-virals used for herpetic uveitis should be kept at therapeutic dose for 7–14 days postoperative, and then reduced to prophylactic levels (acyclovir, 600–800 mg/day and valacyclovir 500–1000 mg/day) for several weeks to months before stopping them [63, 64, 132].

9. Postoperative complications and their management

Postoperative complications after cataract surgery in patients with uveitis are relatively frequent [8]. The reported prevalence of complications is higher in ECCE than in phacoemulsification [78, 79, 133]. The risk for postoperative complications also depends on the type of uveitis and the degree of ocular involvement [8, 12, 85] (**Table 1**). Despite all preventive measurements taken before and during surgery, the most frequent and fear postoperative complication is the outburst of inflammation out of expected proportions [5]. Significant inflammation characterized by >2+ anterior chamber cells, extensive protein exudation with fibrin and plasmoid bodies formation, as well as fibrinoid membranes covering the pupil, and hypopyon may be seen [7, 19, 24, 134]. This aggressive inflammatory response is commonly associated with early postoperative iris synechiae formation and pupillary inflammatory membranes, particularly in disorders like JIA-associated uveitis, and VKH, among others [4, 6, 131, 135]. The best way to deal with this unexpected postoperative inflammatory response consists on avoiding it by previous absolute control of inflammation and the implementation of perioperative measurements discussed before. Nevertheless, in those cases in which a significant inflammatory reaction occurs, an adjustment to the systemic prednisone dose and the administration of atropine 1% will help to control the inflammation [52–54].

Other immediate postoperative complications that may be seen are hyphema and significant pigment dispersion throughout the anterior segment [19, 24]. Pigment dispersion is related to a variety of factors including, surgical trauma, small pupil, and age [24, 83, 91]. In both cases, regular tonometry is mandatory for opportune detection of severe OHT related to clogging of the trabecular meshwork by ghost cells or pigment, respectively [6]. If anti-glaucoma therapy is required, prostaglandin analogs as well as alpha-adrenergic drugs should be avoided as possible because they may exacerbate the inflammatory process [69]. In some patients with corneal stromal edema and Descemet folds due to high IOP, oral carbonic anhydrase inhibitors (e.g., acetazolamide 250 mg, 3–4 times a day) may be administered [69]. If the IOP becomes uncontrollable with medical therapy, filtration surgery or valve implantation should be considered to avoid further optic nerve damage [69, 136]. Finally, an excessive postoperative inflammatory process may produce significant vitreous opacity and membrane formation [5]. Once acute infectious endophthalmitis has been ruled out in such cases, aggressive anti-inflammatory therapy with systemic, periocular, and even intravitreal corticosteroids should be administered [52, 54, 55, 106]. If vitreous condensation and organization persist, a pars plana vitrectomy with or without intravitreal corticosteroid injection should be performed [13, 73, 75, 137].

In the late postoperative period, ocular complications are usually related with recurrent intraocular inflammation occurring from 8.3 to 53% of cases [8, 12, 85, 133]. Recurrent postoperative uveitis may produce anterior and/or posterior iris synechiae which may cause an angle or pupillary block glaucoma, respectively [69].

Certainly one of the most frequent ocular complications observed in this late period is posterior capsule opacification seen in up to 58% of cases [82, 83, 85, 124, 133]. Nd-Yag laser capsulotomy usually resolves this problem, but in some cases retrolental hyaloid-vitreous opacification or significant deposition of pigment and inflammatory debris on the IOL surface may occur therefore, recurrent low-energy Nd-Yag laser and other operative procedures may be needed for polishing the IOL [82, 138]. It must be considered that Nd-Yag laser capsulotomy in patients with uveitis is associated with a higher risk for vision-threatening complications, including OHT, CME, IOL damage or luxation, as well as retinal detachment [40, 139].

Another very important visual-threatening postoperative complication is macular edema occurring from 33 to 56% after ECCE and from 12 to 59% after phacoemulsification [12, 85, 133, 140]. The appearance of CME depends on multiple factors including the cause of uveitis and the type of surgical procedure performed [41]. Treatment of uveitic macular edema (UME) includes the administration of periocular injections of depot corticosteroids [54, 141]. However, as stated before, IVTA has shown to be superior to orbital floor injection for the treatment of UME [55, 142]. OHT is a potential complication of both types of steroid administration and should always be considered, particularly after repeated intravitreal injections [55, 108, 143]. Sustained-delivery corticosteroid devices may also be administered for this purpose [105, 106, 144]. In patients with bilateral UME, steroid-responders or those who do not accept periocular or intravitreal corticosteroid injections, oral prednisone along with oral carbonic anhydrase inhibitor (e.g., acetazolamide 250 mg every 12 hours) may be administered [54]. Epiretinal membrane formation is more commonly seen in patients with chronic

UME with a prevalence ranging from 15 to 56% [12, 145, 146]. Treatment consists of pars plana vitrectomy and internal limiting membrane delamination [73, 146, 147].

Other less common, but serious complications is retinal detachment and hypotony [5, 26]. Hypotony may be related to the retinal detachment per se, or to a low aqueous humor production due to inflammation of the ciliary process, or tractional detachment of the ciliary body due to cyclitic membrane formation [26]. Postoperative hypotony may evolve to pthisis bulbi [10, 88]. Both complications should be attended immediately by retinopexy, and/or posterior vitrectomy with cyclitic membrane and sometimes intraocular lens removal, as well as peri- or intraocular corticosteroid administration [87, 88].

10. Prognosis and visual outcome

The outcome of cataract surgery in patients with uveitis is less predictable than in other causes of cataract. Many factors may contribute to this uncertainty including, pre-existing pathologic changes, intraoperative technical challenges, the impact of postoperative exuberant inflammation, and the reversibility of postoperative complications derived from it [14]. Vision-limiting pathology related to pre-existing uveitis complications, especially macular edema and optic neuropathy are probably the major contributing factors for limited postoperative visual outcome [8, 15, 85].

Different studies suggest that visual prognosis varies according to uveitis subtypes [5, 15, 26]. For instance, the proportion of eyes achieving 20/40 or better vision is better in Fuchs uveitis and worse in Behcet's disease, VKH disease, or sympathetic ophthalmia [20, 27, 47, 148]. In general, diseases that spare the posterior segment have a better prognosis than those affecting it, particularly macular and optic nerve involvement [5, 6, 8, 85]. In addition, acute uveitic entities tend to be associated with better outcome than chronic ones [12].

Uveitic cataract surgery has been associated with worse postoperative visual acuity, higher IOP, and more than double prevalence of UME when compared with non-uveitic cataract surgery [14]. Moreover, the visual outcome following uveitic cataract extraction is not as good as that of age-related cataract surgery with the exception of Fuchs uveitis [27, 149]. Systematic reviews found a successful visual outcome (20/40 or better) in 96% of eyes with age-related cataract surgery compared to 70% in uveitic eyes undergoing either phacoemulsification or ECCE [15, 149]. ECCE and phacoemulsification seem to have similar visual outcomes compared to half less successful rate after pars plana lensectomy [15]. With respect to the comparable visual results reported between ECCE and phacoemulsification, it must be taken into account that most ECCE trials have more exclusion criteria than phacoemulsification studies, favoring better visual outcomes [15, 85, 150].

Finally, regarding IOL implantation, more eyes (71%) undergoing cataract surgery with IOL implantation than eyes left aphakic (52%) achieved a BCVA ≥ 20/40 vision postoperatively [14]. Eyes receiving acrylic IOLs or heparin surface-modified PMMA had better visual outcomes than those receiving non-heparin-PMMA or silicone IOLs [14, 15, 83, 94].

Author details

Alejandro Rodriguez-Garcia[1*] and C. Stephen Foster[2,3,4]

*Address all correspondence to: immuneye@gmail.com

1 Tecnológico de Monterrey, Escuela de Medicina y Ciencias de la Salud, Institute of Ophthalmology and Visual Sciences, Ocular Immunology and Uveitis Service, Monterrey, Mexico

2 Massachusetts Eye Research and Surgery Institute, Waltham, MA, USA

3 Ocular Immunology and Uveitis Foundation, Weston, MA, USA

4 Department of Ophthalmology, Harvard Medical School, Boston, MA, USA

References

[1] Durrani OM. Degree, duration, and causes of visual loss in uveitis. The British Journal of Ophthalmology. 2004;**88**:1159-1162

[2] Hooper PL, Rao NA, Smith RE. Cataract extraction in uveitis patients. Survey of Oph_ thalmology. 1990

[3] Urban RC, Cotlier E. Corticosteroid-induced cataracts. Survey of Ophthalmology. 1986; **31**:102-110

[4] Foster CS, Barrett FR. Cataract development and cataract surgery in patients with juvenile rheumatoid arthritis-associated iridocyclitis. Ophthalmology. 1993;**100**:809-817

[5] Elgohary MA, McCluskey PJ, Towler H, Okhravi N, Singh RP, Obikpo R, Lightman SS. Outcome of phacoemulsification in patients with uveitis. The British Journal of Ophthalmology. 2007;**91**:916-921

[6] Agrawal R, Murthy S, Ganesh SK, Phaik CS, Sangwan V, Biswas J. Cataract surgery in uveitis. International Journal of Inflammation. 2012;**2012**:1-16

[7] Foster CS, Fong LP, Singh G. Cataract surgery and intraocular lens implantation in patients with uveitis. Ophthalmlogy. 1989;**96**:281-288

[8] Yoeruek E, Deuter C, Gieselmann S, Saygili O, Spitzer MS, Tatar O, Bartz-Schmidt KU, Szurman P. Long-term visual acuity and its predictors after cataract surgery in patients with uveitis. European Journal of Ophthalmology. 2010;**20**:694-701

[9] Pershing S, Kumar A. Phacoemulsification versus extracapsular cataract extraction: Where do we stand? Current Opinion in Ophthalmology. 2011;**22**:37-42

[10] Jancevski M, Foster CS. Cataracts and uveitis. Current Opinion in Ophthalmology. 2010;**21**:10-14

[11] Foster CS, Rashid S. Management of coincident cataract and uveitis. Current Opinion in Ophthalmology. 2003;**14**:1-6

[12] Estafanous MF, Lowder CY, Meisler DM, Chauhan R. Phacoemulsification cataract extraction and posterior chamber lens implantation in patients with uveitis. American Journal of Ophthalmology. 2001;**131**:620-625

[13] Walker J, Rao NA, Ober RR, Liggett PE, Smith REA. Combined anterior and posterior approach to cataract surgery in patients with chronic uveitis. International Ophthalmology. 1993;**17**:63-69

[14] Chu CJ, Dick AD, Johnston RL, Yang YC, Denniston AK. Cataract surgery in uveitis: A multicentre database study. The British Journal of Ophthalmology. 2017;**101**:1132-1137

[15] Mehta S, Linton MM, Kempen JH. Outcomes of cataract surgery in patients with uveitis: A systematic review and meta-analysis. American Journal of Ophthalmology. 2014; **158**:676-692

[16] Rosenberg KD, Feuer WJ, Davis JL. Ocular complications of pediatric uveitis. Ophthalmology. 2004;**111**:2299-2306

[17] Thorne JE, Woreta F, Kedhar SR, Dunn JP, Jabs DA. Juvenile idiopathic arthritis-associated uveitis: Incidence of ocular complications and visual acuity loss. American Journal of Ophthalmology. 2007;**143**:840-846

[18] Thorne JE, Woreta FA, Dunn JP, Jabs DA. Risk of cataract development among children with juvenile idiopathic arthritis-related uveitis treated with topical corticosteroids. Ophthalmology. 2010;**117**:1436-1441

[19] Rojas B, Zafirakis P, Foster SC. Cataract surgery in patients with uveitis. Current Opinion in Ophthalmology. 1997;**8**:6-12

[20] Jones NP. Cataract surgery in Fuchs' heterochromic uveitis: Past, present, and future. Journal of Cataract & Refractive Surgery. 1996;**22**:261-268

[21] Loh AR, Acharya NR. Incidence rates and risk factors for ocular complications and vision loss in HLA-B27-associated uveitis. American Journal of Ophthalmology. 2010; **150**:534-542

[22] Tomkins-Netzer O, Talat L, Bar A, Lula A, Taylor SR, Joshi L, Lightman S. Long-term clinical outcome and causes of vision loss in patients with uveitis. Ophthalmology. 2014; **121**:2387-2392

[23] Niederer RL, Sharief L, Bar A, Lightman SL, Tomkins-Netzer O. Predictors of long-term visual outcome in intermediate uveitis. Ophthalmology. 2017;**124**:393-398

[24] Meier FM, Tuft SJ, Pavésio CE. Cataract surgery in uveitis. Ophthalmology Clinics of North America. 2002;**15**:365

[25] Terrada C, Julian K, Cassoux N, Prieur AM, Debre M, Quartier P, LeHoang P, Bodaghi B. Cataract surgery with primary intraocular lens implantation in children with uveitis: Long-term outcomes. Journal of Cataract & Refractive Surgery. 2011;**37**:1977-1983

[26] Quiñones K, Cervantes-Castañeda RA, Hynes AY, Daoud YJ, Foster CS. Outcomes of cataract surgery in children with chronic uveitis. Journal of Cataract & Refractive Surgery. 2009;**35**:725-731

[27] Tejwani S, Murthy S, Sangwan VS. Cataract extraction outcomes in patients with Fuchs heterochromic cyclitis. Journal of Cataract & Refractive Surgery. 2006;**32**:1678-1682

[28] Heinz C, Schoonbrood S, Heiligenhaus A. Intermediate uveitis in children and young adults: Differences in clinical course, associations and visual outcome. The British Journal of Ophthalmology. 2014;**98**:1107-1111

[29] Cuzzani OE, Ellant JP, Young PW, Gimbel HV, Rydz M. Potential acuity meter versus scanning laser ophthalmoscope to predict visual acuity in cataract patients. Journal of Cataract & Refractive Surgery. 1998;**24**:263-269

[30] Fish GE, Birch DG, Fuller DG, Straach RA. Comparison of visual function tests in eyes with maculopathy. Ophthalmology. 1986;**93**:1177-1182

[31] Gupta V, Al-Dhibi HA, Arevalo JF. Retinal imaging in uveitis. Saudi Journal of Ophthalmology. 2014;**28**:95-103

[32] Tran VT, Lehoang P, Herbort CP. Value of high-frequency ultrasound biomicroscopy in uveitis. Eye (Lond). 2001;**15**:23-30

[33] Ciardella AP, Prall FR, Borodoker N, Cunningham ET. Imaging techniques for posterior uveitis. Current Opinion in Ophthalmology. 2004;**15**:519-530

[34] Khairallah M, Jelliti B. Fluorescein angiography in uveitis. Acta Ophthalmologica. 2011; **89**(s248):0-0. DOI: 10.1111/j.1755-3768.2011.4231.x

[35] Kaines A, Tsui I, Sarraf D, Schwartz S. The use of ultra wide field fluorescein angiography in evaluation and management of uveitis. Seminars in Ophthalmology. 2009;**24**:19-24

[36] Bouchenaki N, Cimino L, Auer C, Tao Tran V, Herbort CP. Assessment and classification of choroidal vasculitis in posterior uveitis using indocyanine green angiography. Klinische Monatsblätter für Augenheilkunde. 2002;**219**:243-249

[37] Herbort CP. Fluorescein and indocyanine green angiography for uveitis. Middle East African Journal of Ophthalmology. 2009;**16**:168-187

[38] Klaeger A, Tran TV, Hiroz CA, Morisod L, Herbort CP. Indocyanine green angiography in Behcet's uveitis. Retina. 2000;**20**:309-314

[39] Hassenstein A, Bialasiewicz AA, Richard G. Optical coherence tomography in uveitis patients. American Journal of Ophthalmology. 2000;**130**:669-670

[40] Nazari H, Dustin L, Heussen FM, Sadda S, Rao NA. Morphometric spectral-domain optical coherence tomography features of epiretinal membrane correlate with visual acuity in patients with uveitis. American Journal of Ophthalmology. 2012;**154**:78-86

[41] Bélair ML, Kim SJ, Thorne JE, Dunn JP, Kedhar SR, Brown DM, Jabs DA. Incidence of cystoid macular edema after cataract surgery in patients with and without uveitis using optical coherence tomography. American Journal of Ophthalmology. 2009;**148**:128-135

[42] Copete S, Flores-Moreno I, Montero JA, Duker JS, Ruiz-Moreno JM. Direct comparison of spectral-domain and swept-source OCT in the measurement of choroidal thickness in normal eyes. The British Journal of Ophthalmology. 2014;**98**:334-338

[43] Tan CS, Cheong KX, Lim LW, Sadda SR. Comparison of macular choroidal thicknesses from swept source and spectral domain optical coherence tomography. The British Journal of Ophthalmology. 2016;**100**:995-999

[44] Chee SP, Chan SWN, Jap A. Comparison of enhanced depth imaging and swept source optical coherence tomography in assessment of choroidal thickness in Vogt-Koyanagi-Harada disease. Ocular Immunology and Inflammation. 2016;**2012**:1-5

[45] Kim M, Kim H, Kwon HJ, Kim SS, Koh HJ, Lee SC. Choroidal thickness in Behcet's uveitis: An enhanced depth imaging-optical coherence tomography and its association with angiographic changes. Investigative Ophthalmology & Visual Science. 2013;**54**: 6033-6037

[46] Nakayama M, Keino H, Okada AA, Watanabe T, Taki W, Inoue M, Hirakata A. Enhanced depth imaging optical coherence tomography of the choroid in Vogt-Koyanagi-Harada disease. Retina. 2012;**32**:2061-2069

[47] Lin CP, Yeh PT, Chen PF, Yang CM, Cataract HFR. Extraction surgery in patients with uveitis in Taiwan: Risk factors and outcomes. Journal of the Formosan Medical Association. 2014;**113**:377-384

[48] Ram J, Kaushik S, Brar GS, Gupta A, Gupta A. Phacoemulsification in patients with Fuchs' heterochromic uveitis. Journal of Cataract & Refractive Surgery. 2002;**28**:1372-1378

[49] Bonfioli AA, Curi ALL, Oréfice F. Fuchs' heterochromic cyclitis. Seminars in Ophthalmology. 2005;**20**:143-146

[50] Marak GE. Phacoanaphylactic endophthalmitis. Survey of Ophthalmology. 1992;**36**: 325-339

[51] Kerkhoff FT, Lamberts QJ, van den Biesen PR, Rothova A. Rhegmatogenous retinal detachment and uveitis. Ophthalmology 2003;**110**:427-431

[52] Rodríguez-García A. When should I consider using systemic corticosteroids to treat uveitis? Curbside Consultation in Uveitis: 49 Clinical Questions. In: Curbside Consultation in Ophthalmology Series. C. Stephen Foster (editor). SLACK Incorporated. Thorofare, NJ, USA. 2012:27-30. ISBN: 978-1-55642-998-9

[53] Meacock WR. Steroid prophylaxis in eyes with uveitis undergoing phacoemulsification. The British Journal of Ophthalmology. 2004;**88**:1122-1124

[54] Rothova A. Corticosteroids in uveitis. Ophthalmology Clinics of North America. 2002;**15**: 389-394

[55] Roesel M, Tappeiner C, Heinz C, Koch JM, Heiligenhaus A. Comparison between intravitreal and orbital floor triamcinolone acetonide after phacoemulsification in patients with endogenous uveitis. American Journal of Ophthalmology. 2009;**147**:406-412

[56] Jabs DA, Rosenbaum JT, Foster CS, Holland GN, Jaffe GJ, Louie JS, Nussenblatt RB, Stiehm ER, Tessler H, Russell NVG, Whitcup SM, Yocum D. Guidelines for the use of immunosuppressive drugs in patients with ocular inflammatory disorders: Recommendations of an expert panel. American Journal of Ophthalmology. 2000;**130**:492-513

[57] Donnenfeld ED, Perry HD, Wittpenn JR, Solomon R, Nattis A, Chou T. Preoperative ketorolac tromethamine 0.4% in phacoemulsification outcomes: Pharmacokinetic-response curve. Journal of Cataract & Refractive Surgery. 2006;**32**:1474-1482

[58] Kim SJ, Flach AJ, Jampol LM. Nonsteroidal anti-inflammatory drugs in ophthalmology. Survey of Ophthalmology. 2010;**55**:108-133

[59] Rodríguez-García A, Hernández-Camarena JC, López-Jaime GR, Nava-García JA. Effect of topical nonsteroidal anti-inflammatory drugs on pupillary size during uncomplicated cataract surgery. Journal of Refractive Surgery. 2017;**33**:236-242

[60] Kim SJ, Schoenberger SD, Thorne JE, Ehlers JP, Yeh S, Bakri SJ. Post-cataract prevention of inflammation and macular edema by steroid and nonsteroidal anti-inflammatory eye drops. Ophthalmology. 2014;**121**:1915-1924

[61] Kim SJ, Schoenberger SD, Thorne JE, Ehlers JP, Yeh S, Bakri SJ. Topical nonsteroidal anti-inflammatory drugs and cataract surgery: A report by the American Academy of Ophthalmology. Ophthalmology. 2015;**122**:2159-2168

[62] Walters T, Raizman M, Ernest P, Gayton J, Lehmann R. In vivo pharmacokinetics and in vitro pharmacodynamics of nepafenac, amfenac, ketorolac, and bromfenac. Journal of Cataract & Refractive Surgery. 2007;**33**:1539-1545

[63] Rodriguez A, Power WJ, Neves RA, Foster CS. Recurrence rate of herpetic uveitis in patients on long-term oral acyclovir. Documenta Ophthalmologica. 1995;**90**:331-340

[64] Barron BA, Gee L, Hauck WW, Kurinij N, Dawson CR, Jones DB, Wilhelmus KR, Kaufman HE, Sugar J, Hyndiuk RA, Laibson PR, Stulting D, Asbel PA. Herpetic eye disease study: A controlled trial of oral acyclovir for herpes simplex stromal keratitis. Ophthalmology. 1994;**101**:1871-1882

[65] Najjar DM, Cohen EJ, Rapuano CJ, Laibson PREDTA. Chelation for calcific band keratopathy: Results and long-term follow-up. American Journal of Ophthalmology. 2004;**137**:1056-1064

[66] Stewart OG, Morrell AJ. Management of band keratopathy with excimer phototherapeutic keratectomy: Visual, refractive, and symptomatic outcome. Eye (Lond). 2003; **17**:233-237

[67] Bohnsack BL, Freedman SF. Surgical outcomes in childhood uveitic glaucoma. American Journal of Ophthalmology. 2013;**155**:134-142

[68] Carreño E, Villarón S, Portero A, Herreras JM, Maquet JA, Calonge M. Surgical outcomes of uveitic glaucoma. Journal of Ophthalmic Inflammation and Infection. 2010;**1**:43-53

[69] Siddique SS, Suelves AM, Baheti U, Foster CS. Glaucoma and uveitis. Survey of Ophthalmology. 2013;**58**:1-10

[70] Shimizu A, Maruyama K, Yokoyama Y, Tsuda S, Ryu M, Nakazawa T. Characteristics of uveitic glaucoma and evaluation of its surgical treatment. Clinical Ophthalmology (Auckland, NZ). 2014;**8**:2383

[71] Iwao K, Inatani M, Seto T, Takihara Y, Ogata-Iwao M, Okinami S, Tanihara H. Long-term outcomes and prognostic factors for trabeculectomy with mitomycin C in eyes with uveitic glaucoma: A retrospective cohort study. Journal of Glaucoma. 2014;**23**:88-94

[72] Park UC, Ahn JK, Park KH, Phacotrabeculectomy YHG. With mitomycin C in patients with uveitis. American Journal of Ophthalmology. 2006;**142**:1005-1012

[73] Androudi S, Ahmed M, Fiore T, Brazitikos P, Foster CS. Combined pars plana vitrectomy and phacoemulsification to restore visual acuity in patients with chronic uveitis. Journal of Cataract & Refractive Surgery. 2005;**31**:472-478

[74] Soheilian M, Mirdehghan SA, Peyman GA. Sutureless combined 25-gauge vitrectomy, phacoemulsification, and posterior chamber intraocular lens implantation for management of uveitic cataract associated with posterior segment disease. Retina. 2008;**28**:941-946

[75] Pålsson S, Nyström A, Sjödell L, Jakobsson G, Byhr E, Andersson Grönlund M, Zetterberg M. Combined phacoemulsification, primary intraocular lens implantation, and pars plana vitrectomy in children with uveitis. Ocular Immunology and Inflammation. 2015; **23**:144-151

[76] Shinoda K, O'hira A, Ishida S, et al. Posterior synechia of the iris after combined pars plana vitrectomy, phacoemulsification, and intraocular lens implantation. Japanese Journal of Ophthalmology 2001;**45**:276-280

[77] Ahmad ZM, Hughes BA, Abrams GW, Mahmoud TH. Combined posterior chamber intraocular lens, vitrectomy, Retisert, and pars plana tube in noninfectious uveitis. Archives of Ophthalmology. 2012;**130**:908-913

[78] Chee SP, Ti SE, Sivakumar M, Tan D. Postoperative inflammation: Extracapsular cataract extraction versus phacoemulsication. Journal of Cataract & Refractive Surgery. 1999; **25**:1280-1285

[79] Oshika T, Yoshimura K, Miyata N. Postsurgical inflammation after phacoemulsication and extracapsular extraction with soft or conventional intraocular lens implantation. Journal of Cataract & Refractive Surgery. 1992;**18**:356-361

[80] Oetting TA, Omphroy LC. Modified technique using flexible iris retractors in clear corneal surgery. Journal of Cataract & Refractive Surgery. 2002;**28**:596-598

[81] Lam LA, Lowder CY, Baerveldt G, Smith SD, Traboulsi EI. Surgical management of cataracts in children with juvenile rheumatoid arthritis-associated uveitis. American Journal of Ophthalmology. 2003;**135**:772-778

[82] Dana MR, Chatzistefanou K, Schaumberg DA, Foster CS. Posterior capsule opacification after cataract surgery in patients with uveitis. Ophthalmology. 1997;**104**:1387-1394

[83] Rauz S, Stavrou P, Murray PI. Evaluation of foldable intraocular lenses in patients with uveitis. Ophthalmology. 2000;**107**:909-919

[84] Rahman I, Jones NP. Long-term results of cataract extraction with intraocular lens implantation in patients with uveitis. Eye (Lond). 2004;**19**:191-197

[85] Okhravi N. Assessment of visual outcome after cataract surgery in patients with uveitis. Ophthalmology. 1999;**106**:710-722

[86] Ram J, Gupta A, Kumar S, Kaushik S, Gupta N, Severia S. Phacoemulsification with intraocular lens implantation in patients with uveitis. Journal of Cataract & Refractive Surgery. 2010;**36**:1283-1288

[87] Adán A, Gris O, Pelegrín L, Torras J, Corretger X. Explantation of intraocular lenses in children with juvenile idiopathic arthritis-associated uveitis. Journal of Cataract & Refractive Surgery. 2009;**35**:603-605

[88] Foster CS, Stavrou P, Zafirakis P, Rojas B, Tesavibul N, Baltatzis S. Intraocular lens removal from [corrected] patients with uveitis. American Journal of Ophthalmology. 1999;**128**:31-37

[89] Abela-Formanek C, Amon M, Schild G, Schauersberger J, Kolodjaschna J, Barisani-Asenbaum T, Kruger A. Inflammation after implantation of hydrophilic acrylic, hydrophobic acrylic, or silicone intraocular lenses in eyes with cataract and uveitis: Comparison to a control group. Journal of Cataract & Refractive Surgery. 2002;**28**:1153-1159

[90] Lam DS, Law RW, Wong AK. Phacoemulsification, primary posterior capsulorhexis, and capsular intraocular lens implantation for uveitic cataract. Journal of Cataract & Refractive Surgery. 1998;**24**:1111-1118

[91] Holland GN, Van Horn SD, Margolis TP. Cataract surgery with ciliary sulcus fixation of intraocular lenses in patients with uveitis. American Journal of Ophthalmology. 1999;**128**:21-30

[92] Papaliodis GN, Nguyen QD, Samson CM, Foster CS. Intraocular lens tolerance in surgery for cataracta complicata: Assessment of four implant materials. Seminars in Ophthalmology. 2002;**17**:120-123

[93] Diamond JG, Kaplan HJ. Uveitis: Effect of vitrectomy combined with lensectomy. Ophthalmology. 1979;**86**:1320-1327

[94] Tomlins PJ, Sivaraj RR, Rauz S, Denniston AK, Murray PI. Long-term biocompatibility and visual outcomes of a hydrophilic acrylic intraocular lens in patients with uveitis. Journal of Cataract & Refractive Surgery. 2014;**40**:618-625

[95] Magli A, Forte R, Rombetto L, Alessio M. Cataract management in juvenile idiopathic arthritis: Simultaneous versus secondary intraocular lens implantation. Ocular Immunology and Inflammation. 2014;**22**:133-137

[96] Nemet AY, Raz J, Sachs D, Friling R, Neuman R, Kramer M, Suresh K, Oandi MD, Vidushi S, Assia EI. Primary intraocular lens implantation in pediatric uveitis: A comparison of 2 populations. Archives of Ophthalmology. 2007;**125**:354-360

[97] Ganesh SK, Sudharshan S. Phacoemulsification with intraocular lens implantation in juvenile idiopathic arthritis. Ophthalmic Surgery, Lasers & Imaging. 2010;**41**:104-108

[98] Kotaniemi K, Penttila H. Intraocular lens implantation in patients with juvenile idiopathic arthritis-associated uveitis. Ophthalmic Research. 2006;**38**:318-323

[99] Probst LE, Holland EJ. Intraocular lens implantation in patients with juvenile rheumatoid arthritis. American Journal of Ophthalmology. 1996;**122**:161-170

[100] Lundvall A, Zetterström C. Cataract extraction and intraocular lens implantation in children with uveitis. The British Journal of Ophthalmology. 2000;**84**:791-793

[101] Grajewski RS, Zurek-Imhoff B, Roesel M, Heinz C, Heiligenhaus A. Favourable outcome after cataract surgery with IOL implantation in uveitis associated with juvenile idiopathic arthritis. Acta Ophthalmologica. 2011;**90**:657-662

[102] Okhravi N, Morris A, Kok HS, Menezo V, Dowler JG, Hykin PG, Lightman S. Intraoperative use of intravitreal triamcinolone in uveitic eyes having cataract surgery: Pilot study. Journal of Cataract & Refractive Surgery. 2007;**33**:1278-1283

[103] Dada T, Dhawan M, Garg S, Nair S, Mandal S. Safety and efficacy of intraoperative intravitreal injection of triamcinolone acetonide after phacoemulsification in cases of uveitic cataract. Journal of Cataract & Refractive Surgery. 2007;**33**:1613-1618

[104] van Kooij B, Rothova A, de Vries P. The pros and cons of intravitreal triamcinolone injections for uveitis and inflammatory cystoid macular edema. Ocular Immunology and Inflammation. 2006;**14**:73-85

[105] Larochelle MB, Smith J, Dacey MS. Dexamethasone intravitreal implant in the treatment of uveitic macular edema in the perioperative cataract setting: A case series. American Journal of Ophthalmology. 1999;**166**:149-153

[106] Chieh JJ, Carlson AN, Jaffe GJ. Combined fluocinolone acetonide intraocular delivery system insertion, phacoemulsification, and intraocular lens implantation for severe uveitis. American Journal of Ophthalmology. 2008;**146**:589-594

[107] Arcinue CA, Cerón OM, Foster CSA. Comparison between the fluocinolone acetonide (Retisert) and dexamethasone (Ozurdex) intravitreal implants in uveitis. Journal of Ocular Pharmacology and Therapeutics. 2013;**29**:501-507

[108] Kiddee W, Trope GE, Sheng L, Beltran-Agullo L, Smith M, Strungaru MH, Baath J, Buys YM. Intraocular pressure monitoring post intravitreal steroids: A systematic review. Survey of Ophthalmology. 2013;**58**:291-310

[109] Shah SP, Yarian DL, Prenner J, Friedman ES, Wheatley ES, Fine HF, Mantopoulos D, Roth DB. One-year results of fluocinolone acetonide intravitreal implant for diabetic macular edema in highly treated eyes. Presented at: American Society of Retina Specialists 35th Annual Meeting, Boston, MA. 11-15 August 2017

[110] Holland GN. Intraocular lens implantation in patients with juvenile rheumatoid arthritis-associated uveitis: An unresolved management issue. American Journal of Ophthalmology. 2014;**122**:255-257

[111] Apple DJ. Influence of intraocular lens material and design on postoperative intracapsular cellular reactivity. Transactions of the American Ophthalmological Society. 2000;**98**:257-283

[112] Mondino BJ, Nagata S, Glovsky MM. Activation of the alternative complement pathway by intraocular lenses. Investigative Ophthalmology & Visual Science. 1985;**26**:905-908

[113] Sievers H, von Domarus D. Foreign-body reaction against intraocular lenses. American Journal of Ophthalmology. 1984;**97**:743-751

[114] Majima K. An evaluation of the biocompatibility of intraocular lenses. Ophthalmic Surgery, Lasers and Imaging. 1996;**27**:946-951

[115] Amon M, Menapace R. In vivo documentation of cellular reactions on lens surfaces for assessing the biocompatibility of different intraocular implants. Eye (Lond). 1994; **8**:649-656

[116] Mondino BJ, Rajacich GM. Comparison of complement activation by silicone intraocular lenses and polymethyl-methacrylate intraocular lenses with polypropylene loops. Archives of Ophthalmology. 1987;**105**:989-990

[117] Stavrou P, Murray PI. Heparin surface modified intraocular lenses in uveitis. Ocular Immunology and Inflammation. 1994;**2**:161-168

[118] Percival P. Use of heparin-modified lenses in high-risk cases for uveitis. Developments in Ophthalmology. 1991;**22**:80-83

[119] Kang S, Kim MJ, Park SH, Joo CK. Comparison of clinical results between heparin surface modified hydrophilic acrylic and hydrophobic acrylic intraocular lens. European Journal of Ophthalmology. 2008;**18**:377-383

[120] Ravalico G, Baccara F, Lovisato A, Tognetto D. Postoperative cellular reaction on various intraocular lens materials. Ophthalmology. 1997;**104**:1084-1091

[121] Umezawa S, Shimizu K. Biocompatibility of surface-modified intraocular lenses. Journal of Cataract & Refractive Surgery. 1993;**19**:371-374

[122] Kurosaka D, Ando I, Kato K, Oshima T, Kurosaka H, Yoshino M, Nagamoto T, Ando N. Capsule contraction syndrome. Journal of Cataract & Refractive Surgery. 1999; **25**:930-935

[123] Nishi O, Nishi K, Imanishi M, Tada Y, Shirasawa E. Effect of the cytokines on the prostaglandin E2 synthesis by lens epithelial cells of human cataracts. The British Journal of Ophthalmology. 1995;**79**:934-938

[124] Hollick EJ, Spalton DJ, Ursell PG, Meacock WR, Barman SA, Boyce JF. Posterior capsular opacification with hydrogel, polymethylmethacrylate, and silicone intraocular lenses: Two-year results of a randomized prospective trial. American Journal of Ophthalmology. 2000;**129**:577-584

[125] Lüke C, Dietlein TS, Jacobi PC, Konen W, Krieglstein GK. Massive anterior capsule shrinkage after plate-haptic silicone lens implantation in uveitis. Journal of Cataract & Refractive Surgery. 2001;**27**:333-336

[126] Hollick EJ, Spalton DJ, Ursell PG, Pande MV. Biocompatibility of poly (methyl-methacrylate), silicone, and AcrySof intraocular lenses: Randomized comparison of the cellular reaction on the anterior lens surface. Journal of Cataract & Refractive Surgery. 1998;**24**:361-366

[127] Hollick EJ, Spalton DJ, Ursell PG, Pande MV, Barman SA, Boyce JF, Tilling K. The effect of polymethylmethacrylate, silicone, and polyacrylic intraocular lenses on posterior capsular opacification 3 years after cataract surgery. Ophthalmology. 1999;**106**:49-55

[128] Bellucci R. An introduction to intraocular lenses: Material, optics, haptics, design and aberration. In: Cataract. ESASO Course Series. Güell JL, editor. Basel, Karger; 2013;**3**:38-55. ISBN: 978-3-318-02410-4 (Print) eISBN: 978-3-318-02411-1 (Online). https://doi.org/10.1159/000350902

[129] Leung TG, Lindsley K, Kuo IC. Types of intraocular lenses for cataract surgery in eyes with uveitis. Cochrane Database of Systematic Reviews. 2014;(3):CD007284. DOI:10.1002/14651858.CD007284.pub2

[130] Alio JL, Chipont E, BenEzra D, Fakhry MA, International Ocular Inflammation Society, Study Group of Uveitic Cataract Surgery. Comparative performance of intraocular lenses in eyes with cataract and uveitis. Journal of Cataract & Refractive Surgery. 2002;**28**:2096-2108

[131] Foster CS, Vitale AT. Cataract surgery in uveitis. Ophthalmology Clinics of North America. 1993;**6**:139-146

[132] Schuster AK, Harder BC, Schlichtenbrede FC, Jarczok MN, Tesarz J. Valacyclovir versus acyclovir for the treatment of herpes zoster ophthalmicus in immunocompetent patients. Cochrane Database of Systematic Reviews. 2016;**11**:CD011503

[133] Krishna R. Long-term follow-up of extracapsular cataract extraction and posterior chamber intraocular lens implantation in patients with uveitis. Ophthalmology. 1998; **105**:1765-1769

[134] Pande MV, Spalton DJ, Kerr-Muir MG, Marshall J. Postoperative inflammatory response to phacoemulsification and extracapsular cataract surgery: Aqueous flare and cells. Journal of Cataract & Refractive Surgery. 1996;**22**(Suppl 1):770-774

[135] Moorthy RS, Rajeev B, Smith RE, Rao NA. Incidence and management of cataracts in Vogt-Koyanagi-Harada syndrome. American Journal of Ophthalmology. 2014; **118**:197-204

[136] Merayo-Lloves J, Power WJ, Rodriguez A, Pedroza-Seres M, Foster CS. Secondary glaucoma in patients with uveitis. Ophthalmologica. 1999;**213**:300-304

[137] Kiryu J, Kita M, Tanabe T, Yamashiro K, Miyamoto N, Ieki Y. Pars plana vitrectomy for cystoid macular edema secondary to sarcoid uveitis. Ophthalmology. 2001; **108**:1140-1144

[138] Liesegang TJ, Bourne WM, Ilstrup DM. Secondary surgical and neodymium-YAG laser discissions. American Journal of Ophthalmology. 1985;**100**:510-519

[139] Steinert RF, Puliafito CA, Kumar SR, Dudak SD, Patel S. Cystoid macular edema, retinal detachment, and glaucoma after Nd:YAG laser posterior capsulotomy. American Journal of Ophthalmology. 1991;**112**:373-380

[140] Ganesh SK, Babu K, Biswas J. Phacoemulsification with intraocular lens implantation in cases of pars planitis. Journal of Cataract & Refractive Surgery. 2004;**30**:2072-2076

[141] Choudhry S, Ghosh S. Intravitreal and posterior subtenon triamcinolone acetonide in idiopathic bilateral uveitic macular oedema. Clinical & Experimental Ophthalmology. 2007;**35**:713-718

[142] Maca SM, Abela-Formanek C, Kiss CG, Sacu SG, Benesch T, Barisani-Asenbauer T. Intravitreal triamcinolone for persistent cystoid macular oedema in eyes with quiescent uveitis. Clinical & Experimental Ophthalmology. 2009;**37**:389-396

[143] Young S, Larkin G, Branley M, Lightman S. Safety and efficacy of intravitreal triamcinolone for cystoid macular oedema in uveitis. Clinical & Experimental Ophthalmology. 2001;**29**:2-6

[144] Cunningham Jr ET, de Smet MD, Yeh S, Albini TA, Zierhut M. Sustained-release corticosteroids for uveitis. Ocular Immunology and Inflammation 2015;**23**:421-424

[145] Gilbert C, Hiscott P, Unger W, Grierson I, McLeod D. Inflammation and the formation of epiretinal membranes. Eye (Lond). 1988;**2**(Suppl 6):144-156

[146] Dev S, Mieler WF, Pulido JS, Mittra RA. Visual outcomes after pars plana vitrectomy for epiretinal membranes associated with pars planitis. Ophthalmology. 1999;**106**:1086-1090

[147] Radetzky S, Walter P, Fauser S, Koizumi K, Kirchhof B, Joussen AM. Visual outcome of patients with macular edema after pars plana vitrectomy and indocyanine green-assisted peeling of the internal limiting membrane. Graefe's Archive for Clinical and Experimental Ophthalmology. 2004;**242**:273-278

[148] Berker N, Soykan E, Elgin U, Ozkan SS. Phacoemulsification cataract extraction and intraocular lens implantation in patients with Behcet's disease. Ophthalmic Surgery, Lasers & Imaging Retina. 2004;**35**:215-218

[149] Powe NR, Schein OD, Gieser SC. Synthesis of the literature on visual acuity and complications following cataract extraction with intraocular lens implantation. Archives of Ophthalmology. 1994;**112**:239-252

[150] Foster RE, Lowder CY, Meisler DM, Zakov ZN. Extracapsular cataract extraction and posterior chamber intraocular lens implantation in uveitis patients. Ophthalmology. 1992;**99**:1234-1241

[151] Tugal-Tutkun I, Ötük-Yasar B, Altinkurt E. Clinical features and prognosis of herpetic anterior uveitis: A retrospective study of 111 cases. International Ophthalmology. 2010;**30**:559-565

[152] Miserocchi E, Waheed NK, Dios E, Christen W, Merayo J, Roque M, Foster CS. Visual outcome in herpes simplex virus and varicella zoster virus uveitis: A clinical evaluation and comparison. Ophthalmology. 2002;**109**:1532-1537

[153] Marsh RJ, Cooper M. Ocular surgery in ophthalmic zoster. Eye (Lond). 1989;**3**:313-317

[154] Kaufman AH, Foster CS. Cataract extraction in patients with pars planitis. Ophthalmology. 1993;**100**:1210-1217

[155] Tugal-Tutkun I, Onal S, Altan-Yaycioglu R, Altunbas HH, Urgancioglu M. Uveitis in Behçet disease: An analysis of 880 patients. Ophthalmology. 2004;**138**:373-380

[156] Kadayifçilar S, Gedik Ş, Eldem B, İrkeç M. Cataract surgery in patients with Behçet's disease. Journal of Cataract & Refractive Surgery. 2002;**28**:316-320

[157] Ganesh SK, Babu K, Biswas J. Cataract surgery in patients with Vogt-Koyanagi-Harada syndrome. Journal of Cataract & Refractive Surgery. 2004;**30**:95-100

[158] Ganesh SK, Sundaram PM, Biswas J, Babu K. Cataract surgery in sympathetic ophthalmia. Journal of Cataract & Refractive Surgery. 2004;**30**:2371-2376

[159] Akova YA, Foster CS. Cataract surgery in patients with sarcoidosis-associated uveitis. Ophthalmology. 1994;**101**:473-479

6

Eye Coinfections

Carlos Alberto Pantoja-Meléndez, Victor M. Bautista-de Lucio, Mariana Ortiz-Casas, Jonathan Quevedo-Martínez and Herlinda Mejía-López

Abstract

Ocular infections are an *ophthalmologic* emergency that threatens the eye's integrity, which may result in a poor visual outcome; hence, it requires prompt treatment. The most common microorganisms involved in eye infection are the bacteria, followed by virus and fungi; however the prevalence depends on the geographic location. It is essential to know The etiologic agent of the ocular infection ocular infections and their antibiotic sensitivity because the geographical situation and the urbanization level of the studied population will determine their prevalence. Recently have been described eye coinfections, where at least two microorganisms can infect at the same time and the same anatomic site. Several coinfections have been published, bacteria-bacteria, bacteria-fungus, bacteria-virus, fungus-yeast, fungus-virus, parasite-bacteria, etc. Eye coinfections represent a particular challenge for the ophthalmologists; coinfections are difficult to diagnose because often the clinical characteristic is atypical and mimics different clinical pictures. In addition, eye coinfections respond poorly to antibiotics and usually present an aggressive clinical course. In these circumstances, it is common for patients to receive multiple treatments when they should be receiving a specific treatment. Several risk factors are important to develop coinfections, e.g., trauma, dry eye, use of contact lenses, and comorbidities (diabetes and immunosuppression). Coinfections have been described in keratitis, conjunctivitis, and endophthalmitis. The study of polymicrobial biofilms has been increasing, and in the medical area, the role played by biofilms in confections has been associated with virulence factors; hence, biofilm formation is also considered a determinant virulence factor for pathogenesis in the host. Coinfection diagnosis is an important topic in order to obtain a specific and timely diagnosis. Microbiological and molecular approaches are proposed to identify etiological agents. Delay in diagnosis affects the sensitivity to specific treatments and the evolution of infection. Treatment and prognosis are supported by a specific diagnosis.

Keywords: Coinfection, polyinfections, biofilm

1. Introduction

An infected eye is one of the major causes of corneal blindness after cataract in developing countries [1]. This is mainly induced by bacteria, fungi, yeast, and parasites. However, an increasing number of coinfections, which involve the presence of two or more pathogens, in the same place at the same time, affecting one or both eyes, are being reported. Comparing the single-microorganism infections, in which theoretically there is no competition, the coinfections have been proven to have more mechanisms competing against the host resources. This competition is the main factor influencing the clinical course and evolution of the infection [2].

Eye coinfections represent a particular challenge for ophthalmologists; coinfections are difficult to diagnose because often the clinical picture is atypical and mimics different clinical pictures. In addition, eye coinfections respond poorly to antibiotics and usually present a slow clinical course. In these circumstances, it is common for patients to receive multiple treatments when they should be receiving a specific treatment; this can cause a refractory infection and need for surgical treatments.

Although eye infections are common in immunocompetent patients, coinfection can compromise the immune system of the host [3, 4]. Therefore, the strategies used by each microorganism to survive against different treatments and the self-host immune response have important implications for the diagnosis and prognosis of the infection [5].

This chapter provides a systematic review of the frequency and epidemiological characteristics, with reports of the most common clinical entities, produced by coinfection in the eye.

2. Epidemiological characteristics

2.1. Epidemiological significance

Ocular infectious processes are among the clinical entities that are relevant to the epidemiology. The high incidence of infections in patient care institutions has resulted in high-quality infection control processes and monitoring of various entities of epidemiological relevancy. For example, viral conjunctivitis primarily represents a challenge for management and prevention. Thus, it is common for diseases such as hemorrhagic conjunctivitis and follicular conjunctivitis to be part of the epidemiological surveillance.

The difficulty of the epidemiological surveillance of ophthalmic diseases lies in the limitation of performing a specific etiologic diagnosis of infection, since in practice ophthalmic infections are treated empirically based on the clinical picture and the physician's experience. Ophthalmologists and laboratory staff should not forget that care of patients with endophthalmitis is usually performed at the first level of care, where the general practice is responsible for the greatest amount of attention to this disease. Thus, control programs for conditions such as trachoma are necessary to prevent them from reemerging and being attentive and vigilant regarding emerging diseases.

Within emerging diseases, changes are observed in response to treatment but more important in the modification to the incidence and prevalence to disease. Reports of bacterial strain resistant to antibiotics and changes in the behavior expected of diseases are increasing. Therefore, new mechanisms of resistance of microorganisms, comorbidity states in individuals, new mechanisms of transmission, etc., that explain what changes in the conditions have occurred are sought. One explanation is the presence of more than one causal agent of infectious disease, coinfections.

The mechanisms developed by various microorganisms when present concurrently can alter significantly the clinical presentation, diagnosis, and treatment.

Coinfections resemble clinical pictures presented by other clinical entities and have an adverse effect, as the usual outcome is the use of multi-treatment that fails, causing refractory management and in many cases ending in loss of vision or surgical interventions. This reveals the importance of presenting cases of coinfections of the eye.

Although eye coinfections are not the subject of epidemiological surveillance, they are not as rare as previously thought and can represent 3.88 % of endophthalmitis cases, for example, and more than 50 % in some series of patients with conjunctivitis reported in the literature [6, 7].

3. Agents

Associated microorganisms may occur in different combinations. This association is predominantly bacteria-bacteria and to a lesser extent bacteria-fungus and bacteria-virus.

Acanthamoeba spp. and *Pseudomonas* spp. are associated because of their high resistance to empirical antibiotics and ulceration, which occurs primarily in association with *Acanthamoeba* spp., which is associated with *Legionella* spp., *Streptococcus* spp., herpes virus, *Moraxella* spp., *Candida* spp., etc.

Several viruses, bacteria, or fungi cause eye infections, but the pathogenic agent is modified extensively at presentation as a coinfection especially when the bacterium is coinfecting with different bacteria or a virus. In the case of fungi, when they are present with bacteria, only small changes are observed [3]. The clinical spectrum of keratitis can change when there is a coinfection between bacteria and *Candida* spp., mainly occurs; however, when endophthalmitis involves coinfection of a fungus and Gram-negative bacteria, the result is more unfavorable [6].

4. Risk factors

The core components of the presentation of coinfections are risk factors. However, studies have not shown high causality for association. Coinfections have been diagnosed in patients with no reports of comorbidities (diabetes, immunosuppressive processes, etc.) although coinfections can occur in patients with human immunodeficiency virus (HIV); however, this risk factor was not significant in the patients reported.

One risk factor for coinfection of fungus and bacteria is trauma. Dry eye also seems to be a risk factor.

The most frequently reported risk factor is the use of contact lenses, especially soft lenses. Coinfection with *Acanthamoeba* spp. *and Pseudomonas* spp. has been reported in contact lens-associated keratitis. Poor response to treatment has been observed in young people with greater frequency in women.

5. Challenges

The most important challenge in the emergence of this clinical entity is the identification of a new form of presentation of eye infections. The standard method of causality associates the disease with a single causative agent. However, in this new scenario, more than one causal agent is observed. The new entity must be monitored and addressed as a new disease, which requires a new diagnostic approach, prognosis, and treatment.

6. Keratitis due to coinfections

6.1. Bacteria and fungus

Bacteria and fungus represent the most frequent type of coinfection in the eye (Table 1]. The main microorganisms that produce coinfections are bacteria, such as *Staphylococcus* spp., *Streptococcus* spp., *Pseudomonas* spp., *Haemophilus* spp., *Klebsiella* spp., *Bacillus* spp., and *Corynebacterium* spp. The fungi genera microorganisms include *Aspergillus* spp., *Fusarium* spp., *Curvularia* spp., *Cladosporium* spp., *Bipolaris* spp., *Alternaria* spp., and the yeast *Candida* spp. Most of these microorganisms are normal microbiota in the conjunctival sac or the lids [8]. Their presence depends on the geographic area. However, bacteria and fungus coinfections that have been reported more frequently in a large series of cases are the genera *Staphylococcus* spp. with *Aspergillus* spp. or *Fusarium* spp., [3, 9, 10, 11, 12, 13].

Organisms	**Study type**	**Infection caused**	**Reference**
Bacteria and fungus	Transversal	Keratitis	Gopinathan *et. al.* 2009
	Transversal	Keratitis	Basak *et. al.* 2005
	Transversal	Keratitis	Pate *et. al.* 2006
	Transversal	Keratitis	Bharathi *et. al.* 2002
Bacteria and bacteria	Transversal	Keratitis	Fröhlich *et. al.* 1999
	Transversal	Keratitis	Yeh *et. al.* 2006
	Case	Keratitis	Jones 1981

Organisms	Study type	Infection caused	Reference
Bacteria and yeast	Case	Keratitis	Kim *et. al.* 2006
Filamentous fungus and yeast	Case	Keratitis	Qui *et. al.* 2013
Filamentous fungus and filamentous fungus	Case	Keratitis	Hayashi *et. al.* 2014
Acanthamoeba and bacteria	Transversal	Keratitis	Tu *et. al.* 2009
	Case	Keratitis	Hong *et. al.* 2014
	Case	Keratitis	Dini *et. al.* 2000
	Transversal	Keratitis	Iovieno *et. al.* 2010
	Case	Keratitis	Lone *et. al.* 2009
Acanthamoeba and fungus	Transversal	Keratitis	Froumis *et. al.* 2008
	Case	Keratitis	Gupta *et. al.* 2011
	Case	Keratitis	Slade *et. al.* 2008
Virus and bacteria	Case	Conjunctivitis	Mellman-Rubin *et. al.* 1995
	Case	Conjunctivitis	Tappe *et. al.* 2013
Bacteria and bacteria	Transversal	Conjunctivitis	Iwalokun *et. al.* 2011
Bacteria and bacteria	Transversal	Endophthalmitis	Gharamah *et. al.* 2012
	Transversal	Endophthalmitis	Jindal *et. al.* 3013
	Transversal	Endophthalmitis	Gupta *et. al.* 2002
Bacteria and fungus	Transversal	Endophthalmitis	Long *et. al.* 2014
	Transversal	Endophthalmitis	Gupta *et. al.* 2003
HIV and herpes	Transversal	Retinal necrosis syndrome	Liesegang 2001
HIV and cytomegalovirus	Transversal	Retinitis	Faber *et. al.* 1992
HIV, Epstein-Barr, and cytomegalovirus	Transversal	Retinitis	Freigassner *et. al.* 2002
HIV, cytomegalovirus, and herpes	Case	Retinitis	Skolnik *et. al.* 1989
HIV and several microorganisms (including *Acanthamoeba*)	Case	Keratitis	Tandon *et. al.* 2003
HIV and *Treponema pallidum*	Case	Severe bilateral retinal vasculitis	Albini *et. al.* 2011
Virus and worm	Case	Perilimbal and conjunctival infection and HZV lesson	Seo *et. al.* 2014

Table 1. Main reports of human eye coinfections.

Bacterial and fungal keratitis often is not clinically distinguishable from monomicrobial infections, because they override the pathognomonic picture typical of bacterial or fungal keratitis [14]. Because of the difficulty of clinical diagnosis, other factors are added; many patients use traditional medicine (with the risk of adding other microorganisms to the infection) or initiate topical medication without a medical prescription. These therapeutic interventions delay the specific treatment, and the prognosis of infection is poor [14].

Bacteria and fungus coinfection can be incidental in the first instance. However, this condition favors the development in the participating pathogens of adaptive mechanisms that strengthen their protection versus the immune system host or the antimicrobial drug. This phenomenon is explained by the ability of fungi and bacteria to form biofilms. Studies recently showed that 99 % of microorganisms can form biofilms; only 10 % live as planktonic cells (unicellular cells) [15, 16, 17].

The characteristic that best distinguishes chronic infections from acute infections is the response to treatment with antibiotics. While acute infections can be removed after a short treatment with antibiotics, the biofilm in keratitis coinfections normally fails to be completely eliminated, produces recurrent episodes, and often must be solved with keratoplasty. The etiologic agents form biofilms that can be up to 1,000 times more resistant to antibiotics [17, 18, 19]. The issue of biofilms will be fully explained in the following section.

7. Bacteria and bacteria

Several reports in the literature have described this coinfection. Fröhlich *et. al.* studied patients with and without clinical history of contact lens use and showed that 51 of the 275 samples (18.5 %) from patients with bacteria keratitis were coinfections. The most common pathogens isolated were *Staphylococcus epidermidis* (44 %), *Staphylococcus aureus* (18 %), *Streptococcus* spp. (10 %), *Propionibacterium acnes* (7 %), and *Pseudomonas aeruginosa* (6 %) [20]. Yeh *et. al.* presented a study of 307 samples, of which 21 % were keratitis bacteria-bacteria coinfections with similar bacterial genera [21]. Jones reported coinfections between *Streptococcus pneumoniae* with *Corynebacterium* spp. or *Staphylococcus epidermidis* and isolated three microorganisms from one case, *Staphylococcus aureus* and *Streptococcus pneumoniae, Corynebacterium* spp., and *Micrococcus* spp., and, finally, *Streptococcus equinus* and *Haemophilus influenzae* from another patient.

8. Bacteria and yeast

Coinfections that involve *Candida* spp. or a filamentous fungus are usually difficult to treat, and the prognosis is poor. A coinfection of *Stenotrophomonas maltophilia* (Gram (-) bacteria) and a yeast has been documented. The corneal injury presented as an ulcer that quickly progressed despite treatment with proven sensitivity. The case was treated with penetrating keratoplasty [22].

9. Filamentous fungi and yeast

In a case with clinically distinguishable corneal infiltrates, *Exserohilum mcginnisii* and *Candida parapsilosis*, an unusual coinfection, were isolated. The infection showed torpid evolution with severe damage in the visual area [23]. Katragkou *et. al.* conducted a review that showed *Exserohilum* spp. produces a wide spectrum of diseases, including atopic, cutaneous, subcutaneous, systemic, and corneal infections; the most common factor was immunocompromised status [24]. In addition, *Candida* spp. is an opportunistic pathogen that affects immunocompromised and immunocompetent patients. This genus generates biofilms responsible for resistance to a wide range of antifungal drugs and often affects the cornea [25, 26]. *Exserohilum* spp. and *Candida* spp. can acquire a filamentous form that invades the stroma or produces endophthalmitis and has the capability of assembling biofilms.

10. Filamentous fungus and filamentous fungus

A case of sclerokeratitis produced by *Scedosporium apiospermum* and *Aspergillus cibarius* was recently reported. The case, which was characterized by insidious keratitis and liquefied sclera, was successfully treated with topical and systemic antifungal drugs [27].

11. *Acanthamoeba* spp. and coinfections

Acanthamoeba spp., a protozoon, is a free-living amoeba that can live in diverse environments. It has been isolated from soil, water for domestic use, salt or freshwater sewage, estuaries, hot springs, and swimming pools, among others, which highlight the microorganism's ability to live in extreme heat and pH conditions. Schuster and Visvesvara described *Acanthamoeba* spp. producing keratitis as non-opportunistic and thus occur in immunocompetent humans [28]. Galarza *et. al.*, described this amoeba as *amphizoic* due to its ability to live in the environment and parasitize humans [29].

The life cycle of *Acanthamoeba* spp. includes two stages: the cyst, a form of resistance to adverse environmental conditions, and the trophozoite, the amoeboid free-living stage. Due to the organism's phagocytic condition, *Acanthamoeba* spp. can feed of bacteria, algae, yeast, fungi, etc [30]; but some of these microorganisms have developed mechanisms to avoid intracellular death and take advantage of the amoeba (endosymbiosis). These circumstances make *Acanthamoeba* spp. a vector of almost any type of microorganism; Barket *et. al.*, in studies of the host-parasite relationship, called it a "Trojan horse" [31, 32].

12. *Acanthamoeba* and bacteria

The association of *Acanthamoeba* spp. with other microorganisms is most significant from the ophthalmological point of view. This species can generate corneal injuries that remain for months or years and are difficult to treat with diamine and biguanide drugs in developing countries (chlorhexidine and polyhexamethylene biguanide, respectively) [33].

Some of the bacteria mechanisms within *Acanthamoeba* spp. have been described. Scheid *et. al.*, using an *in vitro* model with electronic microscopy, showed the cycle of a coccoid-like organism in the free-living amoebae *Vannella* spp. The coccoid microorganism is a phagocyte and is transported by phagocytic vacuoles through the cytosol until reaching the amoeba nucleus where the microorganism proliferates and is released by rupture of the host membrane. In the beginning of the life cycle, coccoid microorganisms are phagocytes for other amoeba [34]. In addition, endosymbiont bacteria can replicate only into the amoeba cytosol, can break the cells, and can be ingested by neighboring amoeba [35]. However, the intrusion of bacteria into *Acanthamoeba polyphaga* has consequences for both microorganisms. A protein bellows the amoeba that adheres to the surface of *Legionella pneumophila*. The authors discussed the possibility that the liberation of the bacteria from the amoeba integrates amoeba antigens in its membrane. However, *Pseudomonas aeruginosa* and its liberated products kill *Acanthamoeba* spp. [30, 32, 36]. Another study showed that endosymbiont bacteria favor the growth of different species of *Acanthamoeba*, and all microorganisms isolated from contact lens care solutions contained numerous trophozoites [37].

Acanthamoeba spp. by itself causes severe inflammation in the cornea. Aggressive keratolysis or sclerokeratitis is a common complication. The most frequently reported symptoms are pain, photophobia, and tearing [38]. The association of *Acanthamoeba* spp. with bacteria or a fungus presents a coinfection that can mimic bacterial, fungal, or herpetic keratitis, which can delay the time to diagnosis and increase the pathogenicity of the *Acanthamoeba* spp. infection.

Several molecular methods and electronic microscopy have facilitated the observation of bacteria within *Acanthamoeba*, including *Pseudomonas aeruginosa, Listeria monocytogenes, Mycobacterium* spp., *Escherichia coli, Legionella pneumophila, Chlamydia* spp., and *Aeromonas* spp. They are also capable of producing keratitis themselves [30, 32, 39, 40, 41]. In addition, there are many reports in the literature of cases of *Acanthamoeba* and bacteria coinfection isolated from patients with or without contact lens-associated keratitis [39, 42, 43, 44].

13. *Acanthamoeba* and fungi

This type of coinfection is uncommon. Similar to bacteria, fungi have a complex relationship with *Acanthamoeba* spp. and generate lesions that can be confused with bacterial or herpetic keratitis; the prognosis is discouraging. In all cases reported, penetrating keratoplasty was performed. These coinfections require immediate and aggressive treatment with antifungal and antiamoebic drugs [45, 46, 47, 48, 49].

14. Conjunctivitis due to coinfection

Conjunctivitis is the most common eye infection in the world. Usually, the normal microbiota in the conjunctiva participates in infectious diseases of the ocular surface, and it has been reported that diversity in the conjunctival microbiota varies depending on geographic region or occupational activity [50, 51, 52, 53]. Moreover, the pathogenesis of infectious conjunctivitis depends on the circumstances and intrinsic mechanisms to the microorganism and the host.

Although there are high diversity of microorganisms on the conjunctiva, few coinfections have been reported. This lack of reports could be due to confusing clinical manifestations or the low sensitivity of the methods used or simply because two or more microorganisms are not usually searched in an infection.

In a patient with conjunctivitis, an uncommon relationship between an adenovirus and *Chlamydia* spp. was reported. The study showed three patients positive for *Chlamydia* spp. in a sample of 100 patients with adenoviral conjunctivitis, using polymerase chain reaction (PCR) [54, 55]. Another report showed the presence of adenovirus type 53 with a multiple resistant strain of *Neisseria gonorrhoeae* in a patient with severe bilateral conjunctivitis.

Iwalokun *et. al.*, presented interesting results in a study conducted in Lagos, Nigeria. They analyzed 83 samples from patients with conjunctivitis and isolated 155 bacteria from the samples; the resistance patterns and the plasmid profile were evaluated. The authors found coinfections of two, three, or more pathogens (51.8 % and 18.1 %, respectively) and were able to identify three infection patterns that were significantly different [7]. This work emphasizes the possibility that multiple microorganisms can cause conjunctivitis.

15. Endophthalmitis due to coinfection

Endophthalmitis is an inflammatory intraocular reaction and is the most important complication for an ophthalmologist following surgery, trauma, and between others. The common presentation of the clinical picture is characterized by pain and decreased vision. As previously discussed in the section on keratitis due to bacteria and fungus coinfections, endophthalmitis due to coinfection can be confused with single bacterial or fungal infections. Thus, to facilitate successful interventions, the microorganisms responsible must be identified and antimicrobial sensitivity examined. Studies of several large series have shown the frequency of endophthalmitis due to bacteria and fungus and bacteria and bacteria coinfections.

Depending on patients' geographic region, consecutive case studies have found various incidence rates for this coinfection ranging from 2.4 % to 50 % [56, 57, 58, 59].

The most commonly isolated pathogens are Gram-positive cocci bacteria with filamentous fungi [60, 61]. However, Gram-negative or Gram-positive bacilli related to fungi are also responsible for endophthalmitis [60, 61, 62].

16. Coinfections in immunocompromised patients

The outcome of coinfection is the result of diverse interactions involving the host and the parasite's genetic background and the environment. In these infections, few reports have explained the immune mechanisms implicated, because there is considerable variability in each combination of microorganisms that produces an infection.

The immunological mechanisms that occur in the eye are similar to the rest of the immune system. However, there is more regulation in the silencing response in order to prevent damage from infection and inflammation, and immune mechanisms preserve the functionality of the cornea [63].

In the following, studies that investigated the most common corneal coinfections are reviewed. These reports show the critical role of pathogens and the pathogenesis generated by the host immune response.

Vernal conjunctivitis is an example of how the immune phenotype affects the response to the infection. Patients with vernal keratoconjunctivitis have a family history of atopic diseases such as allergic rhinitis, asthma, and eczema [64]. A theory suggests that patients with a history of atopy are susceptible to intracellular infections because they have a Th2 immune phenotype [65, 66]. Kerr and Stern showed a polymicrobial infection in two patients with vernal keratoconjunctivitis and corneal ulcers [67].

Although regulation of the immune response in the eye is controlled locally, in immunocompromised patients with human immunodeficiency virus (HIV), it is evident that the privilege is broken by the depletion of T CD4+ cells, and infections can occur. In addition, several pathogens can remain latent (herpes virus, bacteria, fungi, parasites). The clinical manifestation produced by the herpes virus can be conjunctivitis, blepharitis, intraocular inflammation, retinitis, or keratitis [68]. In particular, herpes simplex virus types 1 and 2 (HSV-1 and HSV-2] infect 50 % to 90 % of the population infected with HIV, causing ocular herpes and genital orofacial herpes in different geographic regions [69]. Herpetic retinitis has a high incidence; however, few cases have been reported. Faber *et. al.*, studied eyes from 25 cases with AIDS with an immunohistochemical test. *Cytomegalovirus* was found in 60 % of the cases and was related to retinitis, while in another case series, 36.64 % of 131 patients were diagnosed with *Cytomegalovirus* retinitis [70, 71]. Freigassner *et. al.*, documented a case with the Epstein-Barr virus and *Cytomegalovirus* in a patient with AIDS [72]. Other studies showed *Cytomegalovirus* or herpes in isolated cases [73, 74, 75].

Opportunistic microorganisms such as *Toxoplasma* spp., herpes zoster virus (HZV), and *Pneumocystis* spp., participates the least in coinfections.

17. Coinfections produced by strange conjunction of pathogens

Burkholderia ambifaria, *Enterococcus*, and *Staphylococcus aureus* were found in a patient with herpetic stromal keratitis. *Burkholderia ambifaria* is a Proteobacteria, which comprises strains with a virulence potential toward immunocompromised patients [76]. In a report on keratitis, *Acanthamoeba* spp., *Fusarium solani*, and Gram-negative cocci were identified in a patient who had unprotected sexual contact with multiple commercial sex workers [77].

18. Pharmacodynamics of antimicrobials used in eye coinfections

There is little information about the pharmacodynamics of antimicrobials used for coinfections of the human eye. The activity of antimicrobial drugs against yeast, bacteria, and fungi has been evaluated with a standardized microdilution assay in a culture medium [78]. The lowest concentration of an antimicrobial that completely inhibits the growth of any microorganism is known as the minimal inhibitory concentration (MIC), which can be used to determine the sensitivity or resistance.

Based on MICs with microdilutions and the growth radial technique on solid medium using Potato Dextrose Agar (PDA) dishes (using the percent mycelial inhibition) [79], our group reported that *S. aureus* cocultured with *F. solani* or *A. fumigatus* (all isolated from patients) significantly inhibited fungal growth (66.5 % and 55.6 %, respectively). gatifloxacin and moxifloxacin in the cocultures eliminated the bacterial effect on both growth fungi ($p<0.001$). amphotericin B, natamycin, and itraconazole inhibited fungal growth partially or completely, depending on the fungus. In contrast, the effect of amphotericin B or natamycin in the presence of quinolones significantly favored the growth of fungi; this effect was more evident in *F. solani* [80].

Nevertheless, the MIC does not reflect physiological concentrations of drugs because *in vivo* drug concentrations may vary due to many factors such as absorption, metabolism, half-life, elimination, etc. [81, 82, 83]. In addition, in treatments with prophylactic and therapeutic purposes for confections, fortified or coadministered agents are used that may affect the efficacy of the other agent [84, 85].

Attempts to understand the magnitude and type of interactions between drugs have enabled the development in isobolographic analysis of the "gold standard" for drug interactions, which define the interactions as follows: *Additive effect*: The combined effect of two drugs (A and B) equals the sum of the equivalent doses (depending on the relative potency of each drug). *Synergism*: The effect of A and B is greater than that of the two separate drugs. *Antagonism*: The addition of a second drug decreases the effectiveness of the first. *Indifferent*: No interaction between the drugs. The calculation is aided by an isobologram graph. This facilitates visual evaluation of the interaction but requires a separate statistical analysis. The isobolographic analysis for the MIC is more sensitive because the analysis evaluates the dose effects and is the prelude to studies in *in vivo* pharmacodynamics [86].

In coinfections, patients are exposed to simultaneous antifungal and antibacterial therapeutic treatment. Quinolones and antifungals are commonly used in bacteria and fungi or bacteria and yeast coinfections. Nakajima *et. al.*, reported the synergistic effect of DU-9859a fluoroquinolone enhanced the *in vitro* antifungal activity of amphothericin B and fluconazole against *Candida* spp. growth and decreased the load in mice infected with yeast. The last result was also observed in mice infected with *Aspergillus fumigatus* [87]. Similar results were obtained with ciprofloxacin, amphotericin B, levofloxacin, voriconazole, or caspofungin combinations, which has a synergistic effect against *Candida albicans* and *Aspergillus fumigatus* [88]. In another report, ofloxacin had a synergic effect on fluconazole versus a fluconazole-resistant *Candida albicans* strain [89].

Analysis of drug interactions with simultaneous application is still developing. Modified methods have been proposed related to more accurate isobolographic analysis, and *in vitro* models approach physiological conditions. Animal models have also been used. This area will revolutionize therapeutic interventions.

19. Biofilms

An appreciation for the fact that in nature bacteria adhere to many abiotic or biotic surfaces, embedded in an extracellular matrix, and form communities known as "biofilms" has emerged over the past few decades [90]. Biofilm formation conferred on individual bacteria the ability to collaborate and to adapt to a range of harsh environmental conditions and, perhaps most of all, to evade predation by phagocytic microbes. The formation of a biofilm provides a microbe with a small measure of control over the local environment, including fluctuations in temperature, pH, ultraviolet light, starvation, and exposure to toxic agents [91, 92].

Advances in medical biofilm research have led to the understanding that biofilms represent the prevalent form of bacterial life during tissue colonization and may occur in more than 80 % of microbial infections in the body [93].

Members of a biofilm community, which can be of the same or multiple species, show varying stages of differentiation and exchange information, metabolites, and genes with each other. As a result, members of the biofilm community are in a diversity of physiologies influenced by the unequal sharing of nutrients and metabolic by-products, which results in subpopulations with increased tolerance to antimicrobials and environmental stresses, the host immune system, and predatory microorganisms [19, 94, 95, 96, 97, 98].

Canonically, biofilm development has been grouped into five stages that are reflective of conditions in many, but not all, biofilms: (1) reversible aggregation of planktonic cells on a surface, (2) irreversible adhesion, (3) formation of microcolonies, (4) biofilm maturation, and (5) detachment and dispersion of cells [99]. The events that are of special significance for ocular infections and the treatment of biofilm infections will be discussed in greater detail, while the reader is referred to several excellent reviews for details on other biofilm-related subjects [19, 100,101].

The biofilms involve the production of an extracellular matrix (ECM) that embedded the cells and, in some cases, binds the cells together and that can be composed of polysaccharides, lipopolysaccharides, proteins, or extracellular DNA [10]. This process may be active or passive, in that cells on the surface of an adherent colony that are lysed by the ejection of neutrophil antimicrobial factors may encase and protect siblings below in a matrix consisting simply of cell lysate. Whatever the nature of the matrix, its chemical and physical properties contribute to the differentiation of cells within the encased population, a process that can protect the bacteria from the action of antimicrobial agents, host immune responses, bacteriophages, and phagocytic amoeba [19].

As the microcolony grows through cell division or the recruitment of more planktonic cells, the biofilm grows and takes on a three-dimensional structure that often includes open water channels [19, 103].

The three-dimensional organization of the biofilm causes gradients of oxygen, pH, and nutrients, resulting in the development of different microniches [104, 105, 106]. The cell's individual physiological adaptations to these microniches result in physiological heterogeneity [98]. Cells near the surface of the biofilm will be exposed to more nutrients and oxygen and are therefore more metabolically active, while cells in the deep regions will be less active or even dormant. This heterogeneity results in a range of responses to antimicrobial agents, with metabolically active cells at the surface being rapidly killed, while more internal, dormant cells are comparatively unaffected [106]. This, together with potential effects on the diffusion of antimicrobial molecules within the biofilm, causes some cells in a biofilm to be recalcitrant to antimicrobial treatment, with antibiotic susceptibilities reduced by 10- to 1,000-fold compared to their planktonic counterparts [106].

The high local concentration of cells in a biofilm creates an ideal environment for information exchange through cell-to-cell communication and lateral gene transfer. Cell signaling mediated by secreted, accumulating messenger molecules, known as quorum sensing, allows bacteria to sense and respond to their environment and couple cell density and other environmental cues with gene expression in ways that allow adaptive phenotypic responses. Quorum sensing has been shown to be involved in the control of biofilm formation and the production of virulence and colonization factors in a variety of organisms of medical importance [106]. Cell-to-cell signaling is also involved in biofilm dispersion, which is of general and medical interest [107].

20. Practical strategies for coinfection diagnosis

The two leading causes of vision impairment worldwide are uncorrected refractive errors and cataract. Measures for managing those eye abnormalities frequently include the use of contact lenses and the placement of intraocular lenses and have enhanced the quality of life of millions of patients. Although the use of such devices is the great importance for correction of a variety of visual aberrations, these devices also provide a new surface on which many microbial pathogens can form biofilms (Table 2). As a result, device-related ocular infections are an important limitation of the success of such procedures. Moreover, many infections progress to secondary permanent sequelae that may lead to poor visual outcomes and occasionally loss of sight, such as acute bacterial endophthalmitis or corneal ulceration.

In all infection diseases, not only ocular infection, it is important to make sure of the microbiological diagnosis, especially when the coinfections are a large percentage of the total infections. The results will provide a report on the distribution and trends in microbiological and antibiotic sensitivity patterns that will affect the patient's treatment and prognosis. We have developed simple and practical strategies in each phase for ocular infection diagnosis, including the coinfections summarized in Figure 1.

Disease	Main causative agents of infection and/or found in the biofilms	Biofilm localization
Endophthalmitis	Coagulase-negative staphylococci and *Propionibacterium acnes*	Intraocular lens posterior capsule
Keratitis	*Staphylococcus aureus* and other staphylococcal species, *Pseudomonas aeruginosa* and *Serratia* spp. Fungi and *Acanthamoeba* spp. less frequently	Contact lens
	Viridans group Streptococci. Gram-negative bacilli and yeasts less frequently	Corneal stroma (crystalline keratopathy)
Scleral buckle infection	Gram-positive cocci and nontuberculous *Mycobacterium* spp.	Scleral buckles
Lacrimal system infections	*Staphylococcus* spp., *P. aeruginosa,* and *M. chelonae*	Lacrimal intubation devices
	Staphylococcus spp.	Punctual plugs
Periorbital infections	*Staphylococcus* spp. and mixed species biofilms	Sockets and orbital plates

Table 2. Biofilm-associated infections of the eye

A successful microbiological study consists in a correct identification, but, it begins since the pre-analytic phase, where the ophthalmologist plays an important role, so that, in our laboratory, we have improved an initial lesson to emphasize two principal things. The first thing is awareness of the importance to take the ocular sample before the intensive topical antibiotic treatment. It allows us to have greater chance of bacterial growth, although it has been described that scraping may accelerate disease resolution by enhancing antibiotic penetration and the therapeutic debridement of the necrotic tissue [108]. The second thing is that during the lesson we teach to the ophthalmologist the properly way to select, collect, and transport the sample to optimize the analysis and interpretation. For the collection, we prepared kits with all the necessary to take the sample for a molecular and microbiological diagnosis; the kit contains chocolate agar (ChA), Columbia agar (CA), and Brain-Heart Infusion (BHI); these are enrichment mediums for the exigent bacteria growth, like *Streptococcus* spp. and *Kocuria* spp.; the kit also contains Sabouraud dextrose agar (SDA), for fungi growth; different types of applicators (cotton, alginate, and rayon), a glass slide for the frotis, and finally a transport media for the molecular diagnosis are also included. On the other hand, we have accord with the ophthalmologist the conditions for the sample collection and storage that are summarized in Table 3, and especially, we have established the sequence for seeded the sample because of the small amount of material and small numbers of organisms obtainable from the eye: one swab for ChA, CA, and BHI, another swab for SDA, and the frotis for Gram, Wright, and Calcofluor stain. In conclusion, the pre-analytic phase is a continuous team work between the ophthalmologist and the laboratory staff.

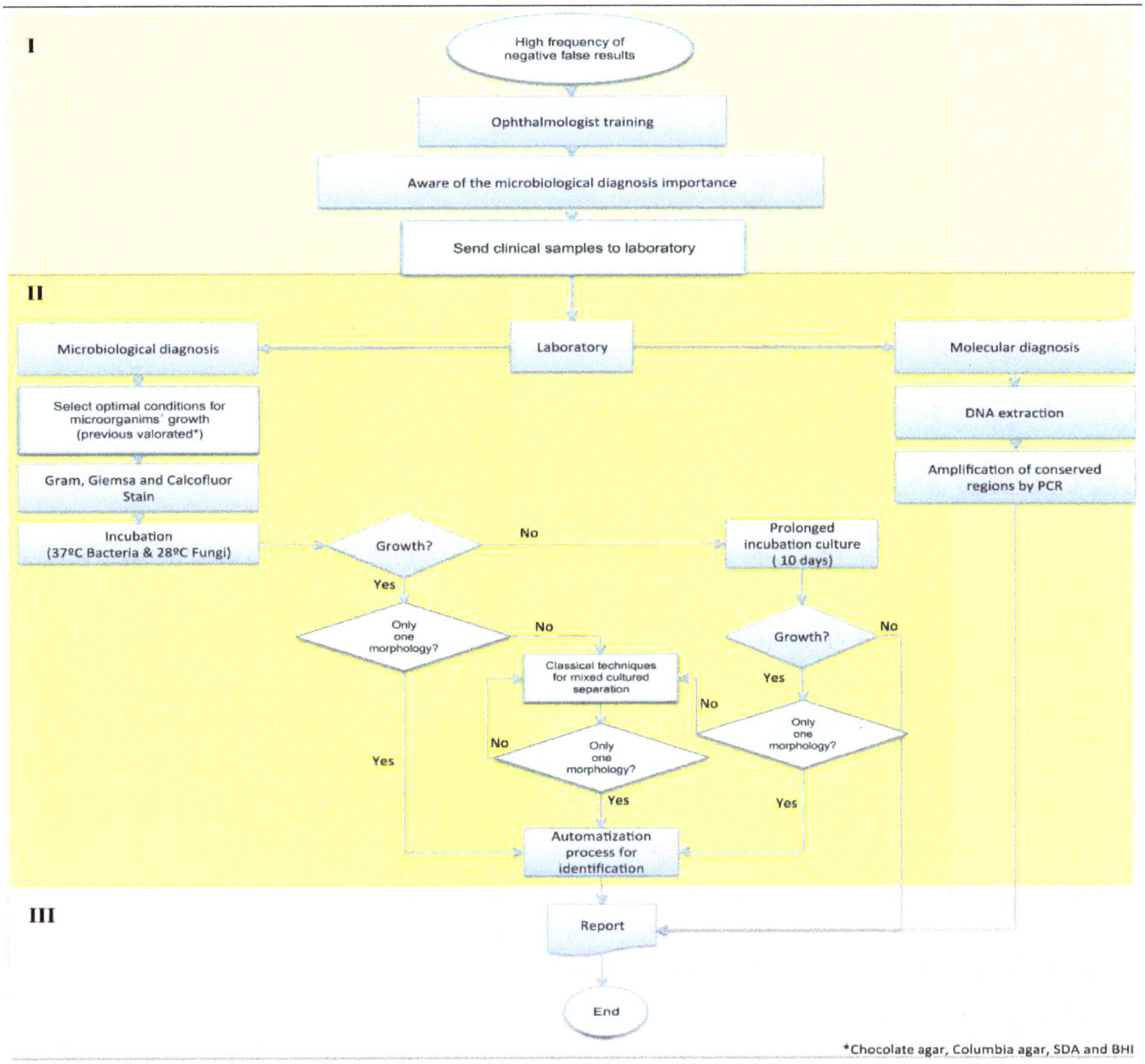

Figure 1. Practical strategies for coinfection diagnosis during the three analytic phases. (I) The pre-analytic phase, when the ophthalmologist is training for selecting, collecting, and transporting the sample, plays an important role. (II) The analytic phase with microbiological and molecular techniques. In the microbiological diagnosis, the laboratory staff's experience is important to discern a pure from a mixed culture; molecular techniques are used to determine non-cultivable microorganisms. (III) The post-analytic phase, the final result in which the partnership between the ophthalmologist and the laboratory staff is reflected in the best outcomes for patients.

In the analytic phase, the sample could be processed by microbiology or by molecular techniques. About the microbiological diagnosis, the agar plates are checked every day, looking for bacterial or fungal growth. We have implemented a prolonged microorganism cultured of up to 15 days, because most of the hospital population includes multi-treatment patients, so that the microorganisms begin to grow until a week of incubation. Most of the times, the microorganisms involved in a coinfection are closely interacting, being impossible the identification in the automatized system (Vitek 2C, bioMérieux, France). The use of simple and classical microbiological techniques has allowed us to separate these interactions, for

Ocular infection	Sample	Equipment	Storage conditions
Keratitis/corneal ulcer	Limit of the corneal ulcer	Alginate applicator	37 °C→ChA, CA, BHI 28 °C→SDA
Conjunctivitis	Upper and lower eyelid conjunctiva	Cotton applicator	37 °C→ChA, CA, BHI 28 °C→SDA
Endophthalmitis and uveitis	Anterior chamber (aqueous humor) Vitreous humor	Sterile syringes	4 °C→ syringes

Chocolate agar (ChA), Columbia agar (CA), Brain-Heart Infusion (BHI), Sabouraud dextrose agar (SDA), 37 °C for bacteria growth, 28 °C for fungi growth, and 4 °C for sample conservation

Table 3. Conditions for the sample collection and storage from ocular infections

example, the sonication (physical separation technique based on ultrasonic waves) and the use of selective media as MacConkey agar (MCk) and mannitol-salt agar (MSA) seeded by a perfect open streak for a good separation of the microorganisms, for positive and negative Gram bacteria, respectively. Talking about the fungi infections, the good sample collected by the ophthalmologists has been sufficient for a fungi growth and a direct observation of the macromorphology and micromorphology for the identification. However, the molecular techniques have revolutionized the ocular infection and coinfection diagnosis; these techniques are more sensitive, specific, and rapid and impact in the best outcome for the patient. The molecular techniques consist in the amplification of conserved regions of the different microorganisms involved in ocular infection, for example, Gram (+)/Gram (−) bacteria; Generic Fungi; herpes viruses I, II, and zoster; Cytomegalovirus; *Chlamydia* sp.; adenovirus; *Mycobacterium tuberculosis* complex (MTC) and no *Mycobacterium tuberculosis* complex (NTC); *Toxoplasma gondii*; and *Acanthamoeba* spp. by polymerase chain reaction (PCR). The PCR helps us for the identification of coinfection caused not only bacteria-bacteria or bacteria-fungi but also coinfection caused by viruses and parasites with bacteria or fungi.

Finally, the post-analytic phase consists of the interpretation of the results. Most laboratories do not report *Staphylococcus epidermidis* and *Staphylococcus aureus*, because they are part of the ocular surface microbiota; however, the laboratory staff of ocular microbiology knows that these microorganisms can be involved directly in the ocular infection, and these two microorganisms have been reported as the microorganisms most frequently isolated in infectious keratitis [109, 110]. It is important to consider the risk factor associated before deciding whether the microorganisms isolated are responsible for the infection or are a contamination.

In conclusion, the diagnosis of infectious disease is best achieved by applying in-depth knowledge of medical and laboratory science by integrating a strategic view of host-parasite interactions. Clearly, the best outcomes for patients are the result of strong partnerships between the clinician and the laboratory specialist [111].

21. Conclusion

The relationship between microorganisms has a long evolutionary history. The ability of microorganisms to interact conferred the possibility to collaborate and to adapt within a wider spectrum of environmental conditions. These circumstances have a direct impact on the clinical presentation as well as the dynamics of infection in the population.

Delay in diagnosis affects the sensitivity to specific treatments and the evolution of infection. The rate of recovery could be slow and morbid, leaving serious sequelae with the risk of loss of vision. Advances in methods for detecting infectious organisms and molecular microbiology have facilitated the recognition of the interactions among pathogens found in coinfections in the human eye. The acute period of coinfection is determinant to identify the coinfecting microorganisms. Awareness in the medical field and particularly in ophthalmology of lesions that do not cover the conditions of a pathognomonic clinical picture should be resolved with molecular biology techniques together with classical techniques of microorganism recognition, until final identification, if possible.

In this chapter, we proposed a strategy for reducing the uncertainty of the presence of two or more microorganisms affecting the eye. This has been implemented in our laboratory and has increased the possibility of isolation and identification.

In addition, the biofilm of each combination of pathogens must be studied molecularly to understand its particular adhesion and aggregation, possible mutations, and strategies for evasion or elimination of antimicrobial. Together with pharmacodynamics, *in vivo* studies will facilitate the application of different antimicrobial dosages to successfully remove coinfecting microorganisms.

Author details

Carlos Alberto Pantoja-Meléndez[1,2*], Victor M. Bautista-de Lucio[1], Mariana Ortiz-Casas[1], Jonathan Quevedo-Martínez[1] and Herlinda Mejía-López[1]

*Address all correspondence to: linda.mejia@institutodeoftalmologia.org

1 Institute of Opthalmology Conde de Valenciana, Mexico

2 National Autonomous University of Mexico, School of Medicine, Public Health Department, Mexico

References

[1] Whitcher J, Srinivasan M. "Corneal blindness: a global perspective". Bull World Health Organ. 2001; 79: p. 214-221.

[2] Birger R, Kouyos R, Cohen T, Griffiths S, Huijben S, Mina M, *et. al.* The potential impact of coinfection on antimicrobial chemotherapy and drug resistance. Trends Microbiol. 2015; 15: p. 106-107.

[3] Frey-Klett P, Burlinson P, Deveau A, Barret M, Tarkka M, Sarniguet A. Bacterial-Fungal Interactions: Hyphens between Agricultural, Clinical, Environmental, and Food Microbiologists. Microbiol Mol Biol Rev. 2011 Dec; 75 (4): 583–609

[4] Russler S, Tapper M, Knox K, Liepins A, Carrigan D. Pneumonitis associated with coinfection by human herpesvirus 6 and Legionella in an immunocompetent adult. Am J Pathol. 1991; 138: p. 1405-1411.

[5] Day T, Graham A, A R. Evolution of parasite virulence when host responses cause disease. Proc Biol Sci. 2007; 274: p. 2685-2692.

[6] Jindal A, Moreker M, Pathengay A, Khera M, Jalali A, Majji A, *et. al.* Polymicrobial endophthalmitis: prevalence, causative organisms, and visual outcomes. J Ophtalmic Inflamm Infect. 2013; 3: p. 6.

[7] Iwalokun B, Oluwadum A, Akisinde K, Niemogha M, Nwaokorie F. Bacteriologic and plasmid analysis of etiologic agents of conjunctivitis in Lagos, Nigeria. J Ophthalmic Inflamm Infect. 2011; 3: p. 95-103.

[8] Huang Y, Yang B, Li W. Defining the normal core microbiome of conjunctival microbial communities. Clin Microbiol Infect. 2016; 16: p. 30065-30069.

[9] Lim N, Lim D, Ray M. Polymicrobial versus monomicrobial keratitis: a retrospective comparative study. Eye Contact Lens. 2013; 39: p. 348-354.

[10] Gopinathan U, Sharma S, Garg P, Rao G. Review of epidemiological features, microbiological diagnosis and treatment outcome of microbial keratitis: experience of over a decade. Indian J Opthalmol. 2009; 57: p. 273-279.

[11] Basak S, Mohanta A, Bhowmick A. Epidemiological and microbiological diagnosis of suppurative keratitis in Gangetic West Bengal, eastern India. Indian J Ophthalmol. 2005; 53: p. 17-22.

[12] Bharathi M, Ramakrishnan R, Vasu R, Meenakshi PR. Aetiological diagnosis of microbial keratitis in South India - A study of 1618 cases. Indian J Med Microbiol. 2002; 20: p. 19-24.

[13] Jones D. Polymicrobial keratitis. Tr Am Ophth Soc. 1981; 79: p. 153-157.

[14] Brand A, Barnes J, K M, Odds F, Gow N. Cell wall glycans and soluble factors determine the interactions between the hyphae of Candida albicans and Pseudomonas aeruginosa. FEMS Microbiol Lett. 2008; 287: p. 48-55.

[15] Seidler M, Salvenmoser S, Muller F. Aspergillus fumigatus forms biofilms with reduced antifungal drug susceptibility on bronchial epithelial cells. Antimicrob Agents Chemother. 2008; 52: p. 4130-4136.

[16] Loussert C, Schmitt C, Prevost M. In vivo biofilm composition of Aspergillus fumigatus. Cell MIcrobiol. 2010; 12: p. 405-410.

[17] Mah T, O'Toole G. Mechanisms of biofilm resistance to antimicrobial agents. Trens Microbiol. 2001; 9: p. 34-39.

[18] Steward P, Costerton J. Antibiotic resistance of bacteria in biofilms. Lancet. 2001; 14: p. 135-138.

[19] Kıvanç SA, Kıvanç M, Bayramlar H. Microbiology of corneal wounds after cataract surgery: biofilm formation and antibiotic resistance patterns. J Wound Care. 2016; 25: 12: p. 14-19.

[20] Fröhlich S, Miño de Kaspar H, Grasbon T, Möhring C, Klauss V, Kampik A. Bacterial keratitis. Microbiological analysis as a principle for therapeutic recommendations. Pphthalmologe. 1999; 7: p. 459-464.

[21] Yeh D, Stinnett S, Afshari N. Analysis of bacterial cultures in infectious keratitis, 1997 to 2004. Am J Opthalmol. 2006; 6: p. 1066-1068.

[22] Kim J, H S, Song J. Infectious keratitis caused by Stenotrophomonas maltophilia and yeast simultaneously. Cornea. 2006; 10: p. 1234-1236.

[23] Qiu W, Yao Y. Mycotic keratitis caused by concurrent infections of Exserohilum mcginnisii and Candida parapsilosis. BMC Ophthalmol. 2013; 13: p. 37-40.

[24] Katragkou A, Z P, Perlin D, Kontoyiannis D, Walsh T, Roilides E. Exserohilum infection Review of 48 cases before the 2012 United States outbreak. The pediatric Infectious Disease Journal. 2005; 24: p. 939-941.

[25] Yokoi N, Okada K, Sugita J, Kinoshita S. Acute conjunctivitis associated with biofilm formation on a punctal plug. Jpn J Opthalmol. 2000; 44: p. 559-560.

[26] Taff HMK, Edward J, Andes D. Mechanisms of Candida biofilm drug resistance. Future Microbiol. 2013; 8: p. 1325-1337.

[27] Hayashi Y, Eguchi H, Toibana T, Mitamura Y, Yaguchi T. Polymicrobial sclerokeratitis caused by Scedosporium apiospermum and Aspergillus cibarius. Cornea. 2014; 33: p. 875-877.

[28] Schuster F, Visvesvara G. Free-living amoebae as opportunistic and non-opportunistic pathogens of human and animals. Int J Parasitol. 2004; 34: p. 1001-1027.

[29] Galarza C, Gutiérrez E, Uribe M, Ramos W, Ortega A, Ávila J, *et. al.* Amebas de vida libre en lesiones cutaneas. Reporte de 4 casos. Dermatol Perú. 2006; 16: p. 36-40.

[30] Scheid P. Relevance of free-living amoebae as hosts for phylogenetically diverse microorganisms. parasitol Res. 2014; 113: p. 2407-2414.

[31] Barker J, Lambert P, Brown M. Influence of intra-amoebic and other growth conditions on the surface properties of Legionella pneumophila. Infec Immun. 1993; 61: p. 3503-3510.

[32] Lim N, Goh D, Bunce C, Xing W, Fraenkel G, Poole T, *et. al*. Comparison of polyhexamethylene biguanide and chlorhexidine as monotherapy agents in the treatment of Acanthamoeba keratitis. Am J Ophthalmol. 2008; 145: p. 130-135.

[33] Scheid P. Mechanism of intrusion of a microspordian-like organism into the nucleus of host amoebae (Vannella sp.) isolated from a keratitis patient. Parasitol Res. 2007; 101: p. 1097-1102.

[34] Scheid P, Hauroder B, Michel R. Investigations of an extraordinary endocytobiont in Acanthamoeba sp., development and replication. Parasitol Res. 2010; 106: p. 1371-1377.

[35] Qureshi M, Perez A, Madayag R, Bottone E. Inhibition of Acanthamoeba species by Pseudomonas aeruginosa: rationale for their selective exclusion in corneal ulcers and contact lens care systems. J Clin Microbiol. 1993; 31: p. 1908-1910.

[36] Bottone E, R M, Qureshi M. Acanthamoeba keratitis: synergy between amebic and bacterial cocontaminants in contact lens care systems as a prelude to infection. J Clin Microbiol. 1992; 30: p. 2447-2450.

[37] Lorenzo-Morales J, Khan N, Walochnik J. An update on Acanthamoeba keratitis: diagnosis, pathogenesis and treatment. Parasite. 2015; 22: p. 10.

[38] Sharma R, Jhanji V, Satpathy G, Sharma N, Khokhar S, Agarwal T. Coinfection with Acanthamoeba and Pseudomonas in contact lens-associated keratitis. Optom Vis Sci. 2013; 90: p. 53-55.

[39] Michel R, Hauroder B. Isolation of an Acanthamoeba strain with intracellular Burkholderia pickettii infection. Zentralbl Bakteriol. 1997; 285: p. 541-547.

[40] Mauger T, Craig E. Combined acanthamoeba and Stenotrophomonas maltophilia keratitis treated with a conjunctival flap followed by penetrating keratoplasty. Cornea. 2006; 25: p. 631-633.

[41] Hong J, Ji J, Xu J, Cao W, Liu Z, Sun X. An unusual case of Acanthamoeba Polyphaga and Pseudomonas Aeruginosa keratitis. Diagn Pathol. 2014; 9: p. 105.

[42] Lone R, Syed K, Abdul R, Sheikh S, Shah F. Unusual case of methicillin resistant staphylococcus aureus and Acanthamoeba keratitis in a non-contact lens wearer from Kashmir, India. BMJ Case Re. 2009; p. 8.

[43] Dini L, Cockinos C, Frean J, Niszl I, Markus M. Unusual case of acanthamoeba polyphaga and Pseudomonas aeruginosa keratitis in a contact lens wearer from Gauteng, South Africa. L Clin Microbiol. 2000; 38: p. 826-829.

[44] Tu E, Joslin C, Nijm L, Feder R, Jain S, Shoff M. Polymicrobial keratitis: Acanthamoeba and infectious crystalline keratopathy. Am J Ophthalmol. 2009; 148: p. 13.

[45] Gupta S, Shrivastava R, tandom R, Gogia V, Agarwal P, Satpathy G. Role of voriconazole in combined acanthamoeba and fungal corneal ulcer. Cont Lnes Anterior Eye. 2011; 34: p. 287-289.

[46] Rumelt S, Cohen I, Lefler E, Rehany U. Corneal co-infection with Scedosporium apiospermum and Acanthamoeba after sewage-contaminated ocular injury. Cornea. 2001; 20: p. 112-116.

[47] Tien S, Sheu M. Treatment of Acanthamoeba keratitis combined with fungal infection with polyhexamethylene biguanide. Kaohsiung J Med Sci. 1999; 15: p. 665-673.

[48] Froumis N, Mondino B, Glaswow B. Acanthamoeba keratitis associated with fungal keratitis. Eye Contact Lens. 2008; 34: p. 185-187.

[49] Slade D, Johnson J, Tabin G. Acanthamoeba and fungal keratitis in a woman with a history of Intacs corneal implants. Eye Contact Lens. 2008; 34: p. 185-187.

[50] Dong Q, Brulc J, Iovieno A, Bates B GA, Miller D, Revanna K, *et. al.* Diversity of bacteria at healthy human conjunctiva. Invest Ophthalmol Vis Sci. 2011; 52: p. 5408-5413.

[51] Dalfré J, Rodrigues J, Donato B, Giancoli A, De Carvalho J, De Andrade D, *et. al.* Fungic microbiota of normal conjunctiva, sugar-cane and anemophilous fungi of the region of Monte Belo- Minas Gerais. Arq Bras Oftalmol. 2007; 70: p. 445-449.

[52] Moreno N, Moreno R, Sousa L. Aerobic bacterial microbiota of the conjunctiva in diabetic patients with normal and altered glycated hemoglobin levels in two regions in Brazil. Arq Bras Oftalmol. 2014; 77: p. 351-354.

[53] Schabereiter-Gurtner C, Maca S, Rölleke S, Nigl K, Lukas J, Hirschl A, *et. al.* 16S rDNA-based identification of bacteria from conjunctival swabs by PCR and DGGE fingerprinting. Invest Ophthalmol Vis Sci. 2001; 42: p. 1164-1171.

[54] Tappe D, Mueller A, WeiBbrich B, Schubert J, Schargus M, Stich A. Severe conjunctivitis due to multidrug-resistant Neisseria gonorrhoeae and adenovirus 53 coinfection in a traveler returning from Thailand. J Travel Med. 2013; 20: p. 403-406.

[55] Mellman-Rubin T, Kowaski R, Uhrin M, Gordon Y. Incidence of adenoviral and chlamydial coinfection in acute follicular conjunctivitis. 1995; 119: p. 652-654.

[56] Galvis V, Tello A, Guerra A, Acuña M, Villarreal D. Antibiotic susceptibility patterns of bacteria isolated from keratitis and intraocular infections at Fundación Oftalmológica de Santander (FOSCAL. Florida Blanca Colombia Biomedica. 2014; 34: p. 23-33.

[57] Gupta A, Gupta V, Dogra M, Panday S, Ray P. Chkraborty A. Spectrum and clinical profile of post cataract surgery endophthalmitis in north India. Indian J Ophthalmol. 2003;51: p.139-145.

[58] Pijl B, Theelen T, Tilanus M, Rentenaar R, Crama N. Acute endophthalmitis after cataract surgery: 250 consecutive cases treated at a tertiary referral center in the Netherlands. Am J Ophthalmol. 2010; 149: p. 482-487.

[59] Gharamah AA, Moharram AM, Ismail MA, Al-Hussaini AK. Bacterial and fungal endophthalmitis in upper Egypt: related species and risk factors. Asian Pac J Trop Biomed. 2012; 2: p. 655-659.

[60] Kunimoto D, Das T, Sharma S, Jalali S, Majji A, Gopinathan U, *et. al.* Microbiologic spectrum and susceptibility of isolates: part II. Posttraumatic endophthalmitis. Endophthalmitis Research Group. Am J Ophthalmol. 1999; 128: p. 242-244.

[61] Long C, Liu B, Xu C, Jing Y, Yuan Z, Lin X. Causative organisms of post-traumatic endophthalmitis: a 20-year retrospective study. BMC Ophthlmol. 2014; 25: p. 34.

[62] Duan F, Wu K, Liao J, Zheng Y, Yuan Z, Tan J, Lin X. Causative Microorganisms of Infectious Endophthalmitis: A 5-Year Retrospective Study. J Ophthalmol. 2016; 2016: 1-7.

[63] Streilen J. Ocular immune privilege: the eye takes a dim but practical view of immunity and inflammation. J Leukoc Biol. 2003; 74: p. 179-185.

[64] Matricardi P, Rosmini F, Riondino S, Fortini M, Ferrigno L, Rapicetta M, *et. al.*Exposure to foodborne and orofecal microbes versus airborne viruses in relation to atopy and allergic asthma: epidemiological study. BMJ. 2000; 320: p. 412-417.

[65] Kurata A. Hygiene hypothesis: why south/north geographical differences in prevalence of asthma and sarcoidosis? Med Hypotheses. 2012; 79: p. 363-364.

[66] von Hertzen LC. Puzzling associations between childhood infections and the later occurrence of asthma and atopy. Ann Med. 2000; 32: p. 397-400.

[67] Kerr N, Stern G. Bacterial keratitis associated with vernal keratoconjunctivitis. Cornea. 1992; 11: p. 355-359.

[68] Rolinski J, Hus I. Immunological aspects of acute and recurrent herpes simplex keratitis. J Immunol Res. 2014; p. 51.

[69] Stric L, Wald A, Celum C. Management of herpes simplex virus type 2 infection in HIV type 1-infected persons. Clin Infec Dis. 2006; 43: p. 347-356.

[70] Faber D, Wiley C, Lynn G, Gross J, Freeman W. Role of HIV and CMV in the pathogenesis of retinitis and retinal vasculopathy in AIDS patients. Invest Ophthalmol Vis Sci. 1992; 33: p. 2345-2353.

[71] Radu L, Serban R, Cornăcel C, Cioboata M, Anghel A. Cytomegalovirus retinitis in HIV/AIDS patients. J Med Life. 2014; 15: p. 237-240.

[72] Freigassner P, Ardjomand N, Radner H, El-Shabrawi Y. Coinfection of the retina by Epstein-Barr virus and cytomegalovirus in an AIDS patient. Am J Opthalmol. 2002; 134: p. 275-257.

[73] Skolnik P, Pomerantz R, De la Monte S, Lee S, Hsiung G, Foos R, *et. al*. Dual infection of retina with human immunodeficiency virus type 1 and cytomegalovirus. Am J Ophthalmol. 1989; 107: p. 361-372.

[74] Rummelt V, Rummelt C, Jahn G, Wenkel H, Sinzger C, Mayer U, *et. al*. Triple retinal infection with human immunodeficiency virus type 1, cytomegalovirus, and herpes simplex virus type 1. Light and electron microscopy, immunohistochemistry, and in situ hybridization. Ophthalmology. 1994; 101: p. 270-279.

[75] Kim J, Singer E, Bonelli L, Klausner J. A case of primary HIV type 1 and cytomegalovirus coinfection presenting with widespread clinical disease. J Int Assoc Provid AIDS Care. 2014; 13: p. 196-199.

[76] Matoba A. Polymicrobial keratitis secondary to Burkholderia ambifaria, enterococcus, and staphylococcus aureus in a patient with herpetic stromal keratitis. Am J Ophthalmol. 2003; 136: p. 748-749.

[77] Tandon R, Vajpayee R, Gupta V, Vajpayee M, Satpathy G, Dada T. Polymicrobial keratitis in an HIV-positive patient. Indian J Ophthalmol. 2003; 51: p. 87-88.

[78] Wayne P. Reference Method for Broth dilution antifungal susceptibility testing of filamentous fungi. 2nd ed. USA; 2008.

[79] Abdelillah A, Houcine B, Halima D, Meriem C, Imane Z, Eddine S, *et. al*. Evaluation of antifungal activity of free fatty acids methyl esters fraction isolated from Algerian Linum usitatissimum L. seeds against toxigenic Aspergillus. Asian Pac J Trop Biomed. 2013; 3: p. 443-448.

[80] Ponce D, Bautista-de-Lucio V, Santacrúz-Valdés C, Climent-Flores A, Rodríguez-Tovar A, Robles-Contreras A, *et. al*. Effect of simultaneous treatment of quinolones and antifungal drugs on fungal-bacterial coculture. In ARVO 2012.

[81] Pradhan L, Sharma S, Nalamada S, Sahu S, DS, Garg P. Natamycin in the treatment of keratomycosis: correlation of treatment outcome and in vitro susceptibility of fungal isolates. Indian J Ophthalmol. 2011; 59: p. 512-514.

[82] Pate J, Jones D, Wilhelmus K. Prevalence and spectrum of bacterial co-infection during fungal keratitis. Br J Opthalmol. 2006; 90: p. 289-292.

[83] Mosquera J, Denning D. Azole cross-resistance in Aspergillus fumigatus. Antimicrob Agents Chemother. 2002; 46: p. 556-557.

[84] Hanet M, Jamart J, Chaves A. Fluoroquinolones or fortified antibiotics for treating bacterial keratitis: systematic review and meta-analysis of comparative studies. Can J Ophthalmol. 2012; 47: p. 493-499.

[85] Jin K, Jeon H, Hyon J, Wee W, Suh W, Shin Y, *et. al.* A case of fungal keratitis and onychomycosis simultaneously infected by Trichophyton species. BMC. 2014; 11: p. 37 90.

[86] Tallarida R. Drug synergism: its detection and applications. J Pharmacol Exp Ther. 2001; 298: p. 865-872.

[87] Nakajima R, Kitamura A, Someya K, Tanaka M, Sato K. In vitro and in vivo antifungal activities of DU-6859a, a fluoroquinolone, in combination with amphotericin B and fluconazole against pathogenic fungi. Antimicrob Agents Chemother. 1995; 39: p. 1517-1521.

[88] Stergiopoulou T, Meletiadis J, Sein T, Papaioannidou P, Tsiouris I, Roilides E, *et. al.* Comparative pharmacodynamic interaction analysis between ciprofloxacin, moxifloxacin and levofloxacin and antifungal agents against Candida albicans and Aspergillus fumigatus. J Antimicrob Chemother. 2009; 63: p. 343-348.

[89] Sasaki E, Maesaki S, Miyazaki Y, Yanagihara K, Tomono K, Tashiro T, *et. al.* Synergistic effect of ofloxacin and fluconazole against azole-resistant Candida albicans. J Infec Chemother. 2000; 6: p. 151-154.

[90] Costerton J, Geesey G, Cheng K. How bacteria stick. Sci Am. 1978; 238: p. 86-95.

[91] Hall-Stoodley L, Costerton J, Stoodley P. Bacterial biofilms: From the natural environment to infectious diseases. Nat Rev Microbiol. 2004; 2: p. 95-108.

[92] Harrison J, Ceri H, Turner R. Multimetal resistance and tolerance in microbial biofilms. Nat Rev Microbiol. 2007; 5: p. 928-938.

[93] Health. NIo. Research on microbial biofilms (PA-03-047). [Online] . 2002; [cited 2015 January 10.] Available from: HYPERLINK "http://grants.nih.gov/grants/guide/pafiles/PA-03-047.html"http://grants.nih.gov/grants/guide/pa-files/PA-03-047.html.

[94] Donlan R, Costerton J. Biofilms: Survival mechanisms of clinically relevant microorganisms. Clin Microbiol Rev. 2002; 15: p. 167-193.

[95] Annous B, Fratamico P, Smith J. Scientific status summary. J Food Sci. 2009; 74: p. R24-37.

[96] Hooshangi S, Bentley W. From unicellular properties to multicellular behavior: Bacteria quorum sensing circuitry and applications. Curr Opin Biotechnol. 2008; 19: p. 550-555.

[97] Stewart P, Franklin M. Physiological heterogeneity in biofilms. Nat Rev Microbiol. 2008; 6: p. 199-210.

[98] Watnick P, Kolter R. Biofilm, city of microbes. J Bacteriol. 2000; 182: p. 2675-2679.

[99] Fux CA, Costerton JW, Stewart PS, Stoodley P. Survival strategies of infectious biofilms. Trends Microbiol. 2005; 13: p. 34-40.

[100] Costerton J, Stewart P, biofilms B. Battling biofilms. Sci Am. 2001; 285: p. 74-81.

[101] Behlau I, Gilmore M. Microbial biofilms in ophthalmology and infectious disease. Arch Ophthalmol. 2008; 126: p. 1572-1581.

[102] H, Wingender J. The biofilm matrix. Nat Rev Microbiol. 2010; 8: p. 623-633.

[103] Sauer K, Camper A, Ehrlich G, Costerton J, Davies D. Pseudomonas aeruginosa displays multiple phenotypes during development as a biofilm. J Bacteriol. 2002; 184: p. 1140-1154.

[104] Hall-Stoodley L, Stoodley P. Evolving concepts in biofilm infections. Cell Microbiol. 2009; 11: p. 1034-1043.

[105] Davies D. Understanding biofilm resistance to antibacterial agents. Nat Rev Drug Discov. 2003; 2: p. 114-122.

[106] Spoering A, Gilmore M. Quorum sensing and DNA release in bacterial biofilms. Curr Opin Microbiol. 2006; 9: p. 133-137.

[107] Kaplan J. Biofilm dispersal: Mechanisms, clinical implications, and potential therapeutic uses. J Dent Res. 2010; 89: p. 205-218.

[108] Allan B, Garth J. Strategies for the management of microbial keratitis. Br J Ophthalmol. 1995; 79: p. 777-786.

[109] Hernandez-Camarena JC, Graue-Hernandez EO, Ortiz-Casas M, Ramirez-Miranda A, Navas A, Pedro-Aguilar L, *et al.* Trends in Microbiological and Antibiotic Sensitivity Patterns in Infectious Keratitis: 10-Year Experience in Mexico City. Cornea. 2015; 34: p. 778-785.

[110] Lichtinger A, Yeung S, Kim P. Shifting trends in bacterial keratitis in Toronto: an 11-18 year review. Ophthalmology. 2012; 119: p. 1785-1790.

[111] Baron E, Miller M, Weinstein M. A Guide to Utilization of the Microbiology Laboratory for Diagnosis of Infectious Diseases: 2013 Recommendations by the Infectious Diseases Society of America (IDSA) and the American Society for Microbiology; 2013.

7

Overview of Common and Less Common Ocular Infections

Shimon Rumelt

Abstract

Infection may occur in any tissue of the eye, orbit, and adnexa. Infection may spread directly through contact and indirectly through blood vessels (especially valveness veins) and nerves. A proper treatment for ocular infections is imperative because it dictates the prognosis. Ocular infections may share identical clinical finding and be caused by different etiologic agents. To obtain the best outcome, a systematic approach for ocular infections is essential. This chapter describes the characteristic clinical features and manifestations of some common ocular infections and the differentiation between them and inflammations and other diseases even without using new imaging modalities such as confocal electron microscopy, anterior segment optical coherence tomography, and laboratory tests including polymeraze chain reaction.

Keywords: diagnosis, treatment, eyelid infections, conjunctiva, cornea, uvea, endophthalmitis, panophthalmitis, intraocular, retina, orbita

1. Introduction

A proper treatment for ocular infections is imperative because it dictates the prognosis. To obtain the best outcome, a systematic approach for ocular infections is essential. This chapter is aimed to describe the characteristic clinical features and manifestations of some common ocular infections and the differentiation between them and inflammations and other diseases even without using new imaging modalities such as confocal electron microscopy and anterior segment optical coherence tomography and laboratory tests including polymerase chain reaction.

Identifying and treating ocular infections can be challenging. Ocular infections may share identical clinical result and be caused by different etiologic agents. The infection is usually named according to the ocular structures involved with the suffix "itis" meaning infectious or noninfectious inflammation.

2. Eyelid infections

Infections of the eyelid include external and internal hordeolum [1]. The first one is abscess localized in the anterior lamella of the eyelid (orbicularis), whereas the internal is located in the posterior lamella (tarsus). Pain and swelling, redness, local tenderness and warmth of the eyelid characterize both. The swelling is well localized. When it is more diffuse, secondary preseptal cellulitis exists.

Preseptal cellulitis is diffuse swelling of one of the eyelids or both [2]. It includes the triad of tenderness (dolor), redness (color) and warmth (calor). The usual cause is eyelid abrasion by trauma. Preseptal cellulitis is distinguished from the more severe orbital cellulitis by the absence of proptosis, limitation of ocular movements and involvement of the optic disc (swelling) because the infection is confined anteriorly by the orbital septum.

Primary herpes simplex infection is characterized by small vesicle on the eyelid that may be accompanied by conjunctival hyperemia [3]. Necrotizing fasciitis is a rapidly progressive infection of the subcutaneous soft tissues that spreads through the fascia and may involve the eyelid and the orbit [4]. The first sign is skin erythema that spreads quickly and changes its color to purple. Later, the skin and subcutaneous tissues may separate from the deep tissues. The patient becomes toxic and suffers of severe local pain. It may be idiopathic or appear after trivial trauma or surgery. The most common causative agents are A streptococci, clostridium (with gas gangrene) and polymicrobial. Since the disease is fatal, early detection and treatment are essential.

Blepharitis is an bilateral inflammation of the eyelid margins that may be caused by infective agents (**Figure 1**) [5]. Seborrheic blepharitis causes scales over the eyelids and may accompany seborrhea. Staphylococcal blepharitis is clinically characterized by collarettes around the eyelash bases that move along the hair shaft as it grows. It is caused by staphylococcal species. Demodex blepharitis is characterized by sleeves along the base of the lash shaft and is caused by *Demodex folliculorum*. The eyelid margins may be erythematous. Patients may complain for ocular irritation, burning sensation, dryness or bouts of dryness and tearing. They may complain of stickiness or ocular tiredness/tense. Blepharitis may be accompanied by conjunctivitis (i.e. blepharoconjunctivitis) and in this case the eyelid margins show identical signs to blepharitis but the conjunctiva is also inflamed.

Phthiriasis palpebrarum is an infestation of the eyelid margins caused by *Phthirus pubis* [6]. Eggs and adults are found near the base of the eyelashes. Patients may complain from irritation. They are usually from nursery homes and the disease is sexually transmitted.

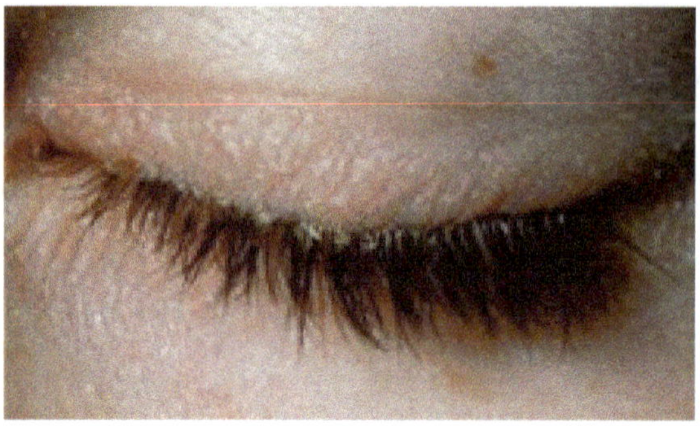

Figure 1. Blepharitis. Note the scales at the base of the eyelashes.

Treatment for localized infection such as hordeolum include warm dry compresses 3–4 times a day for 10 min each and antibiotic ointment until complete resolution is achieved or drainage, if possible. Preseptal cellulitis is treated by antibiotics such as amoxicillin trihydrate 875 mg with clavulanic acid 125 mg (Augmentin®) bid or ceftazidime 1 g/day PO or IV for a week.

Blepharitis can be prevented by eyelid hygiene. Blepharitis is treated by warm dry compresses followed by massage with tetracycline ointment for staphylococcal and seborrhea forms and fusidic acid (Fucithalmic®) for demodex. Topical azithromycin 1% is also very effective. In refractory cases, systemic antibiotics from the tetracycline family such as doxycycline 100 mg 1qd, tetracycline 250 mg qid or azithromycin 200 mg/day PO is added. Terpinen-4-ol, the main component of the essential oil of *Melaleuca alternifolia* (tea tree oil) has been demonstrated for Demodex. Blepharoconjunctivitis is treated similarly with an additional mild topical corticosteroid (such as fluorometholone (FML®) 0/1% qid or loteprednol (Lotemax®) 0.5% qid) for limited period or tear substitutes. Phthiriasis palpebrarum is treated by manual removal of all the mites and ova and treatment of the pubis with yellow mercuric oxide 1%. Necrotizing fasciitis is treated under hospitalization usually in intensive care unit. Treatment includes intravenous penicillin V 500 mg bid or intramuscular benzathine penicillin G 1.2 million units qid, aminoglycoside (e,g., gentamicin 1-1.5mg/kg/day IV tid) and clindamycin 600 mg IV tid in combination with surgical debridement and hyperbaric oxygen. patients that are allergic to penicillin receive either vancomycin 1 g bid and aztreonam 1 g tid with clindamycin instead of penicillin.

3. Conjunctival infections

Conjunctival infections manifested as conjunctival hyperemia [7, 8] (**Figure 2**). Lower eyelid follicles may accompany conjunctivitis. Discharge and preauricular lymphadenopathy may accompany be also present.

Acute conjunctivitis is less than 4 weeks, otherwise it is considered as chronic. Several entities should be mentioned. When conjunctivitis is accompanied by throat pain, fever and malaise, it is suggested as hay fever. When papillae and follicles in both upper and lower eyelids accompany conjunctivitis, adult inclusion conjunctivitis should be suspected. This is a sexually transmitted disease and both mates should be treated. Gonorrhea conjunctivitis is characterized by copious purulent discharge while other agents cause mucopurulent, mucoid or serous discharge. A form of viral conjunctivitis is hemorrhagic conjunctivitis in which conjunctival hyperemia is accompanied by subconjunctival hemorrhages.

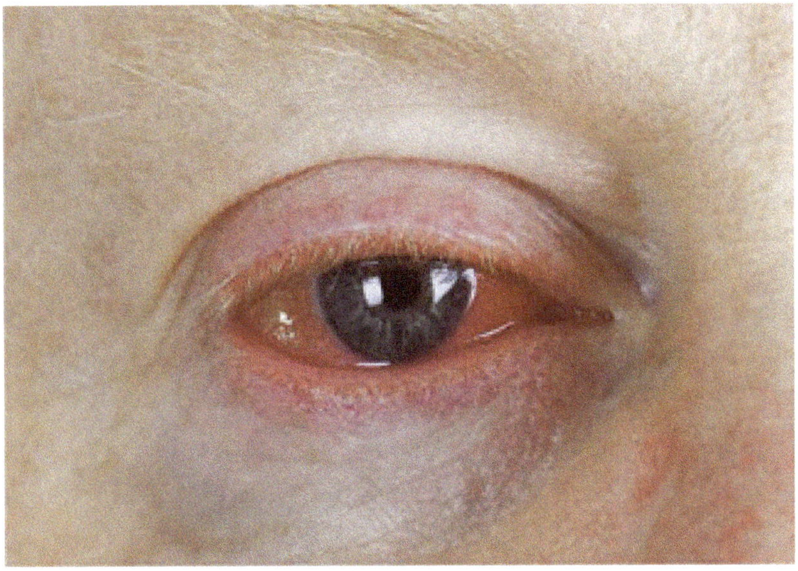

Figure 2. Viral conjunctivitis. Note the conjunctival congestion without corneal or intraocular involvement.

Conjunctival myiasis is conjunctival infestation by larvae of different types of flies depending on the habitat [9]. The larvae are tiny white and move quickly. They cause conjunctival hyperemia and the patient complains of unilateral ocular irritation. Rarely, the larva may migrate into the lacrimal drainage system and cause obstruction.

Infectious agents include bacteria, virus and chlamydia. Most microorganisms cannot invade intact epithelium. The only exceptions are *Neisseria gonorrhoeae, Corynebacterium diphtheria, Haemophilus aegyptius* and Listeria.

Infectious conjunctivitis should be differentiated from noninfectious agents such as allergic conjunctivitis and dry eyes. In neonates occurring in the first month of life, ophthalmia neonatorum is an entity that may be caused by various microorganisms such as chlamydia and less commonly by *Neisseria gonorrhoeae*. Tetracycline 1% or erythromycin 0.5% ointment qid for 3 weeks is effective for prevention and treatment.

Most of the acute viral conjunctivitis forms are self-limited and treatment is aimed to decrease discomfort and prevent secondary infection. Topical antibiotic such as sulfacetamide 10% (Sulfacid®) qid may be applied. In G6PD and sulfa-sensitive patients, other antibiotics such as Gatifloxacin (Zymar®) bid, a quinolon, may be prescribed. It is best to defer topical corticosteroid for a week to ascertain that the conjunctivitis is not herpetic or adenoviral. If no improvement is observed after a week, topical corticosteroid such as fluorometholone (FML®) 0.1% qid may be used for 1–2 weeks in tapered dosage. Patients should be instructed to prevent eye-finger-eye contact (and other contact means) especially with adenoconjunctivitis. The disease is infective between 7 and 10 days. Hay fever is treated by mild topical corticosteroids such as fluorometholone (FML®) 0.1% qid or loteprednol (Lotemax®) 0.5% and nasal decongestant. Adult inclusion conjunctivitis is treated by topical and systemic tetracycline (e.g. doxycycline hyclate 100 mg once a day or tetracycline 250 mg qid). The mate should be treated as well. Myiasis is treated by removal of all the larvae from the conjunctival sac. Instillation of topical cocaine 4% may be added before removing the larvae to decrease their movement.

4. Corneal infections

The general name for corneal infection or inflammation is keratitis. The conjunctiva is usually secondarily involved as conjunctival hyperemia. The clinical manifestations vary and include corneal ulcer, abscess and/or infiltrate [10]. Corneal ulcer is distinguished from abscess and infiltrate by its staining with fluorescein. Abscess and infiltrate do not stain. The clinical findings may overlap between different etiologies.

The diagnosis of all corneal infections is based on scrapping for direct staining with hematoxylin and eosin or Giemsa, and cultures, which should be taken routinely before commencing with empiric broad-spectrum topical antibiotics. The only exceptions for obtaining corneal scarps and cultures are a marginal (near the limbus) smaller than 3 mm width flat ulcer(s) and certain typical findings such as dendrite suggesting herpetic keratitis or bilateral multiple epithelial minute defects (epitheliopathy) suggesting adenoviral (epidemic) keratoconjunctivitis.

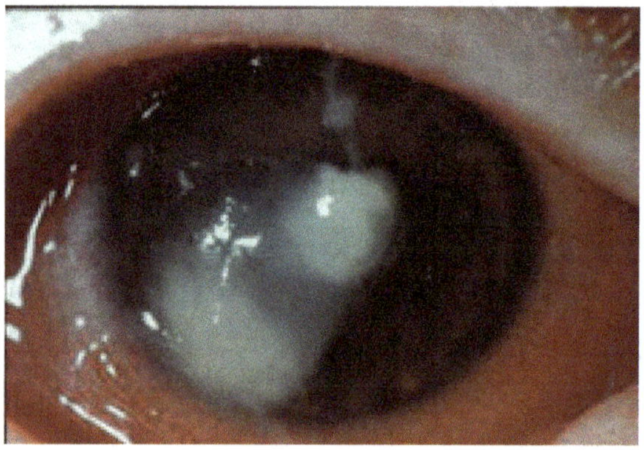

Figure 3. *Pseudomonas aeruginosa* corneal ulcer at the acute stage.

Bacterial keratitis or bacterial ulcer is usually a single solid ulcer with distinctive borders (**Figure 3**). Its size and depth may vary. It may be accompanied by an infiltrate in its base or by localized corneal edema. Infiltrate is white, more dense and distinct and is well localized in contrast to the grayish appearance and less distinctive borders of edema. A grayish, glistening appearance with secretions is a common manifestation of Pseudomonas ulcer. Flare and cells or hypopyon may accompany bacterial ulcer and they may be sterile or infected. If they appear under treatment, they indicate worsening of the infectious process. Any flare or cells in the vitreous in phakic or pseudophakic eyes indicates the development of endophthalmitis. Predisposing factors for corneal ulcer include contact lens wear, ocular trauma, dry eyes and long use of topical antibiotics and/or corticosteroids.

Herpetic keratitis a characterized by dendrites in the secondary infection. In Herpes simplex, dendrites vary in number (usually 1–3). They are coarse with widening of their ends (terminal bulbs) (**Figure 4**). Thus, they differ from Herpes zoster dendrites, which are usually numerous, small, thin and without terminal bulbs (**Figures 5, 6**). Involvement of the tip of the nose (Hutchison's sign) indicates an involvement of the eye on the same side of herpes zoster (**Figure 7**). In repeated Herpes simplex infections, the epithelial defects may form a geographic pattern and may accompanied by corneal vascularization. An important clinical test is corneal sensitivity, which is reduced in recurrent infections. Another finding is patchy sectorial atrophy of the iris that occurs mainly in the midperiphery after herpetic keratouveitis or uveitis.

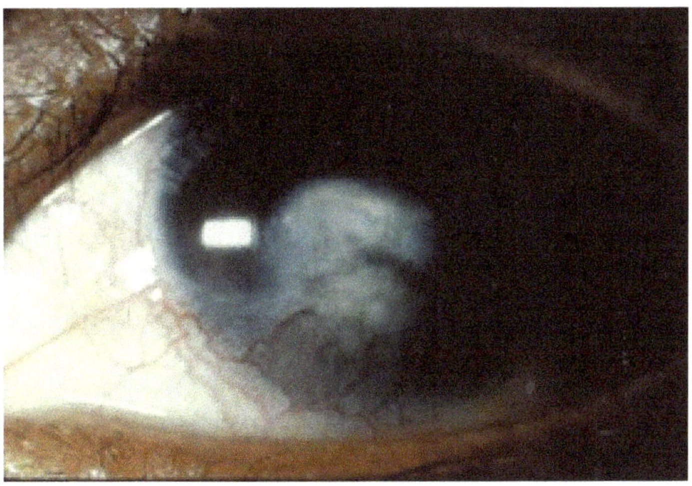

Figure 4. Corneal scar as a result of the ulcer seen in **Figure 3**.

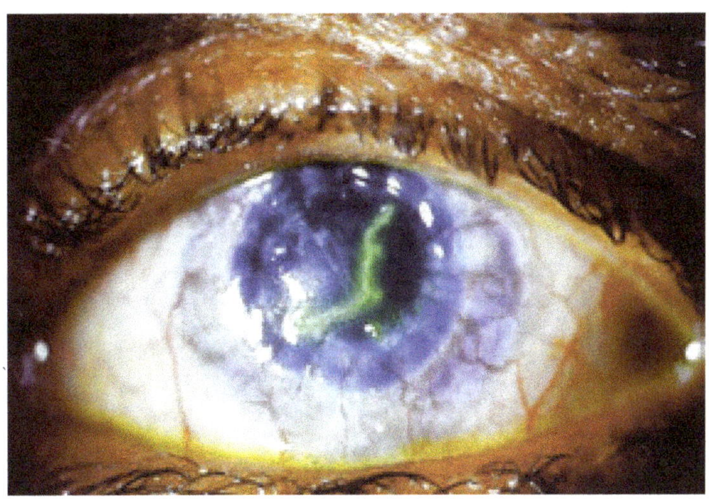

Figure 5. Recurrent herpetic keratitis with dendrite in corneal graft. The dendrite is large and has terminal bulbs.

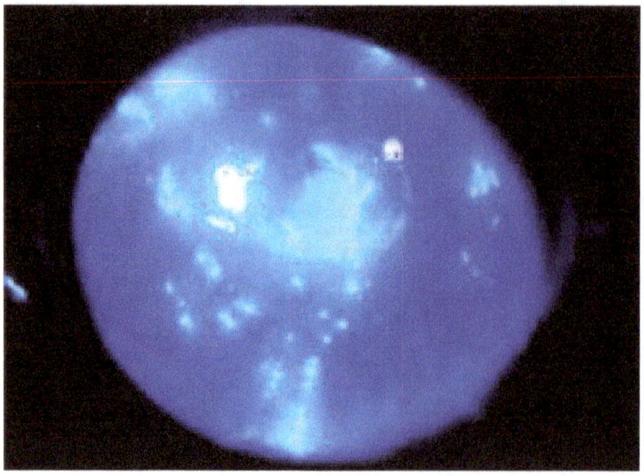

Figure 6. Corneal dendrites in herpes zoster. The dendrites are multiple and very fine. They represent immunologic reaction rather than true infection.

Fungal keratitis appears usually as multiple foci of feathery opacification of the cornea with satellites (**Figures 8** and **9**). Hyphae and yeast may be identified by confocal microscopy in the affected cornea.

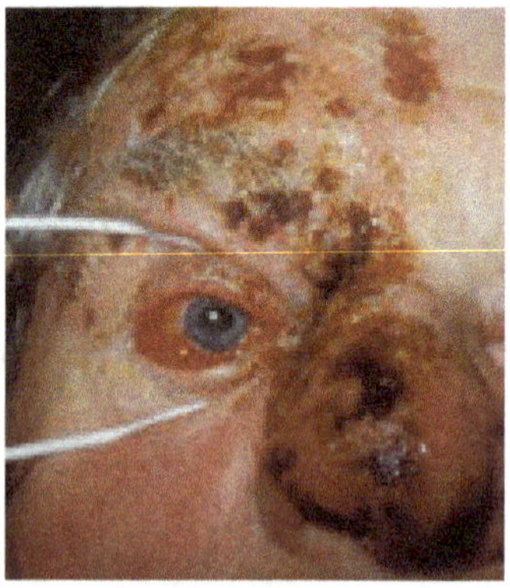

Figure 7. Herpes zoster ophthalmicus. The vesicular rash involves the dermatome innervated by the ophthalmic branch of the trigeminal nerve. Involvement of the tip of the nose indicates involvement of the eye (Hutchison's sign).

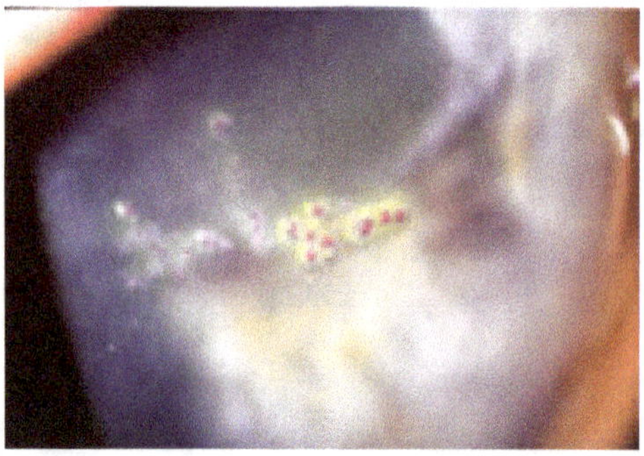

Figure 8. Fungal keratitis. Note the multiple foci.

Acanthamoeba infection may vary in presentation. The earliest clinical signs include multiple corneal epithelial cell swellings (as seen in adenoviral keratoconjunctivitis but here they are unilateral) and/or corneal edema. Late signs include perineural sheathing and stromal ring(s) (**Figure 10**). Acanthamoeba cysts may be identified by confocal microscopy. A history of contact lens wear and/or bathing in pools or sea is common and symptoms of pain are more striking than the clinical appearance. When diagnosis by cultures is impossible especially in recurrent disease, polymerase chain reaction of the involved tissue may establish the diagnosis.

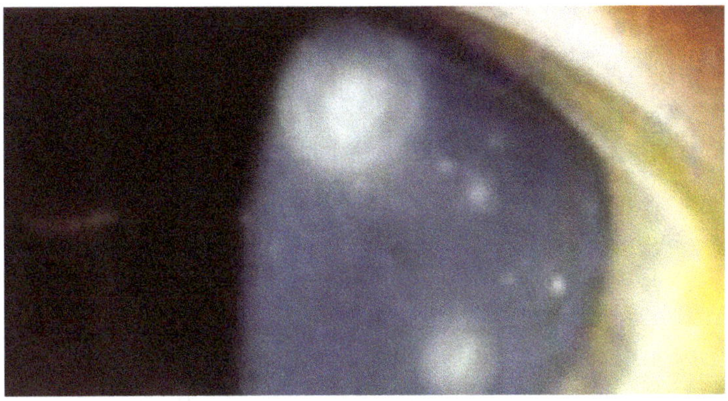

Figure 9. Fungal keratitis with multiple foci and indistinct borders.

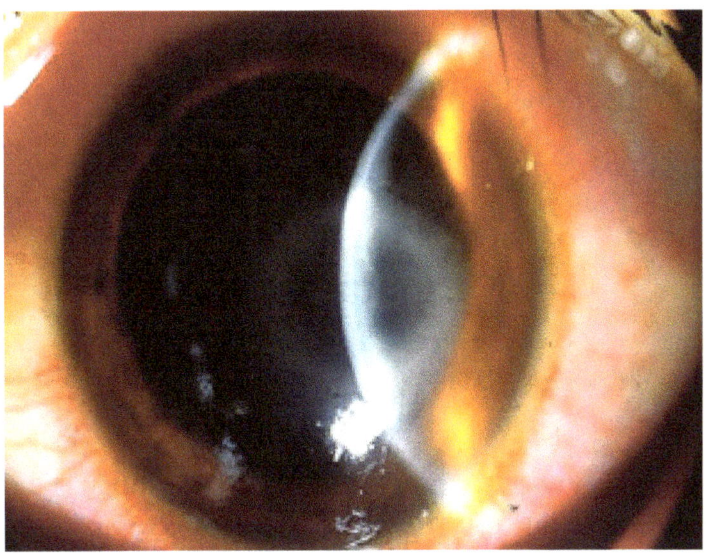

Figure 10. Immune ring in Acanthamoeba keratitis.

Corneal co-infections as other co-infections or mixed infections should be suspected when the course of the disease is atypical or when the condition deteriorates despite of treatment according to cultures and sensitivities. In such cases, repeated cultures should be obtained and broaden accordingly.

All corneal infections may result in either scarring (**Figure 10**) or melting and perforation.

The treatment approach differs between central and peripheral ulcers. Central ulcers are treated with topical antibiotics and are followed frequently to monitor their size and depth. Peripheral ulcers are treated with topical antibiotics and corticosteroids may be cautiously added. Treatment includes broad-spectrum topical antibiotics such as fortified cefazolin and gentamicin or moxifloxacin (Vigamox®) 0.5% every 30 min–1 h until sensitivity is obtained. Then antibiotic treatment is dictated by the sensitivity of the microorganism. In cases of pain and/or flare and cells in the anterior chamber, topical cycloplegic agent (e.g. cyclopentolate hydrochloride 1% tid) is added to decrease the pain originating from the ciliary body and/or prevention of posterior synechiae. Suspicion of infection other than bacteria should be made when no response is achieved or when the condition worsens under treatment. Additional treatment modalities include topical autologous serum, antipolymorphonuclear migration agents such as tetracycline 1% and/ or citrate 10%, which cause decrease of collagenase activity by chelating free calcium ions that are required for collagenase activity. Vitamin A (ascorbic acid) either topically 10% and/or PO (Vitamin A 500 mg bid). Liberal use of partial tarsorrhaphy is useful especially in recurrences of ulcers, exposure, dryness, corneal anesthesia or trophic ulcers and deep ones. All these means should be used in severe ulcer. Topical corticosteroids should be avoided at the acute phase of the keratitis and when the epithelium is not intact because they cause potentiation of collagenase that may lead to perforation and may also promote secondary infection. They may be used in later stage only after the epithelium healed (no corneal staining) to decrease stromal scarring. If descemetocele occurs, several surgical options exist and include anterior corneal grafts such as deep anterior lamellar keratoplasty (DALK) or non-Descemet's membrane endothelial keratoplasty (DMEK). A relatively historic treatment is placement of histoacryl for corneal perforation or descematocele. This promotes healing but also corneal vascularization, which impairs vision. Conjunctival flap (Gunderson operation) is indicated for perforation only for eyes with no potential for vision.

5. Endophthalmitis

The hallmarks of endophthalmitis are flare and white cells both in the vitreous and the anterior chamber [11]. Additional findings may include fibrin in the anterior chamber, hypopyon and retinal periphlebitis. The vision is decreased and ocular pain is noted.

Endophthalmitis is divided to two categories: exogenous (postoperative, bleb-associated and traumatic) and endogenous (source within another organ). Postoperative endophthalmitis may occur following any intraocular surgery including cataract, penetrating keratoplasty, glaucoma, vitrectomy and intraocular injections. Rarely, it may develop by spreading of keratitis or scleritis. In bleb-associated endophthalmitis, the bleb is pale and necrotic. Endophthalmitis should be suspected in any eye after penetrating keratoplasty if epithelial defect or ulcer is present near the corneal-graft interface even if there is corneal edema or signs suggesting corneal graft rejection (presence of flare and cells in the anterior chamber).

Prevention of endophthalmitis before any ocular surgery is by preparation with povidone iodide 5% that includes washing of the ocular periocular and surface. Prevention following penetrating ocular trauma injury is by intravenous broad-spectrum antibiotics (e.g. ciprofloxacin 400 mg bid) for 3 days. The data about treatment of endophthalmitis are based mainly on postoperative (cataract extraction) endophthalmitis. When endophthalmitis is suspected, vitreous samples for smears, cultures and sensitivity should be obtained before commencing antibiotic treatment. Treatment includes intravenous broad-spectrum antibiotics such as vancomycin 1 gr bid and ceftazidime 1 gr tid or moxifloxacin 400 mg/day IV as well as periocular injections and topical. Topical and/or systemic corticosteroids may be added only after the regression of the endophthalmitis.

6. Intraocular infections

Intraocular infections may involve different intraocular structures. Primarily they affect the uveal tissues (choroid, ciliary body and iris), the retina and secondarily the vitreous [12, 13]. Therefore, they may be manifesting as uveitis and/or choroidal and/or retinal lesions and the differential diagnosis is from inflammation (sterile) disorders.

Uveitis may be divided either by location to anterior; intermediate (pars planitis) and posterior, by clinical features: granulomatous versus non-granulomatous and etiology: bacterial, viral, fungal, protozoan and helmintic.

Patients may complain of ocular pain, decreased vision and/or ocular redness. The clinical signs vary. In uveitis, the anterior uvea is affected and white cells and flare are encountered in the anterior and posterior chamber and in the anterior third of the vitreous (behind the lens). Keratic precipitates (inflammatory cells and debris) over the endothelium and hypopyon may exist. The precipitates may be fine as in nongranulomatous uveitis or large and coarse (mutton fat) in granulomatous uveitis. In intermediate uveitis, the pars plana may be covered by inflammatory white band and vitreous veils resembling snowballs may be found. In posterior uveitis, white cells and flare involve the posterior 2/3 of the vitreous. They may be accompanied by retinal, choroidal or chorioretinal lesions. These lesions are key element in clinical diagnosis, which may be made by the involved tissues (retina, choroid or both), location (posterior pole, peripapillary or periphery), size, color and number of lesions (**Table 1**). For definitive diagnosis, laboratory tests are usually required.

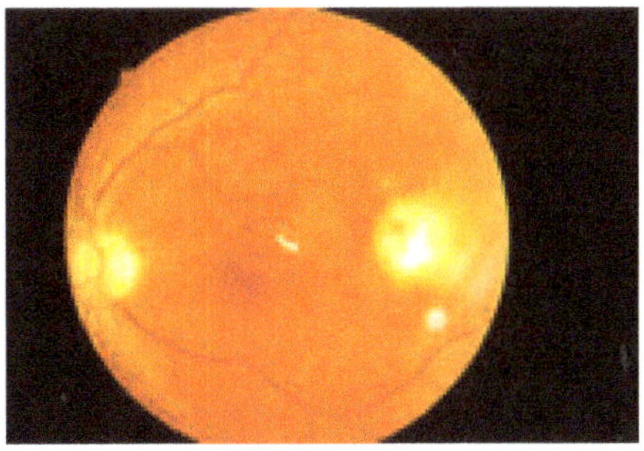

Figure 11. Toxocara retinochoroiditis. Note the active white lesion. It may appear adjacent to a chorioretinal scar.

Treatment should be first aimed at the offending microorganism. Topical and systemic antimicrobial are being used. Topical corticosteroids may be added in the absence of corneal ulcer. Systemic corticosteroids are being added if the offending microorganism is covered and the center of the macula is being threatened or involved by the infectious process.

Diagnosis	Tissue	No. of lesions	Color	Size	Location
Toxoplasmosis (**Figure 11**)	chorio-retina	1–3	White cream—new; usually near black—old scar, vitritis		Posterior pole, peripapillary
Toxocara (**Figure 12**)	Retina	One	White—elevated, TRD	1–2DD	Posterior pole
Tuberculosis	Choroid	1-multiple	Tuberculoma—white, round, elevated, indistinct margins, macular star	0.3–2DD	Posterior pole, midperiphery
Cytomegalovirus (CMV) (w or w/o HIV) (**Figure 13**)	Chorio-retina	Several	White areas with intraretinal hemorrhages, granular borders (Pizza pie)	Several DD	Everywhere
Acute retinal necrosis (herpetic) (**Figure 14**)	Retina	One	Confluent white-yellow, sharp irregular scalloped posterior margins, w or w/o intraretinal hemorrhages later replaced by atrophy and pigmentation	Several DD	Periphery
Syphilis	Sub-retina (chorio-retina)	Multiple, bilateral	Yellowish pale placoid lesions, optic nerve involvement	Variable	Anywhere, a mimicking disease
Cat scratch	Optic disc and retina		Optic disc edema with macular star	1–2 DD	Posterior pole
Candidiasis	Chorio-retina	Multiple	White faint with faint borders	0.5 DD	Posterior pole
Histoplasmosis	Choroid	Multiple	Small round lesions	0.2 DD	Anywhere

Table 1. TRD—traction retinal detachment; DD—disc diameter.

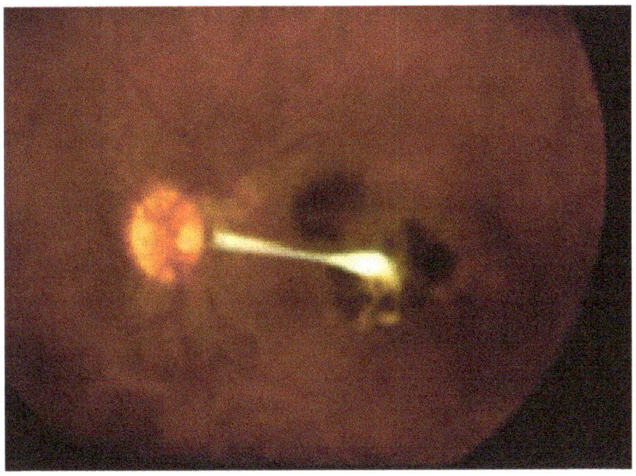

Figure 12. Toxocara chorioretinitis. Note the whitish lesion that may represent shrinked larva. Traction retinal detachment may occur.

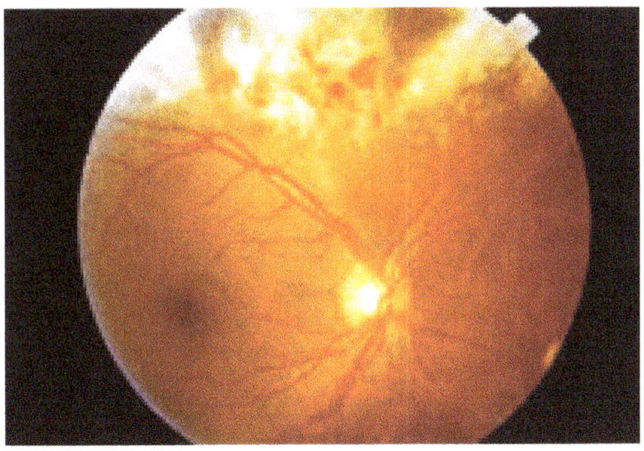

Figure 13. Cytomegalovirus (CMV) retinitis. Note the white lesions and intraretinal hemorrhages.

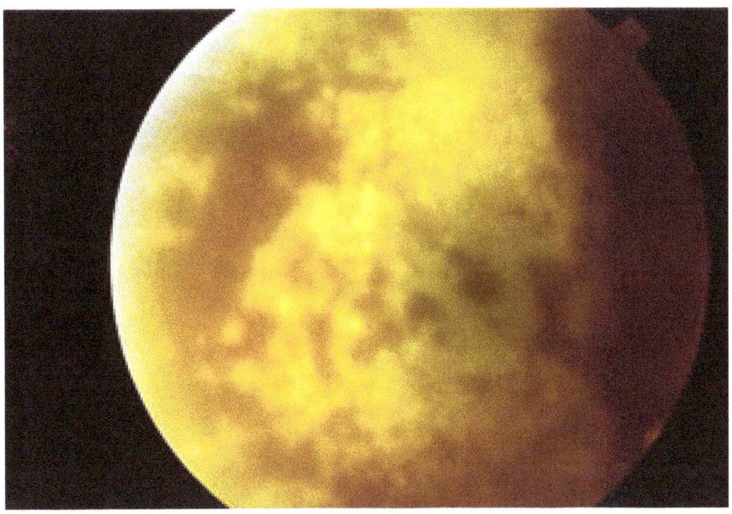

Figure 14. Acute retinal necrosis. Note the whitish lesion without retinal hemorrhages. The lesion is blurred by the inflammation in the vitreous.

7. Orbital infections

The hallmarks of orbital cellulitis include proptosis (exophthalmos) and limited ocular motility and/or involvement of the optic disc (decreased best-corrected visual acuity, positive afferent pupillary defect (Marcus Gunn) and/or swelling of the optic disc) [14, 15] (**Figure 15**). These findings differ from the signs of preseptal cellulitis in which swelling, erythema, heat and sensitivity of the eyelids occur. In both cases, the disease is usually unilateral. Orbital cellulitis in diabetic or immunocompromised patients should be considered as mucormycosis unless otherwise proven. Eschar of the oropharynx or the nose appears late and only in 10% of the patients with mucormycosis. Therefore, it should not be a sign to relay on. Bilateral orbital cellulitis may suggest of cavernous sinus thrombosis and diagnosis is made by computerized tomography. The clinical findings of cavernous sinus thrombosis are exophthalmos, unilateral or bilateral external and internal ophthalmoplegia that are usually accompanied by malaise and systemic fever (**Figure 16**). Nuchal rigidity as part of meningeal signs may also occur. Confirmation of the diagnosis is made by lumbar puncture. In orbital cellulitis and cavernous sinus thrombosis, blood cultures should be obtained when the body temperature increases to or over 39°C. In older patients, blood cultures are being obtained even if the temperature is normal. The source of the infection should be established by physical examination of the nose and mouth and imaging techniques (computed tomography and/or magnetic resonance imaging of the orbits and head. In contrast to preseptal cellulitis that is caused by infection from superficial skin wound, orbital cellulitis is most commonly caused by sinusitis (ethmoidal). Other sources may be upper jaw tooth abscess, otitis, mastoiditis, orbital osteomyelitis or extension from neglected preseptal cellulitis. Contamination may be by direct spreading through natural dehiscence sites and openings (foramina), veins, which are valveless or even nerves.

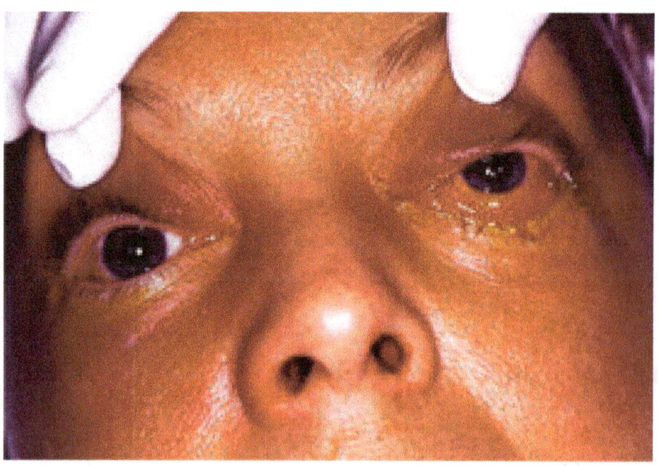

Figure 15. Cavernous sinus thrombosis in a diabetic patient. There was external ophthalmoplegia. The cause was mucormycosis.

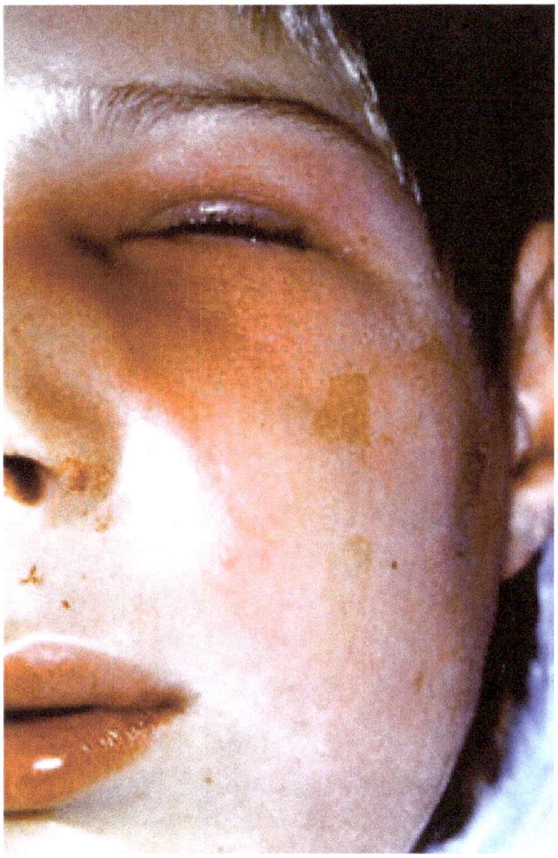

Figure 16. Orbital abscess as a result of tooth abscess. Note the erythema and swelling of both eyelids and chick.

Orbital abscess is a complication of orbital cellulitis (**Figure 16**) [16, 17]. It should be suspected when orbital cellulitis aggravates despite treatment. When aggravation occurs, repeated orbital computerized tomography assists in confirming the diagnosis of orbital abscess. In such a case, drainage of the abscess and continuing systemic antibiotics is required. The source of the infection should also be treated by surgical drainage. In cases of sinusitis, functional endoscopic sinus surgery (FESS) or other procedures with removal of the sinus mucosa may be required to prevent recurrences.

Note: The antibiotic dosage is for adults. The author is not responsible for the dosage or for any use of antibiotics.

Author details

Shimon Rumelt

Address all correspondence to: shimon.rumelt@naharia.health.gov.il

1 Western Galilee, Nahariya Medical Center, Nahariya, Israel

2 Faculty of Medicine, Bar Ilan University, Zefat, Israel

References

[1] Lederman C, Miller M. Hordeola and chalazia. Pediatr Rev 1999;20(8):283–284.

[2] Babar TF, Zaman M, Khan MN, Khan MD. Risk factors of preseptal and orbital cellulitis. J Coll Physicians Surg Pak 2009;19:39–42.

[3] Jackson WB. Blepharitis: current strategies for diagnosis and management. Can J Ophthalmol 2008;43:170–179.

[4] Hakkarainen TW, Kopari NM, Pham TN, Evans HL. Necrotizing soft tissue infections: review and current concepts in treatment, systems of care, and outcomes. Curr Probl Surg 2014;51:344–362.

[5] Raskin EM, Speaker MG, Laibson PR. Blepharitis. Infect Dis Clin North Am 1992;6:777–787.

[6] The Wills eye manual, 6th ed. 2012.

[7] Arfa RC, Grayson's diseases of the cornea, 3rd ed. St. Louis: Mosby. 1991.

[8] Guideline: American Academy of Ophthalmology cornea/external disease panel. Preferred Practice Pattern Guidelines. Conjunctivitis. San Francisco, CA. 2008.

[9] Panadero-Fontán R, Otranto D. Arthropods affecting the human eye. Vet Parasitol 2015; 208: 84–93.

[10] Park J, Lee KM, Zhou H, Rabin M, Jwo K, Burton WB, et al. Community practice patterns for bacterial corneal ulcer evaluation and treatment. Eye Contact Lens 2015;41:12–18.

[11] Rowsey JJ, Jensen H, Sexton DJ. Clinical diagnosis of endophthalmitis. Int Ophthalmol Clin 1987;27:82–88.

[12] Sudharshan S, Ganesh SK, Biswas J. Current approach in the diagnosis and management of posterior uveitis. Indian J Ophthalmol 2010;58:29–43.

[13] Khairallah M, Chee SP, Rathinam SR, Attia S, Nadella V. Novel infectious agents causing uveitis. Int Ophthalmol 2010;30:465–483.

[14] Bergin DJ, Wright JE. Orbital cellulitis. Br J Ophthalmol 1986;70:174–178.

[15] Rumelt S, Rubin PA. Potential sources of orbital cellulitis. Int Ophthalmol Clin 1996;36:207–221.

[16] Harris GJ. Subperiosteal abscess of the orbit. Arch Ophthalmol 1983;101:751–757.

[17] Liao JC, Harris GJ. Subperiosteal abscess of the orbit: evolving pathogens and the therapeutic protocol. Ophthalmology 2015;122:639–647.

8

Glaucoma Surgery and Aqueous Dynamics

Parul Ichhpujani

Abstract

Reduction in intraocular pressure is the only proven method to treat glaucoma. When medical treatment does not achieve adequate intraocular pressure reduction with acceptable adverse effects, laser or incisional surgeries are introduced. In this chapter, we discuss the physiological basis for the established surgical procedures as well as the newer surgical procedures. Most new surgical innovations have been designed according to natural physiology by routing aqueous as nature intended, through the Schlemm's canal. This has been possible because of better understanding of the outflow system and the availability of micro-technology to manipulate it.

Keywords: trabeculectomy, glaucoma drainage device, minimally invasive glaucoma surgery, outflow resistance

1. Introduction

Glaucoma is defined as a group of disorders that result in death of ganglion cells due to axonal damage at the level of the lamina cribrosa of the optic nerve.

Intraocular pressure (IOP) is considered to be the only alterable risk factor for diagnosis and treatment of glaucoma. IOP reduction is attained either by increasing outflow or by reducing aqueous humor production [1]. Therefore, basic understanding of aqueous humor circulation is important for successful management of glaucoma. Aqueous humor pathways have been discussed in detail in a prior chapter in the book. This chapter focuses on the various surgical modalities available to reduce or bypass the outflow resistance.

2. Site of outflow resistance

Evidence suggests that the majority of outflow resistance in the trabecular meshwork is generated in the inner wall endothelium of Schlemm's canal and its underlying matrix in the juxtacanalicular trabecular meshwork [2]. Rosenquist et al. has shown that following trabeculotomy, close to half (49%) of outflow resistance is eliminated at a perfusion pressure of 7 mm Hg [3]. In another study, Grant has shown that nearly two-third (71%) resistance is eliminated at a perfusion pressure of 25 mm Hg [4]. Schuman et al. have shown that 35% of resistance is eliminated at a perfusion pressure at 10 mm Hg, when 1 O'clock hour of the tissue from the outer wall of Schlemm's canal was ablated using the excimer laser [5]. These studies suggest that one-third to half of the outflow resistance lies distal to the inner wall of Schlemm's canal at normal pressure and partly outflow resistance is related to pressure-dependent changes in the outflow pathway. As the intraocular pressure increases, Schlemm's canal collapses and reduces outflow and effective filtration.

3. Restoration of the outflow facility

Excision of sites causing increased outflow resistance would result in restoration of outflow. It is not possible for a surgeon to precisely pinpoint the area which needs to be excised for an individual patient, therefore, logically, surgeons would like to address all aspects of the outflow system.

The current gold standard, trabeculectomy, has done well for many medically refractory glaucoma patients. Despite its efficacy in lowering IOP, ease of the surgical procedure, it is fraught with potential sight threatening issues. Glaucomatologists and bioengineers are leaving no stone unturned to find a better alternative to address the flaws of trabeculectomy.

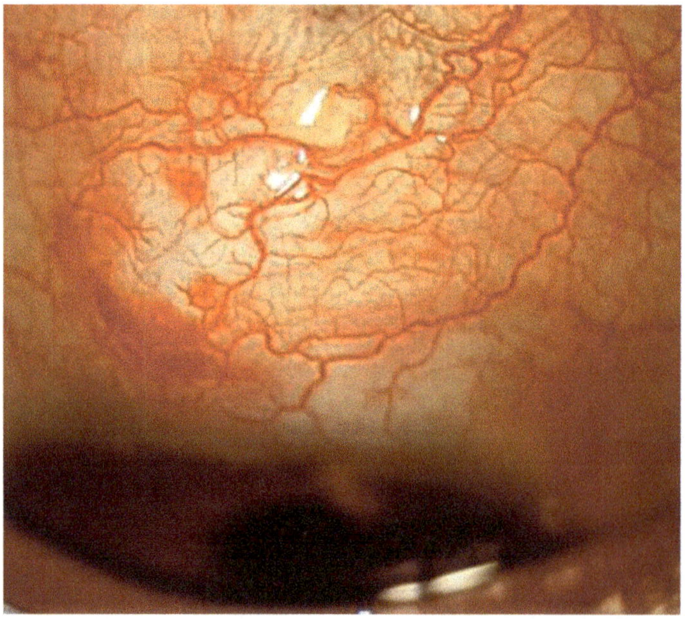

Figure 1. Failing trabeculectomy bleb with corkscrewing of conjunctival vessels secondary to scarring.

3.1. Surgeries addressing trabecular meshwork

- *Trabeculectomy:* Opening a pathway through the meshwork, either by removing tissue or punching a hole (trabeculectomy) encourages aqueous outflow into Schlemm's canal.

  Despite modulation of the subconjunctival space into a porous matrix, the procedure is **not** a physiological bypass and remains dependent on the size of the ostium, tension in the sclera flap, as well as wound healing and its modulation [6].

  A decrease in the hydraulic conductivity of the bleb capsule results in an increase in fluid pressure within the bleb, altering its mechanical and biochemical environment resulting in progressive scarring (**Figure 1**) and consequent bleb failure [7].

  In addition, these incisional surgeries can result in decreased quality of life due to bleb-related foreign body sensation, induced astigmatism, and secondary cataracts.

- *Trabeculectomy with collagen implants:* The development of tissue engineering has offered a plausible solution to reduce postoperative fibrosis and scarring. The use of collagen-glycosaminoglycan copolymers leads to random and relatively loose reorganization of regenerating myofibroblasts, fibroblasts, and the secreted extracellular collagen matrix, resulting in reduced scar formation [8]. These implants offer a potential alternative to antifibrosis agents as they produce more loosely organized, yet more abundant bleb tissue than a bleb created without antimetabolites.

  Ologen (Aeon Astron Corporation, Taipei, Taiwan) (also named iGen) is the commonly available collagen implant, which consists of >90% lyophilized porcine atelocollagen and <10% lyophilized porcine glycosaminoglycan. This implant also acts as a spacer to mechanically separate the subconjunctival and episcleral tissues to prevent fibrosis. The implant is placed subconjunctivally over the scleral flap posteriorly and only a small portion covers the scleral flap (**Figure 2**), else the implant would act as a mechanical tamponade and prevent outflow from the subscleral space [9].

- *iStent:* Trabecular bypass devices such as iStent reduce IOP by bypassing the thin layer of juxtacanalicular tissue, without the need for creating a hole in the sclera and a filtration bleb. iStent bypasses the meshwork, creating a direct route from the anterior chamber into Schlemm's canal (**Figure 3**).

  There is also a second-generation model called the iStent inject (Glaukos Corporation), which has been CE marked for use in Europe. It contains a head facing the anterior chamber that is 230 μm in width with four inlets for the passage of aqueous into the device and out through Schlemm's canal.

  Zhou and Smedley have shown in their cultured autopsy eye perfusion experiments that adding successive bypass shunts produces a step-wise increase in outflow. The first shunt has the maximum IOP reducing effect, reducing IOP from 21.4 ± 3.8 to 12.4 ± 4.2 mm Hg, successive addition of up to four stents placed into SC produced step-wise reduction in system pressure [10].

Hunter et al. showed in anterior segment perfusion models with the iStent inject that outflow facility increases from 0.16 ± 0.05 μL/min/mm Hg to 0.38 ± 0.23 ($P < 0.03$, $n = 7$), and then an additional iStent inject further increased outflow facility to 0.78 ± 0.66 ($n = 2$) [11].

- *Ex-PRESS:* The Ex-PRESS device relies on nonphysiologic subconjunctival flow as its mechanism of IOP lowering. In eyes with prior failed trabeculectomies, Ex-PRESS can help to reestablish the aqueous flow without having to repeat the original procedure [12]. The Ex-PRESS fits easily in the middle ground between a repeat trabeculectomy and a larger glaucoma drainage device like a Baerveldt, Molteno, or an Ahmed tube shunt.
- *Viscocanalostomy:* In viscocanalostomy, inner wall of the endothelium is disrupted and communication is established between the lumen of the canal and the juxtacanalicular space. Bed of canal is scraped with a forceps or trabecular aspiration. This leads to the removal of a homogenous external trabecular membrane in one coherent plane that allows aqueous humor to egress through the remaining inner trabecular layers [13].

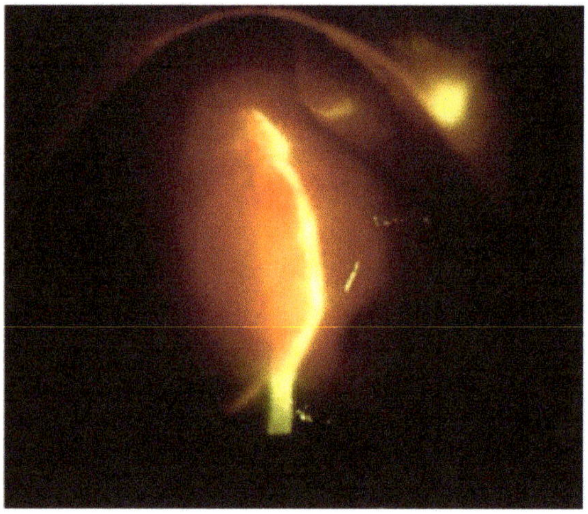

Figure 2. Ologen implant in subconjunctival space.

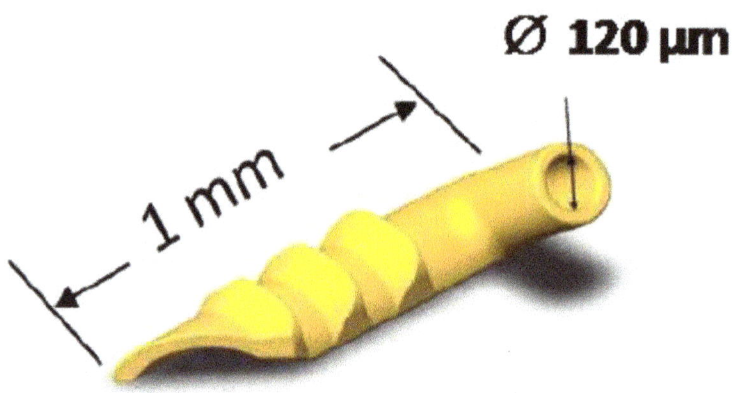

Figure 3. First-generation iStent.

3.2. Surgeries addressing Schlemm's canal

The detailed mechanism of aqueous humor dynamics across the endothelial lining of Schlemm's canal from the Juxtacanalicular trabecular meshwork (JCT) via giant vacuoles and pores has been discussed in detail in a prior chapter. The number of giant pores and vacuoles is less in glaucomatous eyes as compared to normal eyes, thus accounting for the increase in outflow resistance [14].

- *Viscocanalostomy:* Dilating Schlemm's canal with viscoelastic material may remove the stenosis-related resistance, as discussed earlier.
- *Canaloplasty:* Canaloplasty is an ab externo procedure that entails 360° intubation of Schlemm's canal (**Figure 4**), along with suture-assisted distension of the canal in order to restore physiologic outflow via the conventional pathway without the formation of a fistula or bleb. Potentially, the suture tension may increase TM permeability, similar to the action of pilocarpine [15] as well as help to maintain a patent canal lumen, similar to the intraocular tensioning suture [16].

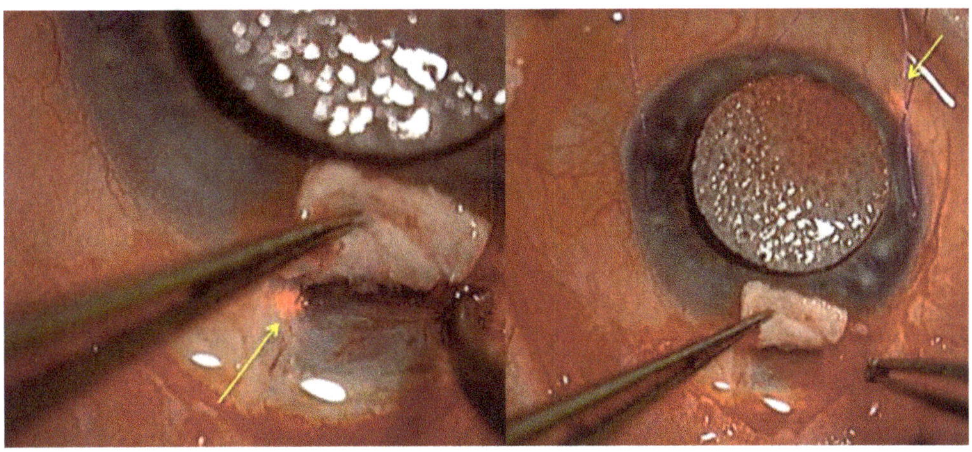

Figure 4. Nonpenetrating Schlemm's canaloplasty using the iScience cannula.

3.3. Surgeries addressing collector channels

The collector channels connecting the aqueous veins and the distal part of the outflow pathways originate in the outer wall of Schlemm's canal. These collector channels are not evenly distributed around Schlemm's canal circumferentially. The outflow is closer to areas with larger collector channels.

- *Minimally invasive glaucoma surgery (MIGS):* The advent of microinvasive glaucoma surgery has brought new dimension to glaucoma treatment. Minimally invasive glaucoma surgery is likely to provide medication-sparing, conjunctival-sparing, ab interno, more physiological approach to IOP reduction for patients with mild-to-moderate glaucoma that is safer than traditional incisional glaucoma surgery.

MIGS stents, e.g., iStent, Hydrus, give better results when positioned close to a patent collector channel, thus increasing the possibility of surgical success.

- *Canaloplasty:* Schuman et al. have shown that when the IOP is elevated, trabecular meshwork herniates into the ostia of collector channels and reduces the passage for aqueous outflow. Cannulating the whole of Schlemm's canal, as in canaloplasty, and injecting viscoelastic material may "pop" open these herniations and enable 360° access to collector channel ostia for the egressing aqueous [17].

3.4. Surgeries addressing episcleral venous system

Theoretically, IOP should directly correlate with the episcleral venous pressure (EVP). However, when the entire TM is removed, 25% of total resistance still remains, underscoring the importance of EVP measurement in an accurate and reproducible way [18]. Episcleral venous pressure is highly variable and may range from 3 to 14 mm Hg. In addition, if the pressure gradient differential is low and resistance is also located distally in the episcleral venous system, restorative outflow surgery has less chance of being effective than if the pressure gradient differential is high.

In cases with elevated episcleral venous pressure, incisional filtration surgery can help lower the IOP, but it is associated with a high incidence of choroidal effusion or hemorrhage.

Preoperative IOP reduction may be attained by intravenous mannitol and other systemic antiglaucoma medications. Additionally, the flow through the scleral flap may be adjusted to allow for a higher IOP in the early postoperative period. Using a releasable suture allows controlled reduction of IOP. Drainage implants may also be a good choice if the flow through the implant is kept to a minimum in the early postoperative period.

Another way of classifying various surgical procedures depends on how the procedure influences the aqueous dynamics.

3.4.1. Surgeries that bypass conventional aqueous outflow pathway

- Trabeculectomy
- Nonpenetrating deep sclerectomy
- Glaucoma drainage devices:

  Most conventional shunts consist of a tube designed to shunt aqueous from the anterior chamber to a distal plate via a tube to the posterior subconjunctival space, from where aqueous is directly absorbed into the sclera and episcleral vasculature to enter the orbital circulation, bypassing both the conventional and uveoscleral pathways. The primary tube-plate junction includes a rim through which the tube empties onto the explant plate surface to avoid closure of the tube orifice following eventual encapsulation of the device by fibrosis [19].

- Viscocanalostomy, canaloplasty

- Trabeculotomy
- Goniotomy
- Ab interno trabeculotomy or Trabectome surgery:

  Selective removal of the TM and inner wall of SC is performed using the Trabectome; while leaving the rest of the outflow system (outer wall of SC, collector channels, and aqueous veins) relatively intact. A strip of TM and inner wall of SC spanning 80–100° is ablated and removed under direct gonioscopic visualization. The simultaneous aspiration of tissue debris reduces the inflammatory stimuli and opportunity for scarring among shards of incised or ruptured tissues remaining after traditional goniotomy or trabeculotomy [20].

3.4.2. Surgeries that increase the uveoscleral outflow

- ExPRESS shunt
- iStent
- Suprachoroidal gold SOLX shunt:

  This shunt is an ab externo suprachoroidal trans-limbal shunt and works as a "controlled" cyclodialysis, draining aqueous into the suprachoroidal space. The anterior end of this 24-karat gold device is placed into the anterior chamber over the sclera spur via a scleral incision and the posterior end positioned in the suprachoroidal space (**Figure 5**). It includes several channels through its body. Aqueous flows both through the channels in the body of the shunt and around its body [21].

- Cypass:

  This mini shunt is placed in the supraciliary and suprachoroidal space to increase uveoscleral outflow by creating a small cyclodialysis (**Figure 6**) [22].

  Along the length of the stent are microholes that allow for circumferential egress of aqueous into the suprachoroidal space and the distal end of the stent allows longitudinal egress of fluid.

- Hydrus:

  Hydrus is implanted using s a preloaded injector via a clear corneal incision and is inserted into and sits within Schlemm's canal, wherein it extends 3 clock hours. It does not block the collector channel ostia in the posterior portion of Schlemm's canal as it has a scaffold design, and it has a 1 mm inlet portion, which resides within the anterior chamber. As a standalone procedure, it can be inserted through a 1–1.5 mm corneal incision. Once inserted into Schlemm's canal, it can dilate it by four to five times the natural width of the canal [23].

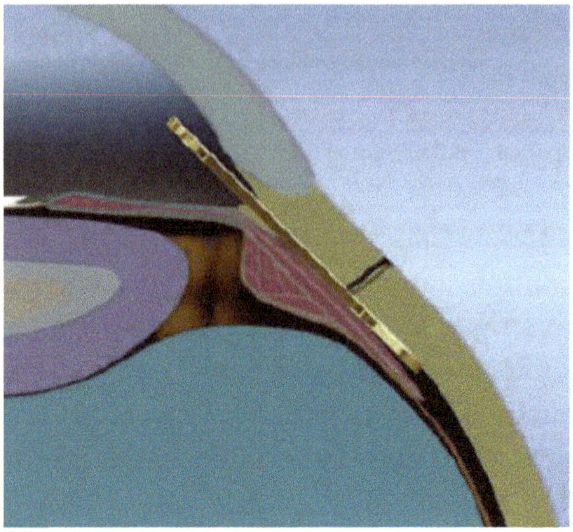

Figure 5. Gold SOLX shunt in suprachoroidal space.

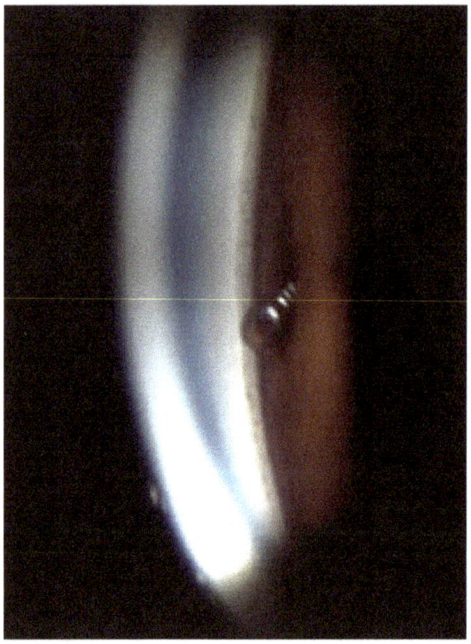

Figure 6. CyPass shunt *in situ*.

3.4.3. Surgeries that decrease aqueous production

Cycloablative procedures reduce IOP by destroying the ciliary body epithelium that produces aqueous humor. Modalities include:

- Contact (transscleral) cycloablation
    - Cyclocryotherapy [24]

- Diode/Nd:YAG [25]

- Noncontact cycloablation
  - Nd:YAG/Diode

- Transpupillary argon green cyclophotocoagulation

- Endoscopic ablation

  In endoscopic cyclophotocoagulation (ECP), the laser is applied under direct endoscopic view causing localized shrinkage of the ciliary processes due to thermal coagulation (**Figure 7**). This causes an initial reduction in blood supply to the ciliary processes, and a consequent reduction in aqueous production. Partial reperfusion of the ciliary body over 4–6 weeks means that the rates of hypotony and phthisis are lower than those associated with other methods of cyclodestruction.

  Earlier cycloablative procedures were reserved only for refractory cases, but recent studies have shown that endocyclophotocoagulation can be used for the treatment of mild-to-moderate glaucoma. It is conjunctival-sparing, blebless, and can be combined with cataract surgery [26, 27].

Despite all the aforementioned advances, the quest for a perfectly predictable and physiological glaucoma procedure with rapid recovery and a greater margin of safety is ongoing.

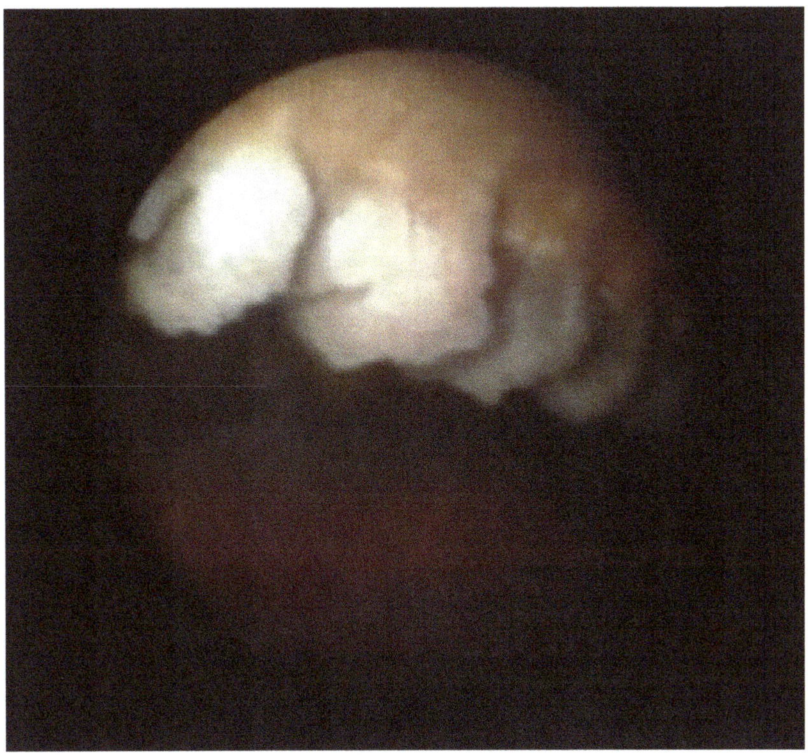

Figure 7. Shrinkage of ciliary processes following ECP.

Author details

Parul Ichhpujani

*Address all correspondence to: itsdrparul@gmail.com

Department of Ophthalmology, Glaucoma Services, Government Medical College and Hospital, Chandigarh, India

References

[1] Ritch R, Shields M, Krupin T. *The Glaucomas: Clinical Science*. 2nd ed. St. Louis: Mosby; 1996.

[2] Goel M, Picciani RG, Lee RK, Bhattachary SK. Aqueous humor dynamics: a review. Open Ophthalmol J. 2010; 4:52–59.

[3] Rosenquist R, Epstein D, Melamed S, et al. Outflow resistance of enucleated human eyes at two different perfusion pressures and different extents of trabeculotomy. Curr Eye Res. 1989; 8:1233–1240.

[4] Grant WM. Experimental aqueous perfusion in enucleated human eyes. Arch Ophthalmol. 1963; 69:783–801.

[5] Schuman JS, Chang W, Wang N, de Kater AW, Allingham RR. Excimer laser effects on outflow facility and outflow pathway morphology. Invest Ophthalmol Vis Sci. 1999; 40(8):1676–1680.

[6] Jea SY, Francis BA, Vakili G, Filippopoulos T, Rhee DJ. Ab interno trabeculectomy versus trabeculectomy for open-angle glaucoma. Ophthalmology. 2012; 119(1):36–42.

[7] Rossier A, Uffer S, Mermoud A. Aqueous dynamics in experimental ab externo trabeculectomy. Ophthalmic Res. 2000; 32:165–171.

[8] Hsu WC, Spilker MH, Yannas IV, Rubin PA. Inhibition of conjunctival scarring and contraction by a porous collagen-glycosaminoglycan implant. Invest Ophthalmol Vis Sci. 2000; 41:2404–2411.

[9] Cillino S, Casuccio A, Di Pace F, Cagini C, Ferraro LL, Cillino G. Biodegradable collagen matrix implant versus mitomycin-C in trabeculectomy: five-year follow-up. *BMC Ophthalmology*. 2016;16:24. doi:10.1186/s12886-016-0198-0.

[10] Zhou J, Smedley G. A trabecular bypass flow hypothesis. J Glaucoma. 2005; 14:74–83.

[11] Hunter KS, Fjield T, Heitzmann H, Shandas R, Kahook MY. Characterization of micro-invasive trabecular bypass stents by ex vivo perfusion and computational flow modeling. Clin Ophthalmol. 2014; 8:499–506.

[12] Buys YM. Trabeculectomy with Ex-PRESS: weighing the benefits and cost. Curr Opin Ophthalmol. 2013; 24(2):111–118.

[13] Smit BA, Johnstone MA. Effects of viscoelastic injection into Schlemm's canal in primate and human eyes: potential relevance to viscocanalostomy. Ophthalmology, 2002; 109(4): 786–792.

[14] Maepea O, Bill A. Pressures in the juxtacanalicular tissue and Schlemm's canal in monkeys. Exp Eye Res 1992; 54:879–883.

[15] Flocks M. The anatomy of the trabecular meshwork as seen in tangential section. AMA Arch Ophthalmol 1956; 56(5):708–718.

[16] Ashton N, Brini A, Smith R. Anatomical studies of the trabecular meshwork of the normal human eye. Br J Ophthalmol 1956; 40(5):257–282.

[17] Lewis RA, von Wolff K, Tetz M, et al. Canaloplasty: circumferential viscodilation and tensioning of Schlemm's canal using a flexible microcatheter for the treatment of open-angle glaucoma in adults: interim clinical study analysis. J Cataract Refract Surg. 2007; 33:1217–1226.

[18] Linner E, Rickenbach C, Werner H. Comparative measurements of the pressure in the aqueous veins and the conjunctival veins using different methods. Acta Ophthalmol (Copenh). 1950; 28:469–478.

[19] Minckler DS, Francis BA, Hodapp EA, Jampel HD, Lin SC, Samples JR, Smith SD, Singh K. Aqueous shunts in glaucoma. A report by the American Academy of Ophthalmology. Ophthalmology 2008; 115:1089–1098.

[20] Minckler DS, Mosaed S, Dustin L, Francis BA. Trabectome (trabeculectomy-internal approach): additional experience and extended follow-up. Trans Am Ophthalmol Soc. 2008; 106:1–12.

[21] Mastropasqua L, Agnifili L, Ciancaglini M, et al. In vivo analysis of conjunctiva in gold micro shunt implantation for glaucoma. Br J Ophthalmol. 2010; 94(12):1592–1596.

[22] Helmut H, Ahmed IK, Grisanti S, et al. Early postoperative safety and surgical outcomes after implantation of a suprachoroidal micro-stent for the treatment of open-angle glaucoma concomitant with cataract surgery. J Cataract Refract Surg. 2013; 39(3): 431–437.

[23] Grover DS, Godfrey DG, Smith O, Feuer WJ, Montes de Oca I, Fellman RL. Gonioscopy-assisted transluminal trabeculotomy, ab interno trabeculotomy: technique report and preliminary results. Ophthalmology. 2014; 121:855–861.

[24] Bellows AR, Grant WM. Cyclocryotherapy in advanced inadequately controlled glaucoma. Am J Ophthalmol. 1973; 75:679–684.

[25] Egbert PR, Fiadoyor S, Budenz DL, et al. Diode laser transscleral cyclophotocoagulation as a primary surgical treatment for primary open-angle glaucoma. Arch Ophthalmol. 2001; 119:345–350.

[26] Siegel MJ, Boling WS, Faridi OS, et al. Combined endoscopic cyclophotocoagulation and phacoemulsification versus phacoemulsification alone in the treatment of mild to moderate glaucoma. Clin Experiment Ophthalmol. 2015; 43:531–539.

[27] Francis BA, Berke SJ, Dustin L, Noecker R. Endoscopic cyclophotocoagulation combined with phacoemulsification versus phacoemulsification alone in medically controlled glaucoma. J Cataract Refract Surg. 2014; 40:1313–1321.

9

Ocular Parasitic Infections

Nancy Malla and Kapil Goyal

Abstract

Eyes are said to be the windows of body, by which this beautiful world is visualized. Human eye has a unique structure and is vulnerable to numerous infections. Whenever anatomical structures are breached, host defenses come into play, but if infection is severe and not treated timely, it could lead to visual impairment or blindness. Parasitic infections are considered, the significant causes of ophthalmic diseases worldwide. In this chapter, an overview of ocular parasitic infections (OPI) is detailed out, with an initial brief introduction followed by description of anatomy of the human eye and various defense mechanisms to provide better understanding of the parasitic infections affecting different parts of human eye. The last part includes individual details of various human ocular parasitic infections.

Ocular infections can be classified based on either the etiological agent or according to the anatomical site of infection. The parasitic etiological agents include mainly protozoa, helminths and ectoparasites. Due to the complex life cycles of parasites and their tendency to cause wide range of pathologic lesions, different parasites/parasitic infections have been addressed separately, including brief epidemiology, clinical features, diagnosis and treatment.

Keywords: Eye, parasitic infections, protozoa, nematodes, cestodes, trematodes, ectoparasites

1. Introduction

The ocular parasitic infections (OPI) are considered significant causes of ocular pathologies worldwide [1]. The common protozoal parasites primarily infecting the ocular tissue(s) are *Acanthamoeba* species and *Toxoplasma gondii* [2–7]. In addition, case studies of eye diseases caused by *Leishmania, Trypanosoma cruzi, Entamoeba histolytica, Hartmannella, Plasmodium falciparum, Microsporidia* and *Giardia lamblia* have been rarely reported [1, 8, 9]. Among the helminths, ocular infections are caused primarily by nematode parasites (*Onchocerca volvulus,*

Loa loa, Toxocara canis and Toxocara cati) [1, 8, 10–12]. In addition, case studies of ocular infections caused by other nematodes (*Angiostrongylus cantonensis, Dirofilaria repens, Trichinella spiralis, Thelazia callipaeda, Baylisascaris procyonis, Wuchereria bancrofti* and *B. malayi*), cestodes (*T.solium cysticercus, Echinococcus granulosus,* and *Multiceps multiceps* larvae) and trematodes (*Fasciola hepatica and Schistosoma* species) have been reported from different geographical areas [1, 8, 13–15]. The ectoparasites infecting the eye include larvae of flies [16] (*Oestrus ovis, Rhinoestrus purpureus, Dermatobia hominis, Chrysomia bezziana, Lucilia* spp., *Cuterebra, Hypoderma, Cochliomyia, Wohlfahrtia, Gastrophilus*), *Phthirus pubis,* hard and soft ticks (belonging to class Arachnida) [1, 17]. Ocular pentastomiasis caused by the larval stage of Pentastomida, the crustacean-related parasites, is reported to cause permanent loss of vision due to the retinal detachment or lens subluxation [18]. Further, with the advent of HIV/AIDS (human immunodeficiency virus/acquired immune deficiency syndrome), few ocular infections have also been reported in HIV-infected patients [19, 20].

Ocular parasitic infections have been widely reported from different geographical areas (Table 1), mainly depending on the endemicity of the parasite(s). The prevalence depends primarily on the geographical distribution of the parasite, socioeconomic environment and immune status of the patient. The common modes of infection are direct contact (blepharoconjunctivitis caused by *Leishmania, Acanthamoeba* keratitis, microsporidial infections, infestation caused by lice and mites) [21–23], through blood stream (Toxoplasma chorioretinitis, retinal involvement in malaria, uveitis caused by *Toxocara)* [1, 23, 24], congenital transmission (Toxoplasmosis) and zoonotic transmission (primarily infectious diseases of animals that can naturally be transmitted to humans) [25]. In addition, few of the helminths that may lead to ocular infection are transmitted by vectors (onchocerciasis, dirofilariasis and thelaziasis), consumption of contaminated food (sparganosis, trichinellosis) and indirectly from the environment (fascioliasis, ascariasis and echinococcosis).

Adult and/or larval stages of the parasites may reside in human ocular tissues externally or in the ocular globe. The clinical symptoms and signs vary, depending on the etiological agent and the ocular tissue/part involved. However, local defense mechanisms and host immune responses play role in establishing the infection. The pathology in the eye can occur due to direct damage by the infecting pathogen, indirectly by toxic products, immune mediated or ectopic localization by ectoparasites. The clinical diagnosis usually mimics other pathologies due to numerous etiologies both infectious and non-infectious, which can cause conjunctivitis, keratitis, uveitis and endopthalmitis [26]. Thus, a high index of clinician suspicion is required for infective parasite etiology in patients having inflammation in the eye. In addition, eye can be involved in various systemic disorders and thorough ocular examination along with history of travel to the endemic area, risk factors and other associated medical illness that help in establishing the preliminary diagnosis. However, confirmatory diagnosis is usually achieved by direct demonstration of parasite in clinical samples and/or pathological changes observed by either slit lamp or biopsy examination [1, 8, 27, 28]. The antigen and antibody detection in ocular fluids and/or serum usually substantiates the clinical diagnosis in few parasitic infections (Toxoplasmosis, malaria, leishmaniasis, ocular gnathostomiasis, cysticercosis, toxocariasis, echinococcosis) [1, 10, 29, 30]. Molecular techniques including detection of parasite DNA by polymerase chain reaction (PCR) have added new dimensions in the diagnosis and species identification [31–36]. The treatment of choice is mostly surgical excision, while in few infections, medical treatment is usually advised either in conjunction with surgical procedure (onchocerciasis, dirofilariasis [37], cysticercosis [38], echinococcosis [39], myiasis, infections due to ticks and mites) or for inoperable patients. Although surgical excision is usually reserved for worms that are large, it is also recommended for space-occupying lesions of the orbit. Drug resistance is posing problem for the effective medical treatment, thus necessitating the discovery of new antiparasitic drugs [32]. Prevention and control measures differ in various infections and usually include proper health education and awareness of various risk factors. The various experimental animal models for few of the ocular infections have been successfully established to study the pathogenic mechanisms, drug efficacy and local immune responses [40, 41].

Although issues mainly are the timely diagnosis and treatment, yet many challenges need to be considered/addressed.

2. Anatomy

Diagrammatic representation of human eye depicting significant ocular parasitic infections is shown in Figure 1.

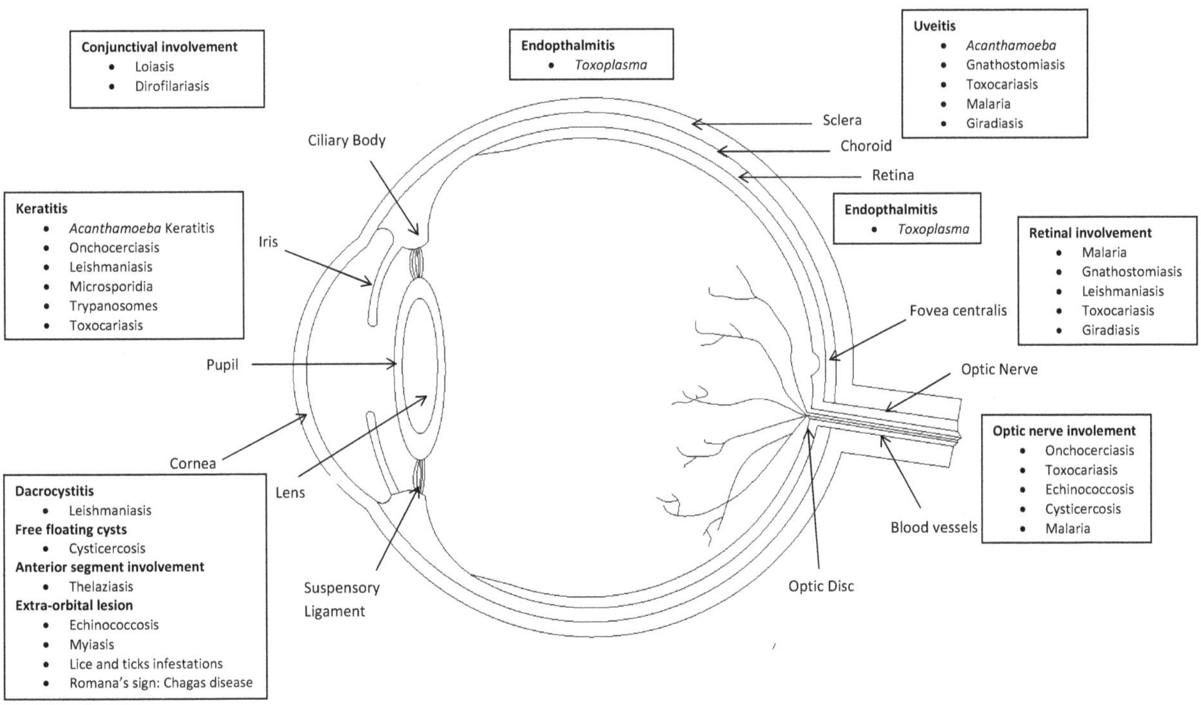

Figure 1. Human eye anatomy depicting significant ocular parasitic infections.

2.1. Orbits

The eye balls along with extraocular muscles, nerves, blood vessels and fat are situated in the bony cavities known as orbits. The periosteal covering of the bony orbit fuses with orbital septum and duramater. Abscess due to infectious agent can localize in the space beneath the periostium. The paranasal sinuses are separated from it by the floor, medial wall and roof of the orbit and may act as the source of orbital infection. Lamina papyracea are the thinnest bony walls, which separate orbit from ethmoidal sinuses. Thus, any breach in it causes the ingress of sinus microbiota to orbital tissue leading to infection. Orbital cellulitis can also be caused by direct extension of the infection from the ethmoidal sinuses to the orbital cavity. The lateral wall of the sphenoidal sinus constitutes the medial wall of the optic canal and infection of the former can percolate to the latter causing optic nerve damage and visual loss. There are various apertures present in the orbital cavity, which provides the route of communication with the adjacent structures. The superior and inferior orbital fissures, the lacrimal fossa, nasolacrimal duct and the optic canal constitute such important apertures [1, 42–46].

2.2. Blood supply

The ophthalmic artery and its branches constitute main arterial supply of orbit. The majority of the venous drainage occurs through superior ophthalmic vein, which drains into cavernous sinus that is located just posterior to the orbital apex. Veins from the facial region and many anterior ophthalmic veins anastomose and drain into cavernous sinus through superior orbital vein. Thus, cavernous sinus is prone to infection from facial region and also from the orbital region through the superior ophthalmic vein leading to a serious complication.

2.3. Eyelids

The eyelids impart two protective anatomical barriers, i.e., orbital septum and conjunctiva. Former divides the orbit from the eyelid into preseptal and postseptal spaces and provides a physical barrier to infectious agents and latter one is reflected back on itself, which provides protection by hindering the free movement of the material posteriorly from the anterior surface of the globe.

2.4. Lacrimal system

Lacrimal system consists of lacrimal gland, accessory gland and excretory system. Tears are secreted by lacrimal gland, which flows over the cornea and finally drain into nasal cavity by nasolacrimal duct through lacrimal sac. Any obstruction to the nasolacrimal duct can lead to regurgitation of the accumulated fluid onto the ocular surface leading to increased chances of infection.

2.5. Layers of eye ball

The basic structure of eye ball or globe consists of three concentric layers. The outermost covering is composed of sclera and cornea. The middle covering is composed of uveal tract, consisting of choroid, ciliary body and iris. The inner most covering is retina. The sclera is almost avascular except for the presence of superficial small blood vessels. The choroid is a highly vascular structure and provides nutrition and oxygenation to the retina beneath it. Due to these qualities, choroid serves as a fertile area for the proliferation of various pathogens, which spread by hematogenous route.

2.6. Anterior and posterior chambers

Anterior segment of the eye in front of the vitreous humor comprises anterior one-third of the eye and is further divided into anterior chamber and posterior chamber. Anterior chamber is the space between posterior surface of cornea and the iris, whereas posterior chamber is the space between iris and the front of vitreous. The aqueous humor is produced by non-pigmented ciliary epithelium in the posterior chamber and drains through the pupillary aperture into the anterior chamber. Cornea is composed of well-organized collagen fibrils, which is avascular in nature. Lens is also an avascular crystalline structure, which continues to grow throughout life. Thus, aqueous humor fills these spaces and provides nutrition to the surrounding structures.

2.7. Vitreous humor

It is a gel-like substance present in front of retina and posterior to the lens in the posterior segment of the eye. It is optically clear and is composed of collagen framework interspersed with hyaluronic acid. During intraocular inflammation, it becomes hazy and may cause impairment of vision.

2.8. Retina and optic nerve

Retina constitutes the innermost covering of the eye ball and captures the light energy with the help of rods and cones. The outer half of the retina is supplied by central retinal artery, whereas inner half receives its blood supply from the choroid.

The optic nerve is formed by axons of the inner cell layer that exits the globe. It is covered by all the three meningeal coverings, which are direct extensions of the brain coverings. Thus, it is vulnerable to infections originating from both within cranial vault and within orbits.

3. Ocular defense mechanisms

The surface of the eye is well protected by both mechanical and immunological defense mechanisms. To breach the defense mechanism, some form of trauma is essential. The eyelids provide mechanical protection to the surface of eyeball. The eyelashes protect against airborne particles and trauma by initiating blink reflex. The cornea is also sensitive to tactile sensation and helps in the initiation of blink reflex, which is provided by dense sensory nerve endings. The lids direct the tears, particulate debris, allergens and microbes to the lacrimal excretory system by its sweeping action over the anterior surface of the eyeball. Bell's phenomenon also provides protection to cornea as globe is turned upwards and slightly outwards during eyelid closure to avoid corneal exposure [47]. Meibomian glands secrete lipids, which provide stability to the tear film. The epithelial surface of the cornea and conjunctiva provides anatomical barrier to the pathogens. This function is further strengthened by the impermeability provided by the basement and cellular junctional complexes of the cornea. Indigenous flora of the eye also provides protection by creating a competition for colonization by the pathogens.

Immune defense mechanisms are provided by the vascular supply of the eye. Any breach in the anatomical defense system initiates the ocular inflammatory response, which helps in vasodilation and exudation of immunologically active substances and cells [1, 8, 48–52].

3.1. Defenses of the tear film

There are three layers of the tear film: oil, aqueous and mucous. Majority of the tear film is composed of aqueous layer and pH of the tear film helps in neutralization of toxic substances. Flow of tears help in mechanical flushing of the foreign particles and allergens into the lacrimal excretory system. Mucosal layer helps in entrapment of pathogens. Tear film contains various immunological active substances such as lactoferrin, lysozyme, β-lysin, ceruloplasmin, complement and immunoglobulins.

3.2. Conjunctival defenses

The conjunctival associated lymphoid tissue lies beneath the conjunctiva. It consists of both B and T lymphocytes. B and T cell precursors mature when exposed to foreign particles or allergens, then migrate to regional lymph nodes for further development, and thereafter return to the conjunctiva through blood stream to produce specific immunoglobulins and cellular defense responses.

3.3. Corneal defenses

Although the cornea is avascular, it is provided by limited defense mechanisms in the form of Langerhans cells (dendritic cells) and immunoglobulins. The surface of the cornea is covered by mucous glycoprotein, which helps in cross-linkage of the IgA and protects the anterior surface of the cornea. Immune defense mechanisms are activated whenever injury occurs, leading to recruitment of the polymorphonuclear cells, lymphocytes and fibroblasts.

3.4. Cellular immune responses

Langerhans cells are situated along the peripheral margin of the cornea and conjunctiva. These cells possess receptors, which help in phagocytosis and processing of certain antigens for presentation. Langerhans cells stimulate B and T cells to elicit a strong cellular immune response. During inflammation Langerhans cells migrate toward the cornea, causing increased release of inflammatory substances.

3.5. Leukocyte defense

Polymorphonuclear leukocytes are the hallmark of acute inflammation and are associated with oxygen-dependent pathways for the generation of free radicals that help in killing of the invading pathogens. Another immune defense mechanism operated by the production of defensins is antimicrobial proteins active against wide range of pathogens.

3.6. Defensins

Ocular surface is constantly exposed to environment and foreign bodies, thus there are greater chances of infection. However, robust innate immune system at ocular surface protects the eye from infection. There are several peptides of defensins and cathelicidin families that are present in tear film and secreted by corneal and conjunctival cells. These are not only antimicrobial in nature but also help in the recruitment of immune cells and thus provide a link to adaptive immunity. The important defensins present in human eye are hBD-1 (human beta defensins), hBD-2, hBD-3, CAP37 (Cathelicidin-related antimicrobial peptide), LL37 (type of cathelicidin) and HNP-1, 2, 3 (human neutrophil defensins) [53].

4. Protozoan eye infections

4.1. Toxoplasmosis

Toxoplasmosis is caused by obligatory intracellular protozoan parasite known as *Toxoplasma gondii.* The mode of infection is either by the ingestion of oocysts shed in feces of the cats or other Felidae (definitive host) or by the consumption of tissue cyst present in the raw or uncooked meat. Life cycle of *Toxoplasma* includes three stages that are oocysts, tachyzoites and bradyzoites. It completes its life cycle in two phases, one as an intestinal phase in its homologous host, such as cats and another as an extraintestinal phase in its heterologous host, such as mouse, man and other animals. When cats feed on mouse brain containing tissue cysts of *T. gondii*, a large number of oocysts are released in the infected cat's feces. After 1–5 days, oocysts get matured and become infective to man and other animals. After ingestion, oocysts liberate sporozoites, which penetrate intestinal mucosa and reach to distant organs such as brain, eyes, liver, spleen, lymph nodes, heart, skeletal muscles and placenta by blood and lymphatic stream. *Toxoplasma* tissue cysts also occur in the skeletal muscles of the intermediate host such as sheep and pigs (Figure 2) [54]. In addition, developing fetus can acquire the infection transplacentally from the mother during pregnancy. Rarely, infection may also result from consumption of drinking water contaminated with oocysts. The ocular infection can be either congenital or acquired.

Approximately, one-third of the world's population is thought to be infected by *T. gondii.* It is common in hot and humid climates such as Central America, Asia and the Caribbean region (Table 1, Figure 3). In Europe, toxoplasmosis is common and the highest prevalence rates have been reported in France. Various risk factors such as geographical region, meat consumption, personal habits, animal reservoir and climatic conditions play a significant role in the transmission of infection. In recent years, due to indoor keeping of livestock and improvement in hygiene standards, the risk of acquiring infection has decreased tremendously in the developed nations. However, in the developing nations, risk has increased due to population growth, urbanization trends and increase in meat consumption. Drinking water, seawater and

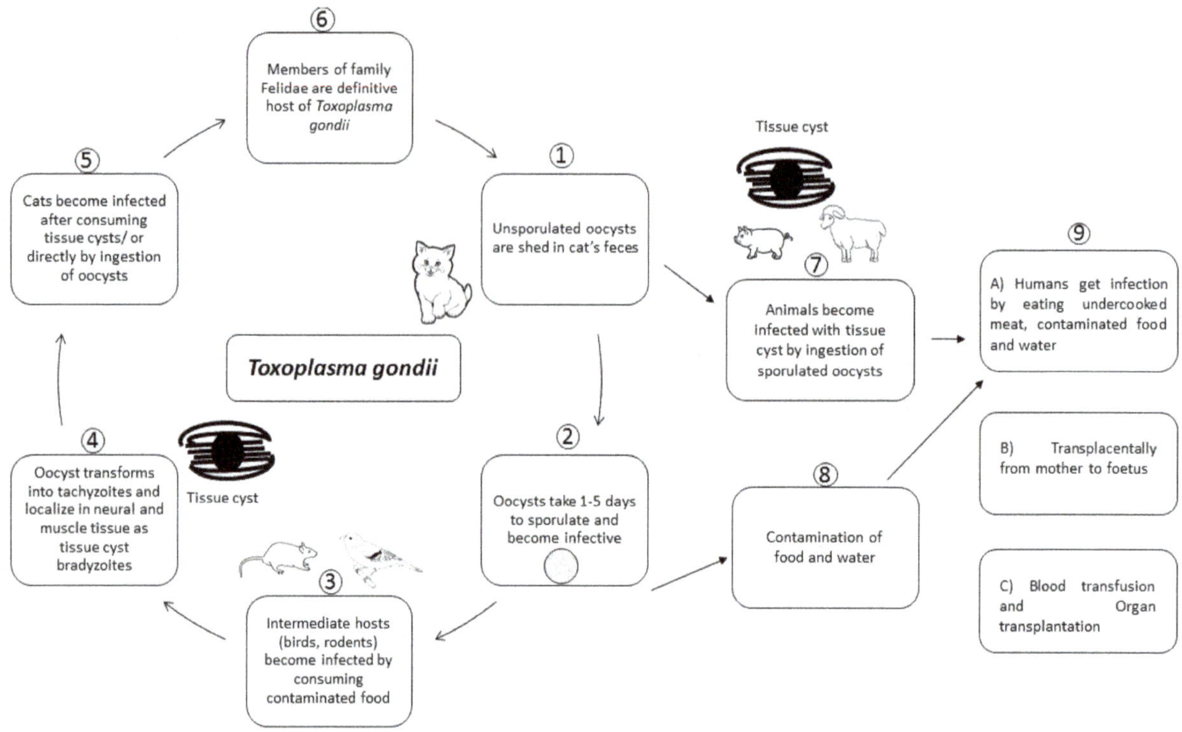

Figure 2. Life cycle of *T. gondii* (Diagrammatic representation).

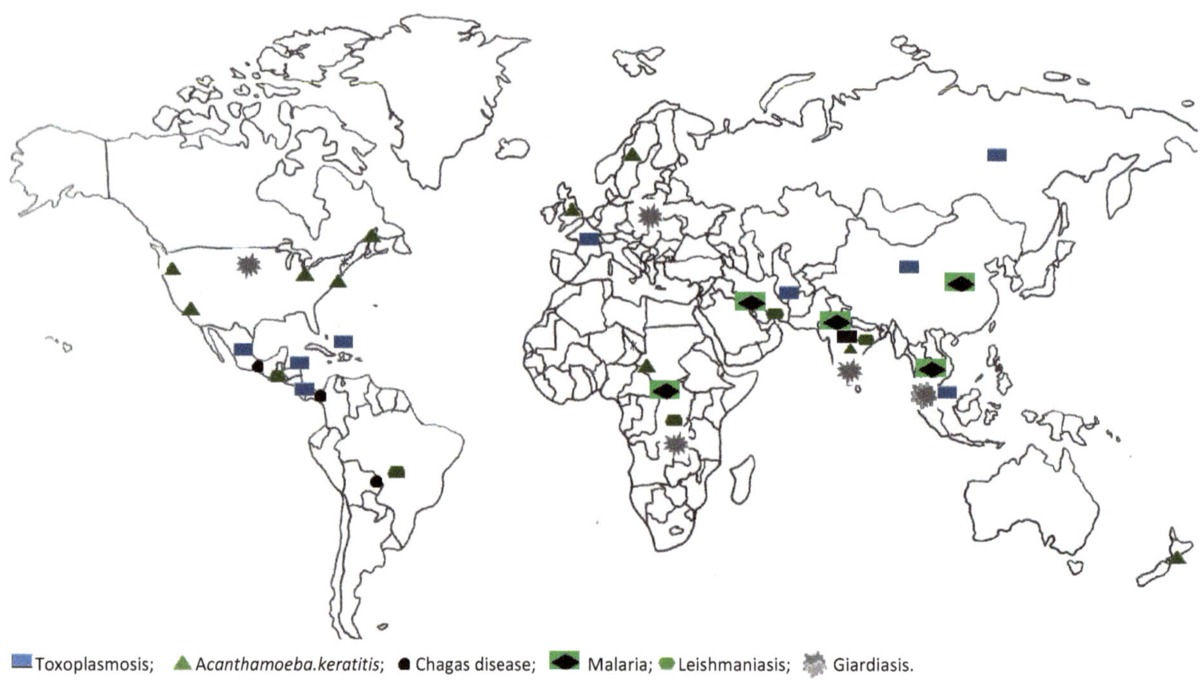

Figure 3. World map showing geographical areas endemic for ocular protozoal infections.

seafood contaminated with oocysts when consumed may account for many unreported cases. Therefore, exact prevalence would be much higher than reported in the literature [55–58].

Ocular toxoplasmosis usually manifests in immunocompromised *T. gondii*-infected individuals and in neonates who acquire infection transplacentally [4]. The main target organs in congenital toxoplasmosis are the brain, eyes and placenta. *T. gondii* disseminates through the blood stream, lodges at particular site(s) and develops into tissue cysts. The dendritic cells and macrophages act as "Trojan horses" to guide the parasite through blood-brain barrier to reach at its target site in brain [59]. Inside the host cell, it protects itself from the toxic host molecules by hiding inside the parasitophorous vacuole (structure produced by apicomplexan parasites that allows the parasite to develop inside host cell and protects from phagolysosomes). There are three main clonal lineages of *T. gondii*. Type I strains being the highest virulent, whereas types II and III are moderately virulent. However, at present more than 130 "atypical" genotypes are known, but their exact role in pathogenesis is not well established. Host genetic factors such as polymorphism in Toll-like receptors (TLR) (TLR2, 5 and 9) are also known to play a role in the susceptibility to and severity of ocular toxoplasmosis [60, 61].

Congenital ocular toxoplasmosis usually involves both the eyes, whereas acquired ocular toxoplasmosis is usually unilateral [62, 63]. Chorioretinitis is caused by necrotizing inflammation due to the rupture of an older cyst. Intense form of choriretinitis may occur in newborns and patients infected with HIV. In addition, congenital toxoplasmosis patients may present with wide range of ocular symptoms such as strabismus, nystagmus and blindness. Acute, acquired infection may result in photophobia, scotoma and loss of central vision. Ptosis may occur due to oculomotor nerve involvement.

Diagnosis of ocular toxoplasmosis in children with congenital infection is established by recognizing distinctive clinical findings such as focal necrotizing retinitis, vitritis, anterior uveitis and cataract [64] However, in cases with atypical presentation or having severe fulminant disease, diagnosis is usually established by analyzing the intraocular fluid for the presence of specific antibodies or the presence of parasite DNA by molecular techniques such as PCR or real-time PCR [65, 66]. PCR is performed by targeting the *Toxoplasma* B1 gene or other multiple repeat sequences [67–69]. Though, in general, PCR with amniotic fluid is known to have significantly high sensitivity (64%) and specificity (100%) for the diagnosis of toxoplasmosis [70], sensitivity of only 53 and 83% has been documented for the diagnosis of ocular toxoplasmosis [71]. PCR can be performed on either aqueous humor or vitreous fluid, but aqueous humor can be collected more easily. However, the DNA burden in aqueous humor is low, and in rare instances a confirmation would necessitate vitreous sampling [72].

Antibody detection in serum samples is widely used for establishing the diagnosis of toxoplasmosis [73–76], while its role is limited in establishing the diagnosis of the ocular toxoplasmosis. A rising titer of specific IgG over a period of 3 weeks helps in establishing the diagnosis [77]. The detection of specific antibodies in intraocular fluids by the enzyme-linked immunosorbent assay (ELISA) is the most commonly used test for the diagnosis of toxoplasmosis. The Goldmann-Witmer coefficient (GWC) calculation is a common method to estimate the local versus systemic *Toxoplasma*-specific IgG. This index helps in measuring the intraocular levels of specific antibodies against *Toxoplasma*. It is expressed as the level of *Toxoplasma*-specific IgG relative to the level of total IgG in the aqueous humor as a fraction of the level of *Toxoplasma*-specific IgG relative to the level of the total IgG in the serum. A value of 2 or above is considered as an evidence of intraocular infection. Toxoplasma specific IgG antibodies are produced in response to the actively multiplying tachyzoites at local site of infection [72, 78] The presence of *T. gondii*-specific IgM is the hallmark of a recently acquired systemic or, possibly, ocular infection. However, high rate of false-positive results due to the persistence of antibodies, decreases its utility as a diagnostic marker for recent ocular toxoplasmosis. In patients with reactivated ocular toxoplasmosis, it is not useful as *T. gondii*-specific IgM antibodies are either absent or present in very low quantity [79]. Saliva samples have also been tested for the detection of specific antibodies for the diagnosis of toxoplasma encephalitis in immunocompromised individuals, but it may play a limited role in ocular toxoplasmosis [74].

An algorithm for the laboratory confirmation of clinically suspected cases of ocular toxoplasmosis has been reported [72]. Reactivated form of ocular toxoplasmosis is considered in patients with typical lesions of toxoplasmic retinochoroiditis, specific IgG seropositive, specific IgM seronegative and responding to anti-*Toxoplasma* treatment. However, if patients are specific IgM seropositive, then additional laboratory tests are required. If doubt persists about diagnosis, paired serum and aqueous samples are required to be tested in parallel. The clinical diagnosis along with laboratory evidence is documented in 60-85% of cases and thus, laboratory evidence is lacking in 15-40% of clinically suspected patients. Analysis of aqueous humor is useful in patients presenting with atypical ocular lesions or not responding to specific treatment [72].

In immunocompetent individuals, toxoplasma retinochoroiditis usually resolves within 2–3 months [80]. Classic therapy or triple therapy with a combination of pyrimethamine, sulfadiazine and systemic corticosteroids is recommended for lesions involving or near to fovea, an area critical for vision. Classic therapy is usually associated with significant side effects, therefore other drugs such as trimethoprim-sulfamethoxazole, clindamycin, atovaquone and azithromycin are being evaluated for the treatment of ocular toxoplasmosis [81].

Trimethoprim-sulfamethoxazole (Bactrim) appears to be a safe and effective substitute for sulfadiazine, pyrimethamine and folinic acid for the treatment of ocular toxoplasmosis.

Progressive and recurring necrotizing retinitis, with vision-threatening complications such as retinal detachment, choroidal neovascularization and glaucoma, may occur at any time during the clinical course if the infection is not treated on time. Congenital toxoplasmosis can lead to cataract. The aim of the treatment is to arrest parasite multiplication during the active period of retinochoroiditis and to minimize damage to the retina and optic disc [64].

Animal model(s) can be used to study various aspects of ocular toxoplasmosis [40].

4.2. *Acanthamoeba* keratitis

Acanthamoeba keratitis (AK) is caused by *Acanthamoeba* spp., a free-living protest parasite [82]. The word "acanth" in Greek means "spikes" and has been added as a prefix to "amoeba" to denote the spine-like structures present on its surface. The parasite is present ubiquitously in the environment and exists in two forms, trophozoite and cyst forms. In humans, it can enter through eye, nasal passage or ulcerated broken skin (Figure 4). Infection of the eye can cause blinding keratitis and life-threatening granulomatous encephalitis. Various risk factors contributing to the development of *AK* are (1) wearing of contact lenses for long time, (2) poor personal hygiene, (3) cleaning of lenses with contaminated water and (4) formation of biofilm on contact lenses [82].

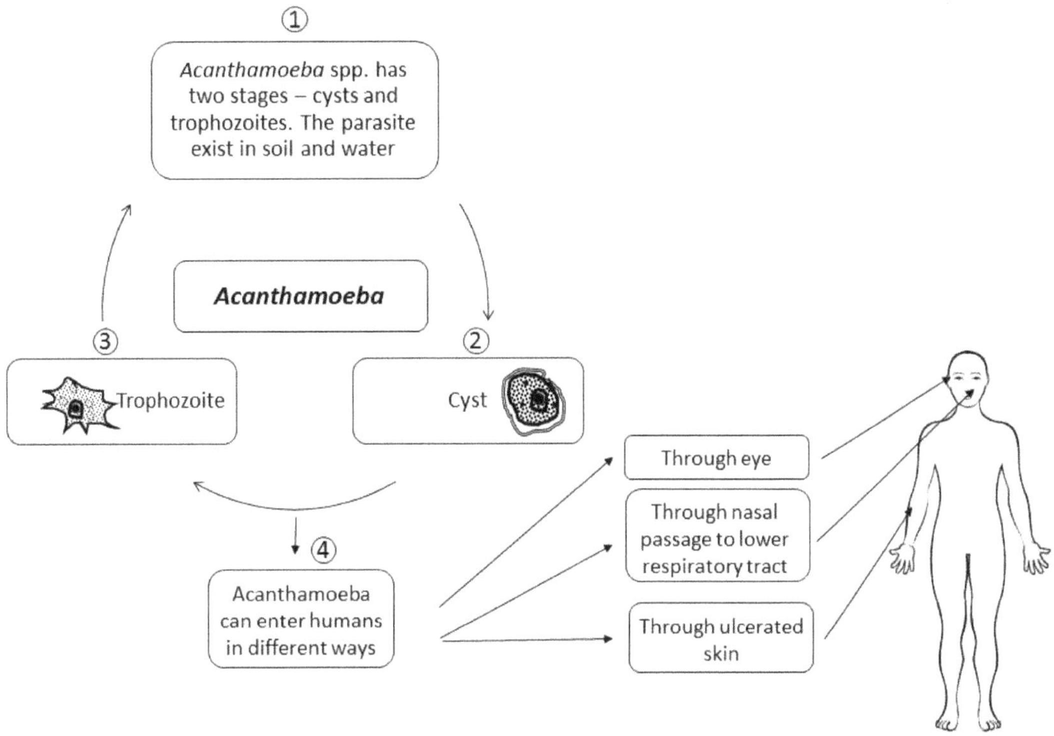

Figure 4. Life cycle of *Acanthamoeba* (Diagrammatic representation).

Acanthamoeba keratitis is common among the contact lens users, and its geographic distribution is depicted in Table 1 and Figure 3. However, in India the infection is reported even in non-contact lens users [7]. The incidence of *Acanthamoeba* keratitis in developed nations varies from 1 to 33 cases per million contact lens wearers. In developing nations where contact lens users are limited, the other suggested risk factors are trauma, exposure to contaminated water, use of traditional eye medicine, low socioeconomic background, splashing contaminated water into the eye following dust fall and corneal injury with mud [7, 22, 83]. The pathogenesis of *Acanthamoeba* involves following sequential events, i.e., breach in the epithelial barrier, invasion of stroma by amoeba, depletion of keratocytes, induction of inflammatory response, photophobia and finally necrosis of stroma leading to blindness [82].

The diagnosis of AK is difficult as it is usually confused with symptoms of bacterial, fungal or viral keratitis. However, history of contact lens use together with a history of excruciating pain is a strong indication toward the diagnosis of AK. For establishing the clinical diagnosis with high sensitivity, in vivo confocal microscopy can be used, which is a non-invasive procedure. The *Acanthamoeba* cysts appear as hyper-reflective, spherical structures that are well defined because of their double wall. However, trophozoites are difficult to distinguish from leukocytes and keratocyte nuclei [84, 85]. Laboratory confirmation is established by direct demon-

Ocular protozoal infections	Geographical distribution
Toxoplasmosis	Worldwide particularly in Central America, Asia, Caribbean region, Europe particularly in France
Acanthamoeba keratitis	Worldwide significantly in Chicago, San Francisco, Boston, Philadelphia, Sweden, Portland, New Zealand, United Kingdom, India, Africa
Chagas disease	Central and South America
Malaria	Africa, Central & South America, Middle East and Asia
Leishmaniasis	Africa, Mediterranean region, Middle East, Central and South America, parts of Asia
Microsporidiosis	Worldwide
Giardiasis	Southeast Asia, South Africa, Europe and USA
Ocular nematode infections	
Onchocerciasis	Africa, South America, Arabian peninsula
Loiasis	Central and West Africa
Dirofilariasis	Asia, Africa and Europe
Gnathostomiasis	South East Asia particularly Thailand, China, Japan and India, Central and South America particularly in Mexico, Guatemala, Peru and Ecuador
Thelaziasis	Asia Pacific region - China, India, Thailand, Indonesia, Japan and Korea
Toxocariasis	Worldwide particularly in Asia, Japan, Korea, Ireland, Alabama
Ocular cestode infections	
Cysticercosis	Indian subcontinent, Central and South America, Africa and Far East
Echinococcosis	South America, Middle East, Mediterranean countries, India and Australia
Ocular trematode infections	
Fascioliasis	France, Spain, Italy, Austria, Belgium, United Kingdom, Algeria, Tunisia, Iran, Uzbekistan, Korea, China, Argentina, Chile, Peru, Brazil, Guatemala
Schistosomiasis	Sub-Saharan Africa, China, South Asia
Philopthalmosis	Europe (Yugoslavia), Israel, Asia (Thailand, India, Sri Lanka, Japan) and America (i.e., Mexico, and the United States)
Clinostomum lacramalitis	Thailand
Fascioliasis	Iran
Alaria mesocercariasis	San Francisco, California
Ocular infections by ectoparasites	
Myiasis	Worldwide with greater abundance in poor socioeconomic regions of tropical and subtropical countries, Mediterranean basin and Middle East
Phthiriasis palpebrum	Case reports from Tunisia, Taiwan, India, Pakistan, China, Korea, Lebanon, Israel, Brazil, Turkey, United Kingdom, Belgium, Italy, Cyprus, United States of America (USA)
Tick infestation	Case reports from Ireland, Turkey and USA

Table 1. Ocular parasitic infections and geographical distribution

stration of parasite by immunofluorescence microscopy or by isolating the parasite in culture. Although culture remains the gold standard, it is tedious and time consuming. Multiplex real-time PCR assays (multiplex assays targets more than one region and simultaneously can detect two or more target regions) have also been developed for the detection of different pathogenic free-living amoeba and/or different genotypes of *Acanthamoeba*. Although molecular techniques have high sensitivity and specificity, these are only available at apex laboratories and also require a well-established molecular laboratory [86]. Newer techniques such as Matrix-Assisted Laser Desorption Ionization Time-Of-Flight (MALDI-TOF) and ^{1}H-NMR spectroscopy [87] are also being tested for the rapid identification of *Acanthamoeba* in the clinical specimens [88].

Chances of recovery are good if the pathogen is restricted to cornea epithelium but can lead to vision loss, if it invades stroma leading to necrosis and intense inflammation. Medical treatment, if started early, can lead to a significant improvement within 2–3 weeks [89].

Preventive measures include thorough and adequate disinfection of contact lenses. It is recommended to remove contact lenses before any activity involving contact with water, including showering, using a hot tub, or swimming. Hands should be washed with soap and water and dried before handling contact lenses. Contact lenses should not be rinsed with tap water and should be cleaned and stored as per manufacturer's guidelines. It is suggested that the increased awareness about the other predisposing factors (corneal injury, fall of foreign body in eye) among the general public may enable early and frequent recognition and proper management of AK in patients other than contact lens wearers [7].

4.3. Chagas disease

Chagas disease or American trypanosomiasis is caused by *Trypanosoma cruzi* [90]. It is a chronic systemic disease, included in the WHO's list of most neglected tropical diseases. Approximately, 8 million people are known to be affected in Latin America (Table 1, Figure 3) [8]. The life cycle of the parasite is passed in two stages involving trypomastigotes and amastigotes forms as depicted briefly in Figure 5. *T. cruzi* passes its life cycle in two hosts: one in man or the reservoir host and other in the transmitting insect. The infection is transmitted by the blood-sucking triatomine bugs when infective metacyclic trypomastigotes in bug's feces are released onto the skin of humans. These infective trypomastigotes enter the human host when bite wound is either scratched or rubbed, or through permissive mucosal or conjunctival surfaces. Parasites circulate in the human body affecting various tissues and organs. If the initial bite of the triatomine bug is near the orbit, it may lead to severe palpebral and periorbital edema (Romana's sign) [91]. It causes a painless edema and constitutional symptoms of fever, malaise and anorexia are common. Ocular involvement (posterior uveitis) in congenital Chagas disease is recently reported. Although ocular fundus examination has been unobtrusive, small parafoveolar retinal pigment epithelium defects have been reported in 7.6% of chagasic patients [92].

The diagnosis of acute Chagas disease is established by the direct demonstration of trypomastigotes in the blood/buffy coat preparation. Parasites can also be isolated by direct culturing of blood on NNN medium (Novy, MacNeal, Nicolle's medium). It may take 7 to 10 days for culture to become positive. Diagnosis may also be established by xenodiagnosis. During acute phase, the role of serology is limited in the diagnosis as antibodies take time to

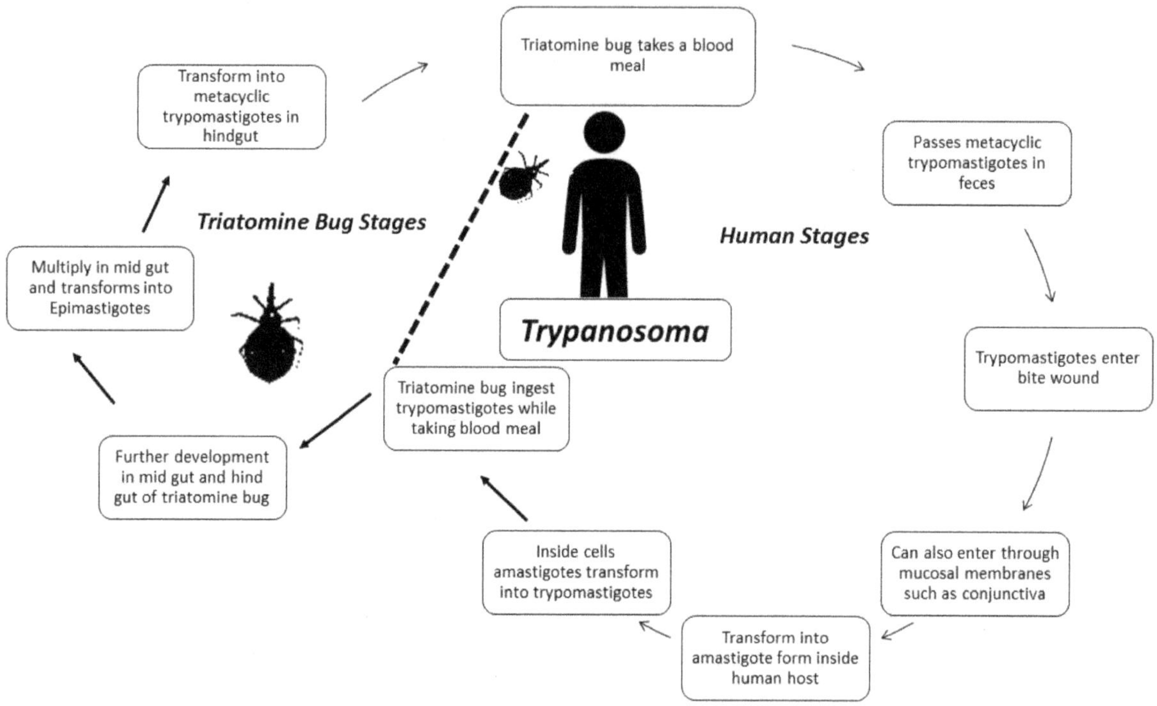

Figure 5. Life cycle of *Trypanosoma cruzi* (Diagrammatic representation).

develop and false positive results have also been known to be associated with serological tests due to cross-reaction of antibodies to non-pathogenic *Trypanosoma rangeli* [8, 91]. Furthermore, detailed examination by the ophthalmologist may aid in establishing the diagnosis. However, accumulation of retinal pigment epithelium defects have been shown in patients with intra-ocular involvement of intermediate and chronic Chagas disease in Paraguay/South America, but overall fundus examination has shown to be unobtrusive [92, 93].

Acute cases of Chagas disease are treated by nifurtimox and benznidazole. Benznidazole is given as 5–7.5 mg/kg per day orally in two divided doses for 60 days. Nifurtimox is given as 8–10 mg/kg per day orally in three or four divided doses for 90 days [91, 94].

Within few weeks, symptoms of acute Chagas disease such as Romana's sign fade away, but infection persists. The average life-time risk of developing complications of chronic phase is around 30%. It may take more than 20 years to develop chronic complications. However, trypanocidal therapy did not significantly reduce cardiac clinical deterioration through 5 years of follow-up as documented by randomized trial of benznidazole for chronic Chagas' cardiomyopathy [95, 96].

4.4. Leishmaniasis

Leishmaniasis is caused by protozoan parasite that belongs to genus *Leishmania*. Humans get infection by the bite of phlebotomine sand flies. There are different clinical forms of leishmaniasis, such as visceral leishmaniasis (VL), cutaneous, diffuse cutaneous and mucocutaneous caused by different species of *Leishmania*. Worldwide, approximately 1.3 million new cases occur every year with a mortality of 20,000 to 30,000 persons per annum [97]. While taking the blood meal, infected sandfly injects promastigotes into humans. Further in the human body, the promastigotes are transformed into amastigote forms, and these are engulfed by tissue macrophages. Amastigote forms replicate inside the cells and further spread either systemically or through cutaneous route, depending on the species of the parasite (Figure 6). Ocular involvement due to leishmaniasis has been reported from various countries such as India, Sudan, Italy, Norway, Turkey and Iran (Table 1, Figure 3) [98–103]. Anterior uveitis is the most common ocular manifestation in VL, which can occur during the course of infection and can further progress to glaucoma [104, 105]. Focal retinal whitening, cotton wool spots, hemorrhages and increased vessel tortuosity have also been reported on fundus examination [106–110]. In severe cases, flame-shaped lesions also appear, which denote hemorrhage from the anterior capillaries of the nerve fiber layer. These findings have also been correlated with anemia and thrombocytopenia as these hemorrhages usually get resolved with treatment, leading to improvement in anemia/thrombocytopenia. Optic neuropathy has been reported due to mucosal leishmaniasis. Eyelid involvement has been documented in cutaneous and mucocutaneous leishmaniasis [111, 112]. Severe involvement can progress to ptosis and ectropion secondary to cutaneous leishmaniasis leading to keratopathy and altered vision [112]. However, eyelid is rarely involved by leishmaniasis and is reported in approximately only 2.5% of cases with cutaneous leishmaniasis [113]. The most common aspect of eyelid leishmaniasis is chalazion-like lesions, but other forms such as ulcerous, phagedenic, cancer-like forms and unilateral chronic granulomatous blepharitis may be observed. Chronic dacryocystitis has been reported in patients suffering from mucocutaneous leishmaniasis, which can effect formation of tear film, leading to dryness of eyes [114]. Endo-ocular lesions have been observed in patients having disseminated cutaneous leishmaniasis. A report from Brazil documented the presence of *Leishmania* in the aqueous humor along with iridiocyclitis [115]. Although ocular manifestations are not very common, it is suggested that a person with ocular manifestation from endemic country should undergo fundus examination for early diagnosis [116].

Diagnosis of leishmaniasis can be achieved by the direct demonstration of parasites in the tissue smears and/or biopsy samples, culture technique(s), antigen and/or antibody detection and molecular technique(s). However, each technique has its own merits and demerits. Amastigotes can be easily identified in the cutaneous and mucocutaneous lesions but are not easily identified in cases with ocular disease [103, 117, 118]. Molecular techniques such as PCR/real-time PCR can identify the genome of parasite with greater sensitivity (100%) and specificity (100%) [119, 120]. The treatment of leishmaniasis depends on several factors such as clinical form of the disease. The antileishmanial drugs include pentavalent antimony, sodium stibogluconate, liposomal Amphotericin B, miltefosine and paromomycin [118, 121].

Ocular lesions do not heal without treatment and could lead to vision loss if conjunctiva is involved due to severe ulceration. Healing occurs without visual impairment if treatment is initiated early during the course of infection and vigorous treatment is required to prevent blindness [121, 122].

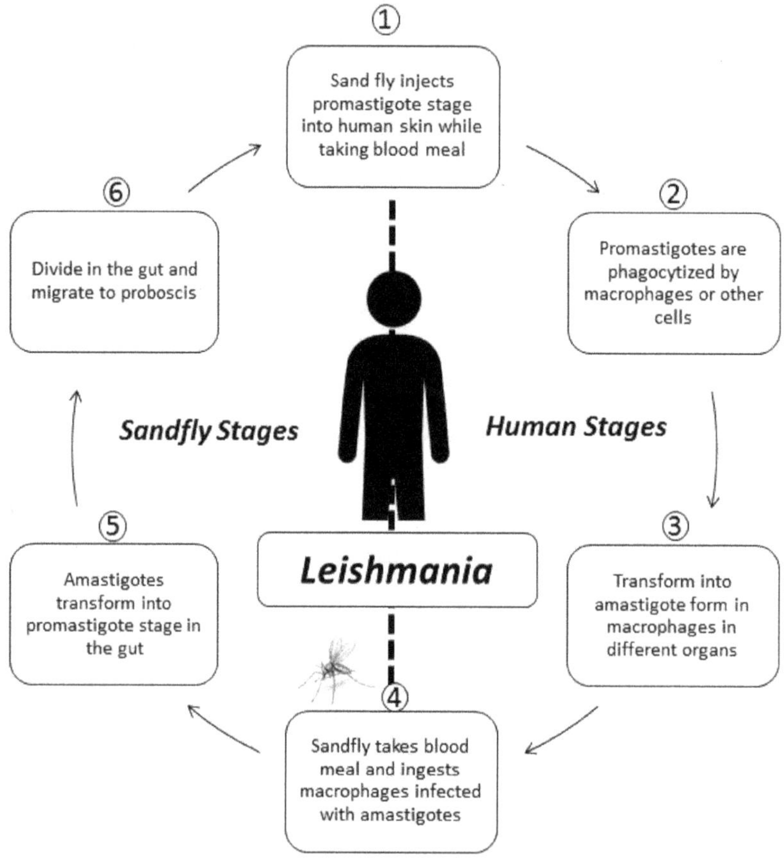

Figure 6. Life cycle of *Leishmania* (Diagrammatic representation).

4.5. Malaria

Malaria is caused by the parasites of Genus *Plasmodium* and is transmitted by the bite of female anopheles mosquitoes. The malarial parasite passes its life cycle in humans and mosquitoes. Inside human host, *Plasmodium* undergoes exoerythrocytic and erythrocytic schizogony as shown briefly in Figure 7. Malarial parasite multiplies by asexual method (schizogony) while residing inside liver cell and the red blood cells. After the parasites have undergone erythrocytic schizogony for a certain period, some of the merozoites give rise to gametocytes, which are taken up by mosquitoes during their blood meal. The gametocytes further develop into sporozoites that are infective to man. Sporozoites when introduced into humans are not directly infective for red blood cells, but undergo development initially in hepatic cells (exoerythrocytic schizogony) and later on invade red blood cells to complete erythrocytic schizogony. As per World Malaria Report 2014 [123], an estimated 3.3 billion people are at risk of developing malaria (Table 1, Figure 3). Complications of severe malaria due to *P. falciparum* mainly occur due to the sequestration of malarial parasite in the microvasculature leading to occlusion and hypoxia. Most of the ocular manifestations occurring in malaria are a result of the same mechanism. Sequestration is further amplified by auto agglutination and resetting [124, 125].

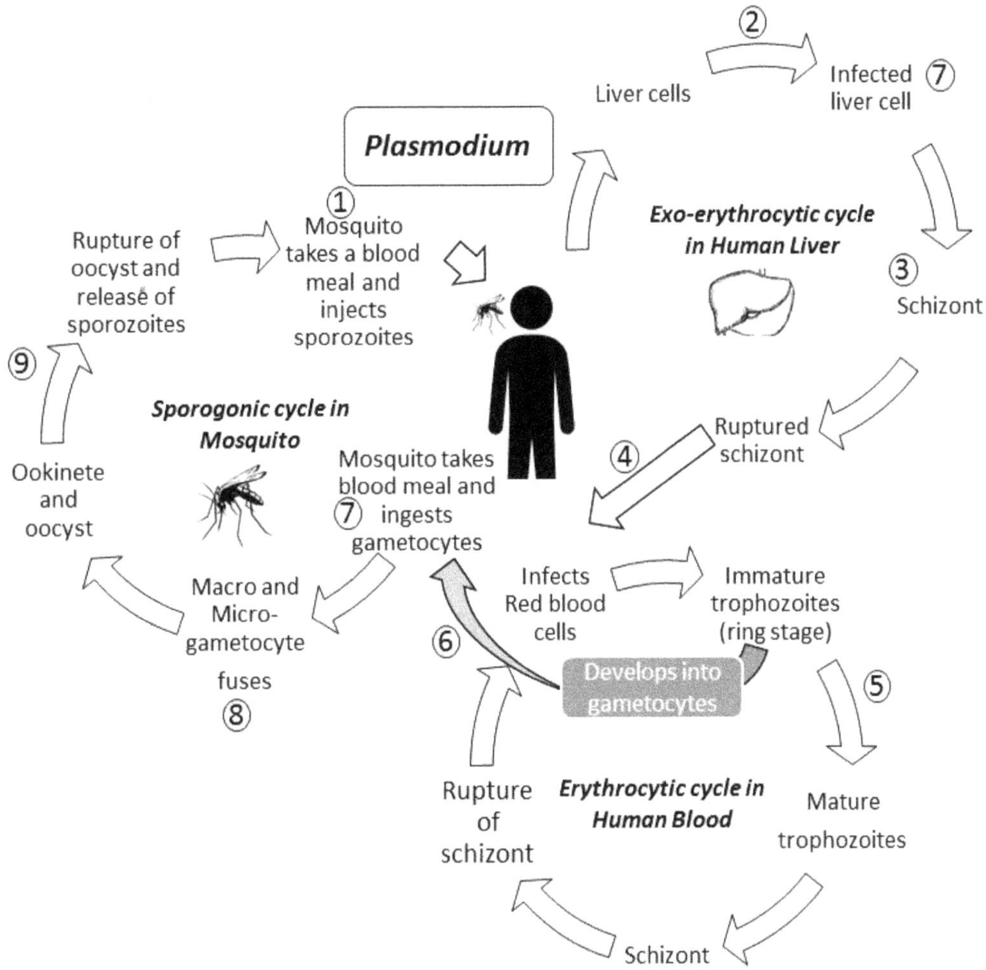

Figure 7. Life cycle of *Plasmodium* (Diagrammatic representation).

Wide range of ocular symptoms has been reported in patients suffering from malaria. Uncomplicated malaria is usually not associated with significant ocular findings but rarely may be associated with edema and hyperemia of the eyelids, chemosis of conjunctiva, conjunctival hemorrhage and anterior uveitis [126]. On the other hand, severe ocular manifestations may occur in cerebral malaria due to *P. falciparum* leading to visual field defects, cortical blindness, optic neuritis, papilledema and optic atrophy [127]. Ocular motor disturbances have also been reported. Occasionally, infarcts in brainstem may cause changes in pupillary reaction and disorders of eye movements. Patients with cerebellar syndromes may present as nystagmus [128, 129]. Characteristics features such as retinal whitening consisting of irregular patchy areas may be localized or diffused in all segments of retina [130]. Blood vessel changes manifest as discoloration (white or orange) occurring mainly in the peripheral fundus, whereas white-centered retinal hemorrhages may manifest as malaria retinopathy. Discoloration of retinal vessels occurs due to the absence of hemoglobin in parasitized erythrocytes, sequestered within retinal vasculature and thus cannot reflect normal red color. Retinal changes in cerebral malaria are considered as poor prognostic markers [131]. The prevalence of any retinopathy, papilledema, hemorrhages, vessel changes, macular whitening and peripheral whitening has been reported in 61, 15, 46, 32, 46 and 44%, respectively, among children with cerebral malaria in Malawi [132].

Diagnosis of malaria is established by light microscopy or by rapid antigen detection kits. Light microscopic examination of Giemsa-stained peripheral blood smear is considered as gold standard for the diagnosis of malaria with a threshold of about 50–100 parasites/μL [133]. However, in addition, ocular examination may provide clue to the diagnosis as specific retinal changes can be seen directly [129, 134, 135].

Treatment depends on the species of *Plasmodium* causing infection. Artemisinin combination therapy is recommended for malaria due to *P. falciparum.* Artemisinin combination therapy includes short-acting artemisinin derivative and long-acting antimalarial (sulphadoxine-pyrimethamine, lumefantrine). Chloroquine along with primaquine is recommended for malaria due to *P. vivax.* Ocular toxicity [136] is very well documented with chloroquine therapy. This includes corneal changes (cornea verticillata) and corneal deposits. Toxic maculopathy and scotoma has also been reported. Quinine overdose has also been known to cause decreased vision, retinal and macular degeneration, mild scotomas and color vision defects [136].

If not treated, malarial retinopathy is associated with serious consequences as reports indicate that the severity of retinopathy is related to prolonged death and coma. After antimalarial treatment and resolution of coma in severe malaria, malarial retinopathy resolves after some time [132, 137].

4.6. Microsporidiosis

Microsporidiosis is the term used to denote the infection caused by microsporidia belonging to phylum Microspora [23]. Microsporidia were once thought to be protists but are now known to be fungi. Although it is classified as a protozoal disease in ICD-10, their phylogenetic placement has been resolved to be within the fungi [138]. Microsporidiosis is considered as an opportunistic infection in AIDS/HIV-infected individuals and is prevalent worldwide (Table 1) [1]. Microsporidia are small, unicellular, spore forming, obligate intracellular pathogens. Important genera responsible for ocular manifestations are Encephalitozoon and Nosema. Another species, Septata, has also been reported to cause keratoconjunctivitis [139]. The prevalence of microsporidiosis ranges from 2 to 50% among severely immunocompromised, HIV-infected patients found in North America, western Europe and Australia. The prevalence data for microsporidiosis is limited among non-HIV-infected persons [9].

1. The life cycle of parasite involves three stages (Figure 8):
2. The resistant spore (infective form)
3. The spore injects the infective sporoplasm into the host cell. Inside the host cell, sporoplasm undergoes multiplication either in the cell cytoplasm or inside parasitophorous vacuole. Microsporidia develop to mature spores by sporogony that are released by disruption of cell membrane. The free mature spores are the infective forms.

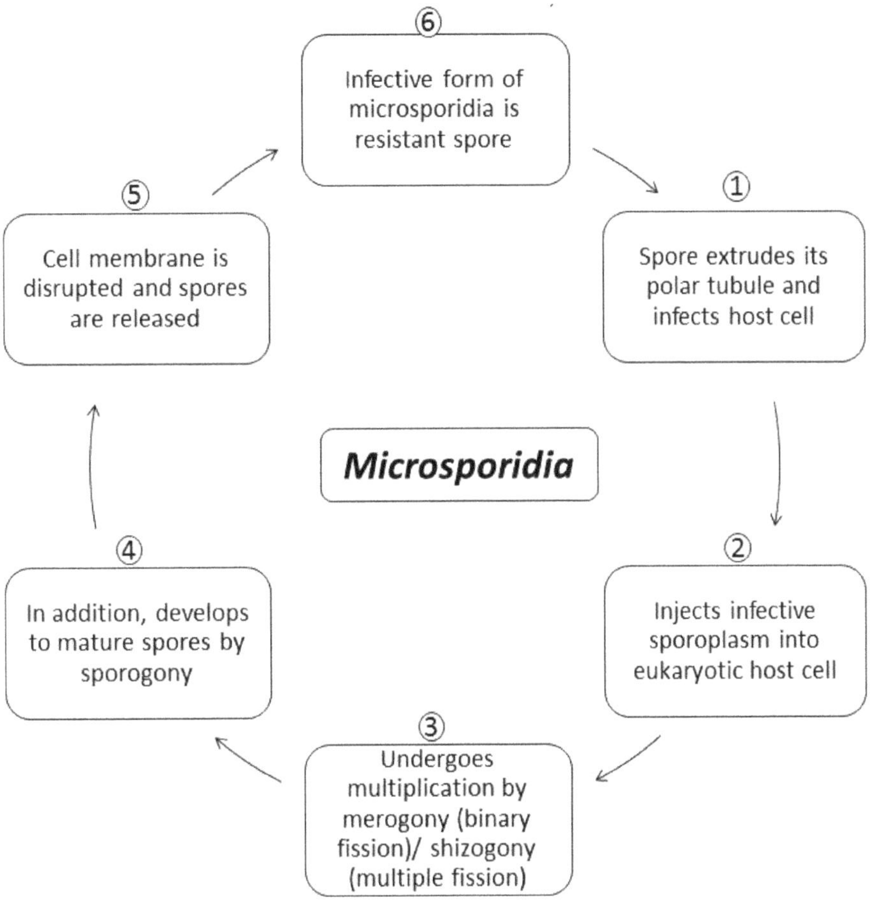

Figure 8. Life cycle of *Microsporidia* (Diagrammatic representation).

Ocular manifestations caused by *Microsporidia* are mainly limited to conjunctiva and cornea. Corneal involvement may lead to punctate epithelial keratitis, hyphema, necrotizing keratitis and corneal ulcer. Symptoms include foreign body sensation, photophobia and decrease in visual acuity [23].

Diagnosis is established by direct demonstration of the spores by microscopy or electron microscopy of the corneal scrapping or biopsy specimens. Isolation of the parasites in culture has also been attempted [140]. There are no reports on use of serological tests to detect antibodies in serum or tears in ocular microsporidiosis [9]. Lesions usually heal after 1–2 weeks as it is self-limiting. Treatment of microsporidial keratoconjunctivitis with polyhexamethylene biguanide does not offer any significant advantage but treatment with topical fumagillin showed significant improvement [141–143].

4.7. Giardiasis

Giardiasis is caused by *Giardia duodenalis* (syn. *G. lamblia* or *G. intestinalis*) [144]. The infection is transmitted by ingestion of contaminated water/food or directly by feco-oral route. The parasite exists in trophozoite and cyst forms as shown in Figure 9. In the trophozoite stage the parasite multiplies in the intestine of man by binary fission. When conditions become unfavorable in the small intestine, encystment occurs and cysts are released along with feces. After ingestion, within 30 minutes, cyst hatches out trophozoites that further multiply in the small intestine. It is found both in developing and developed nations (Table 1, Figure 3). Although it mainly causes diarrhea and malabsorption, in one-third of the patients, it can also result in long-term extra intestinal manifestations [145].

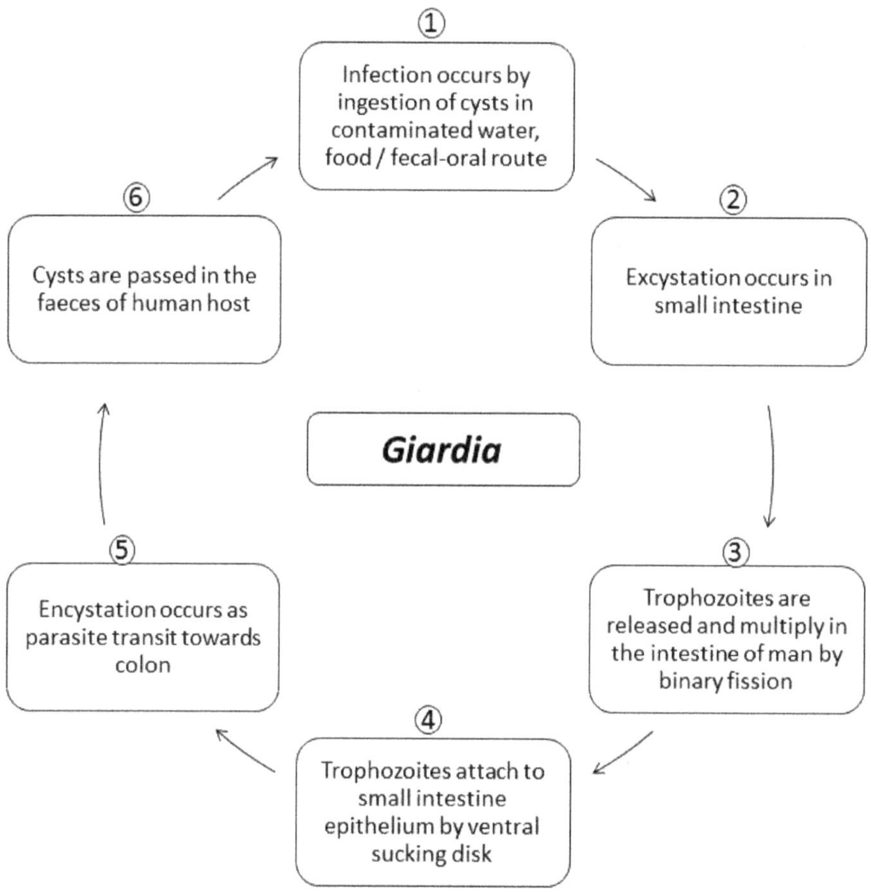

Figure 9. Life cycle of *Giardia lamblia* (Diagrammatic representation).

Barraquer was the first to report the ocular manifestation (iridiocyclitis, choroiditis and retinal hemorrhages) in patients who were suffering from diarrhea due to *G. duodenalis*. Retinal changes in the form of "salt and pepper" degeneration have been reported in children suffering from giardiasis. Corsi et al. [146] reported salt and pepper retinal changes in 19.9% of the patients with giardiasis. This occurs due to the damage of the retinal cells and subsequent release of pigment granules in retina giving an appearance of blackish dots on a background of light yellow pink retina. The exact mechanism(s) by which giardiasis leads to ocular manifestations is still unknown, although possibility of direct invasion by the parasite is excluded (137). Further studies are desired to exactly pinpoint the mechanism by which retinal manifestations follow the occurrence of intestinal giardiasis. Alterations in the retinal pigment layer are most common but do not cause functional changes in retina, and these lesions do not progress or regress with time [146].

The diagnosis is established by direct demonstration of the parasite in the fecal samples by microscopy. Concentration techniques of the samples yield higher sensitivity. Nitroimidazole group of drugs are highly effective against *G. duodenalis.* Most commonly used drugs are metronidazole for 5–7 days or ornidazole/tinidazole in single dose [147]. Treatment of intestinal infection is recommended if present, but no specific treatment is required for ocular manifestations related to retina [146].

5. Nematode infections

5.1. Onchocerciasis

Onchocerciasis, also known as "river blindness", is caused by *Onchocerca volvulus,* the filarial nematode. It is transmitted from person-to-person by the repeated bites of infected blackflies (*Simulium* species). These blackflies are mostly found near the flowing rivers and streams and transmit the infection to the people residing in nearby remote villages [148]. The life cycle of the parasite passes between black flies and humans as shown in Figure 10. While taking a blood meal, stage 3 larvae present in infected blackfly are transmitted onto human skin and penetrate into bite wound. In subcutaneous tissue, these larvae develop into adult filariae. Adult worm produces hundreds of thousands of embryonic larvae (microfilariae) that may persist for 3-5 years in the human host. These embryonic larvae migrate to the skin, eyes and other organs. The microfilariae are ingested by the female blackfly when it bites infected humans and develop further in the blackfly. During subsequent bites, it transmits infection to new human host [148, 149].

Onchocerciasis mainly occurs in tropical countries and majority of the cases (99%) have been reported from sub-Saharan Africa. It is also found in some countries of the Middle East and Latin America such as Brazil, Guatemala, Mexico and Venezuela (Table 1, Figure 11). Approximately, 25 million people are known to be affected by onchocerciasis worldwide, and it is known to cause visual impairment and blindness in approximately 800,000 and 300,000 people, respectively [148, 150]. The inflammatory response initiated against dying microfilariae causes gradual and progressive loss of vision due to sclerosal keratitis [149, 151]. Apart from causing keratitis, clinical features may also manifest as iridiocyclitis, chorioretinitis and optic atrophy. Autoimmune mechanisms have also been postulated to cause inflammation in the posterior eye. Accumulation of retinal and retinoic acids, strong eosinophilic response and immune reaction against *Wolbachia* antigens [152] released by dying microfilariae also contributes to the ocular pathogenesis [153].

The filarial parasites of major medical importance in humans contain the symbiotic bacterium *Wolbachia,* and reports have revealed that targeting of these bacteria with antibiotics results in a reduction in worm viability, development, embryogenesis and survival. *Wolbachia* is present as an intracellular bacteria symbiont in all the developmental stages of *Onchocerca volvulus.* Clearance of the endosymbionts by antibiotic treatment causes inhibition of worm development. *Wolbachia* contributes directly to the metabolic activity of the nematode. Various

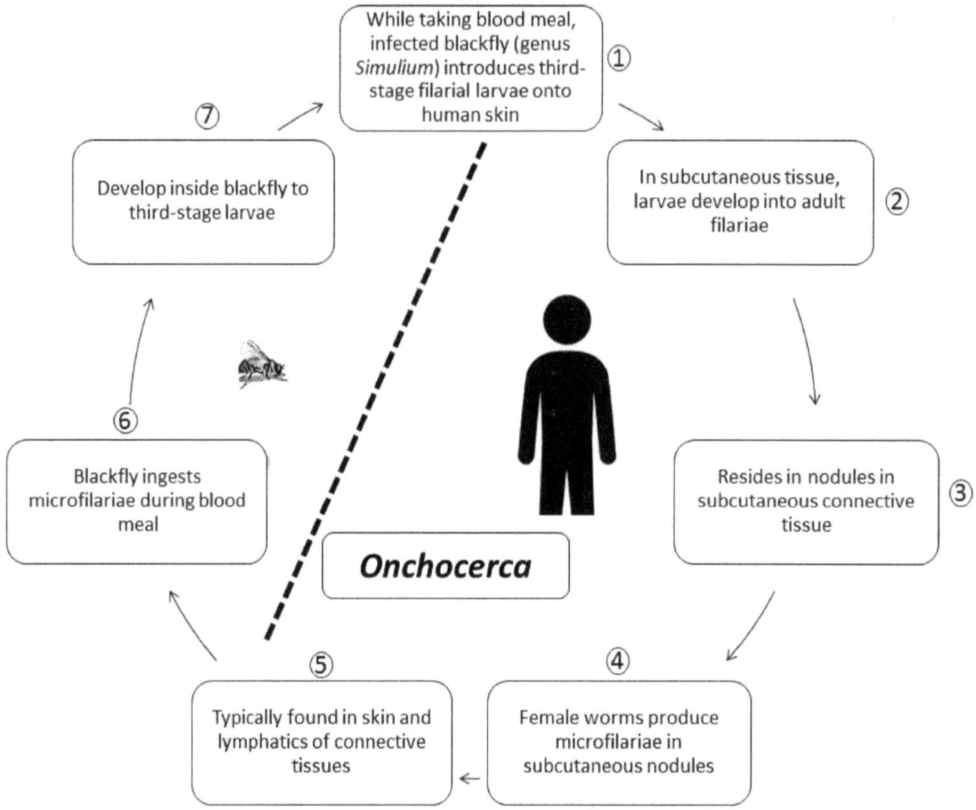

Figure 10. Life cycle of *Onchocerca volvulus* (Diagrammatic representation).

biochemical pathways such as heme, nucleotide and enzyme co-factor biosynthesis are intact in *Wolbachia* but absent or incomplete in nematode [154].

Diagnosis is difficult to establish in light infections. Skin snips can be subjected to microscopy for visualizing the larvae, but it yields very low sensitivity. Infections of the eye can be diagnosed with direct demonstration of the parasite by slit-lamp examination or by demonstrating the parasite in sclerocorneal punch biopsy. Newer techniques such as skin-snip PCR can establish the diagnosis if larvae are not visualized [155]. Antibodies can be detected by ELISA or EIA, but these tests cannot distinguish between past and current infections [156, 157]. Skin-snip PCR has 84–91% sensitivity and 100% specificity [149]. The sensitivity and specificity of serum antibody detection has been reported to be 78–99% and 95–100%, respectively [149]. A promising antigen detection by dipstick assay was recently developed, but its specificity was found to be low in high endemic areas due to cross reaction with urine filarial antigen [158, 159]. Xenodiagnosis (exposing possible infected tissue to a vector and then examining the vector for the presence of microorganism) has also provided clue in some cases.

If the infection is not treated on time, it can progress toward blindness [160]. Drug of choice for the treatment is ivermectin, given 150 to 200 μg /kg body weight, every 6 months to prevent the skin damage and blindness. Treatment with ivermectin has been shown to decrease visual field loss and severity of keratitis. Ivermectin only kills the larvae but not the adult worms. Doxycycline can be used to kill the adult worm. The mechanism of action is that it kills the

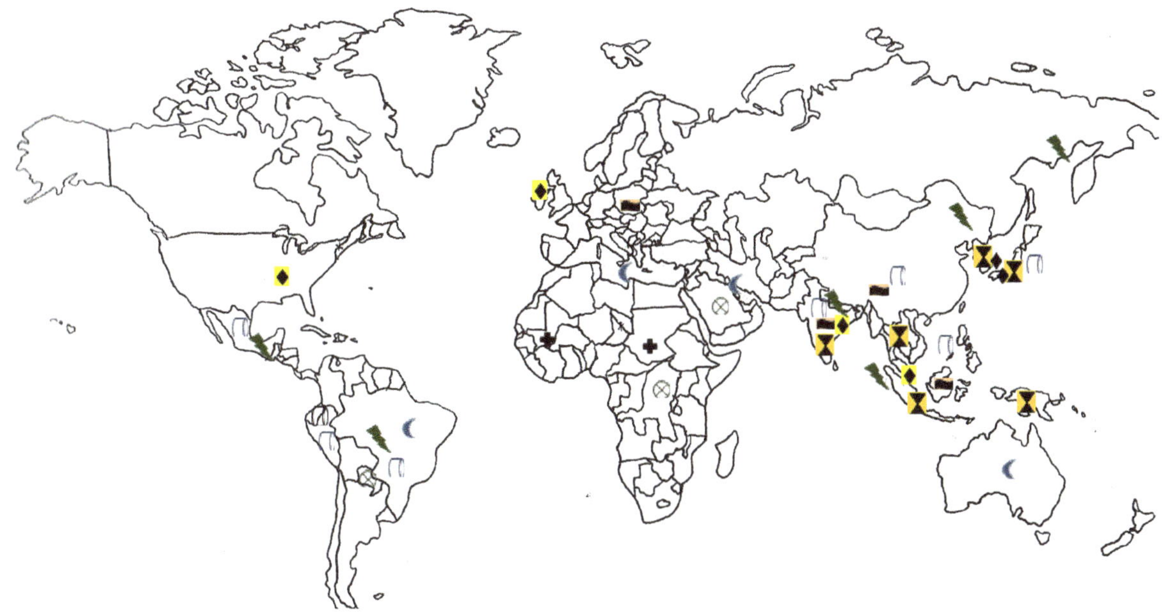

⊗ Onchocerciasis; ✚ Loiasis ▬ Dirofilariasis; Gnathostomiasis; ⧗ Thelaziasis ♦ Toxocariasis; Cysticercosis;
☾ Echinococcosis;

Figure 11. World map showing geographical areas endemic for ocular nematode and cestode infections.

Wolbachia bacteria residing in the worm, on which the adult worm depends for its survival. Treatment with a 6-week course of doxycycline has been shown to kill more than 60% of adult female worms and to sterilize 80–90% of females 20 months after treatment. Thus, treatment with ivermectin is advised one week prior to treatment with doxycycline to provide relief to patient [148, 161].

The best method to get the protection from insect bite is the use of insect repellent. Community-directed treatment with ivermectin (CDTI) along with vector control measures is the main approach to control onchocerciasis. Ivermectin kills microfilariae and also prevents adult worms from producing more microfilariae for few months following treatment, so reduces transmission [148].

5.2. Loiasis

Loiasis is caused by *Loa loa,* the African eyeworm. It is transmitted by the bite of tabanid flies, belonging to the genus *Chrysops.* It affects approximately 3 million people, residing in certain rain forests of Central and West Africa (Table 1, Figure 11) [162, 163]. The tabanid flies most commonly bite during day time and are more common during rainy season. The smoke of wood fires and movement of people attract them. These flies are more commonly found near rubber plantations and are attracted by the well-lit homes. The larvae are passed from flies to humans when humans are bitten by these flies [162]. The larvae develop into adults in the human host over one year and migrate through cutaneous and subcutaneous tissue (Figure 12). Migration of the adult worm is painless, but it is associated with mild tingling sensation. It may involve the nasal area, bulbar conjunctiva and eyelids [164].

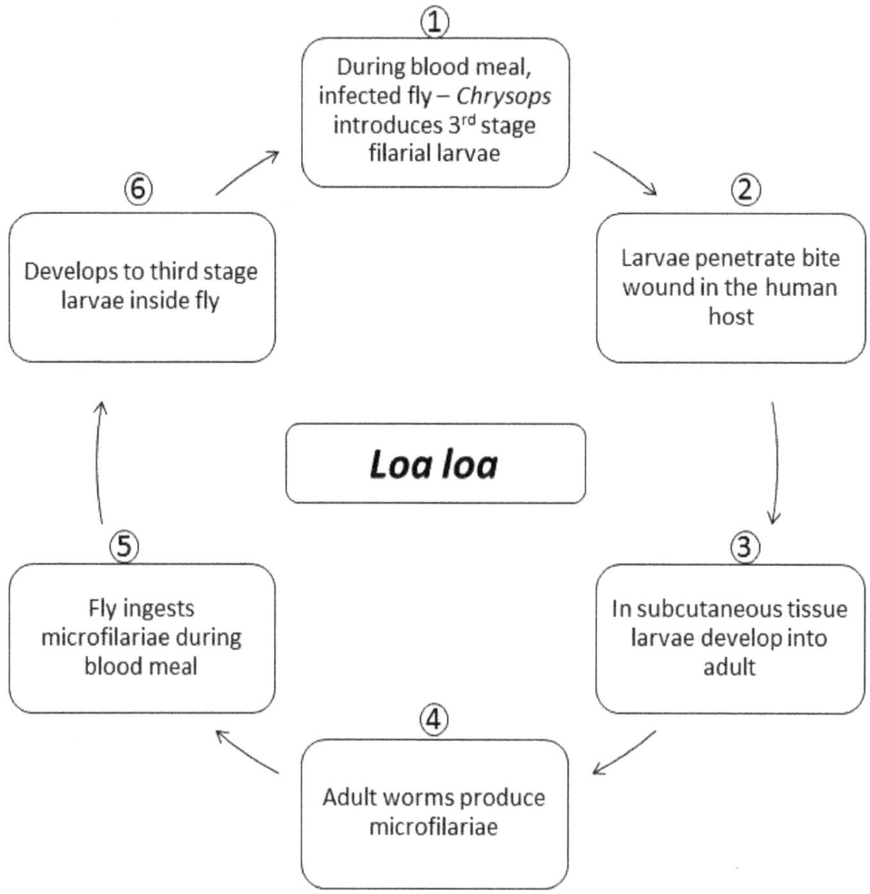

Figure 12. Life cycle of *Loa loa* (Diagrammatic representation).

Ocular manifestations may occur due to the presence of both microfilariae and adult worms. The adult worms may survive up to 15 years and have been found in the conjunctiva, vitreous, eyelid and anterior chamber. Calabar swellings [165] may occur as a result of localized angioedema due to intense atopic reaction. Retinal hemorrhages may occur due to aneurysmal dilatation of the retinal vessels due to the invasion of the retinal and choroid vessels by the microfilariae present in blood stream. Perivascular inflammation can also be present, and ocular examination under slit lamp examination is useful in establishing the diagnosis.

The diagnosis is usually confirmed by the direct demonstration of the microfilariae in the blood by visualizing Giemsa-stained slides under the microscope. However, many of the individuals having visible worm in the eye may test as amicrofilaraemic [166]. Blood should be drawn during the midday as this time coincides with the periodicity of the microfilariae in the blood. The microfilariae can also be demonstrated in unstained blood smear. Adult worm extraction establishes the diagnosis in patients having conjunctival involvement [167]. Antibody detection [168] may aid in establishing the diagnosis, but its presence cannot differentiate between recent and past infection. Eosinophilia and high IgE also indicate active infection [169].

Eye worm if not treated causes very little damage to eye as it lasts less than one week (often just hours). Surgical removal relieves eye symptoms, in addition medical treatment is required

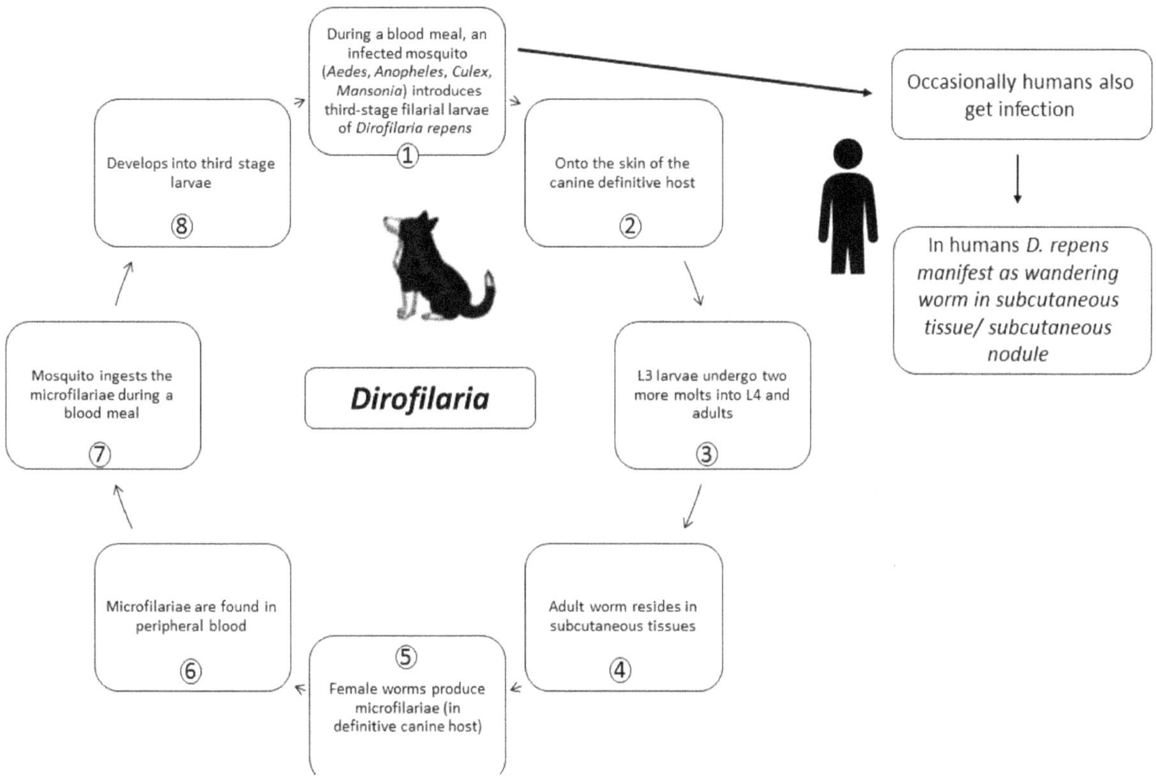

Figure 13. Life cycle of *Dirofilaria repens* (Diagrammatic representation).

for treating loiasis [170]. Therapy involves manual removal of adult worms and administration of diethylcarbamazine (DEC), which kills both adult worms and microfilariae.

5.3. Dirofilariasis

Dirofilariasis is caused by nematodes belonging to the genus *Dirofilaria.* The various species of *Dirofilaria* that are natural parasites of domestic and wild animals are *D. immitis, D. repens, D. tenuis* and *D. ursi* [37]. It is prevalent worldwide and is an important zoonotic infection. It is being reported in increasing numbers from Mediterranean countries such as Italy and have also been reported from France, Greece, Spain, Croatia, India, Serbia, Denmark, Russia and Tunisia (Table 1, Figure 11). The parasite passes its life cycle in canids as definitive host as shown in Figure 13. Mosquitoes act as intermediate host and vector for the transmission of infection from animals to human host. Mosquitoes take up microfilariae along with blood meal from the infected host, develop inside the mosquitoes and are subsequently transmitted to other hosts while taking a fresh blood meal. Larvae migrate from the subcutaneous tissue to the right side of the heart and/or to other parts of the body where maturation takes place. Depending on the site of lodgment, it can cause pulmonary, cardiovascular, subcutaneous or ocular infection [28].

There are several cases that document ocular involvement due to dirofilariasis [37, 171–173]. Ocular symptoms depend on the site of infection. Eyelid involvement [174] leads to edema, pain, pruritus and congestion of conjunctiva, whereas intraocular [175] involvement leads to foreign body sensation, diplopia, photophobia and floaters.

Diagnosis can be established by the direct demonstration and identification of the adult worm. Intraocular presence of the parasite can be confirmed by ophthalmoscopy. Serological techniques are not useful in establishing the diagnosis due to the cross reaction with other parasitic helminths, particularly *Toxocara canis*. Recombinant proteins proved to exhibit 100% sensitivity and 90% specificity by ELISA for the diagnosis of pulmonary dirofilariasis [176].

Without treatment, worm remains in eye causing symptoms due to its presence [177]. Surgical excision is the treatment of choice; however use of diethylcarbamazine (DEC) has also been reported with some success [37, 178].

5.4. Gnathostomiasis

Gnathostomiasis is a food-borne zoonotic parasitic infection, caused by ingestion of raw or undercooked freshwater fish, pork, chicken, frog and snake [179, 180] contaminated with the third-stage larvae of *Gnathostoma* species. The life cycle of the parasite passes in pigs, cats and wild animals as definitive host, whereas small crustaceans act as first intermediate host and fish, frog or snake act as second intermediate host as depicted in Figure 14. In the infected person, larvae migrate through viscera and reach internal organs and subcutaneous tissues. Depending on the location of lodgment, it can cause cutaneous, visceral, ocular or cerebral gnathostomiasis. Majority of the cases have been reported from East Asia (Thailand, China, Japan and India) and Central and South America (Mexico, Guatemala, Peru and Ecuador) (Table 1, Figure 11). However, sporadic cases have been reported worldwide [181]. *Gnathostoma spinigerum* is the most common species causing infection in humans.

Ocular manifestations occur due to the migration of the parasite and its metabolites, leading to inflammatory response. Conjunctiva and corneal infection may lead to congestion of the conjunctiva and corneal ulceration, respectively. Intraocular involvement may lead to glaucoma, uveitis, retinitis and vitreous hemorrhage [182, 183]. In severe cases, retinal detachment has also been reported due to the fibrinous scarring along the migratory path.

Diagnosis is difficult to establish and high index of suspicion is required. Patients may present with marked eosinophilia [184] and elevated IgE levels [185]. ELISA for specific antibody detection and histopathological examination of the biopsy samples may assist in establishing the diagnosis [186–188]. ELISA for antibody detection reported to have low sensitivity, ranging from 59 to 87%, with a specificity of 79–96% [189, 190]. If parasite is not removed, it leads to persistence of visual disturbances such as floaters. Surgical treatment is curative and only modality available [191].

5.5. Thelaziasis

Thelaziasis is caused by nematode *Thelazia callipaeda*, transmitted to humans by drosophilid flies [192]. It is also known as oriental eyeworm due to its geographical distribution in Asia Pacific region (China, India, Thailand, Indonesia, Japan and Korea) and Russia [12, 193] (Table

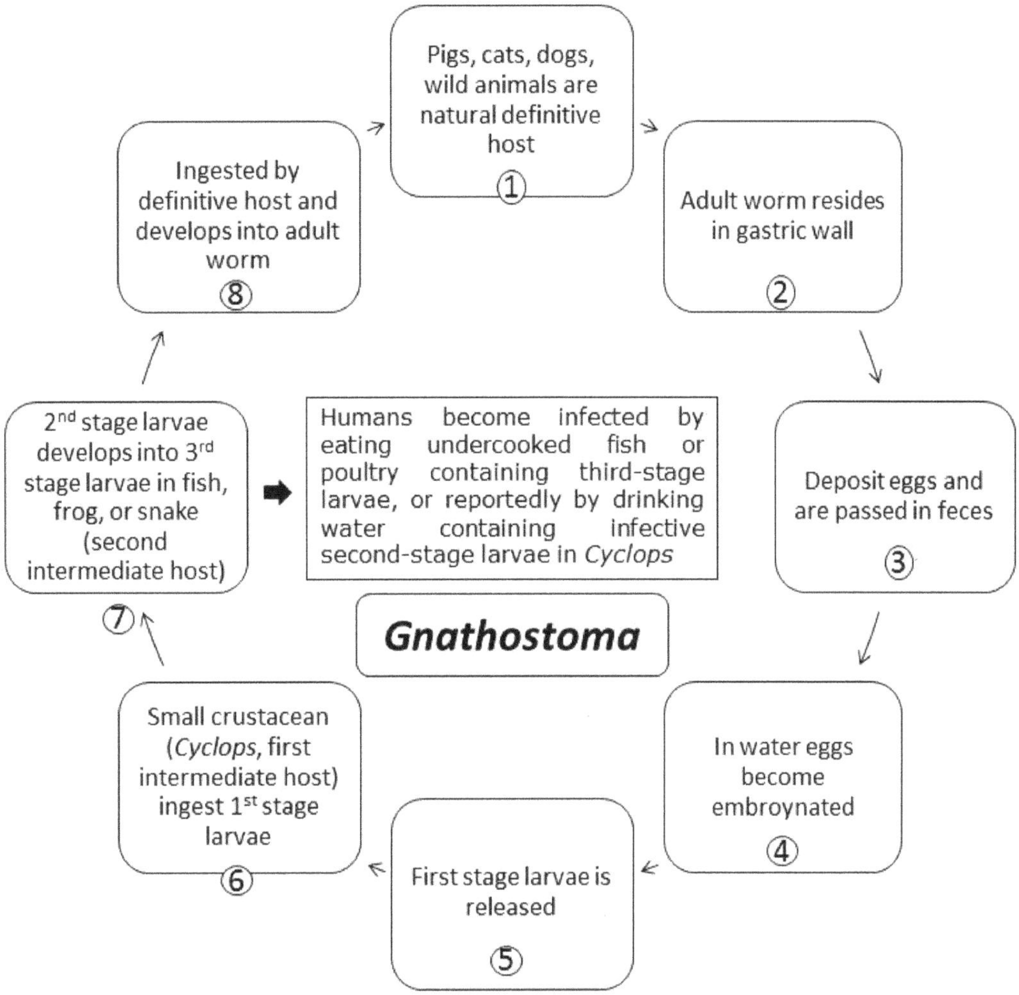

Figure 14. Life cycle of *Gnathostoma* (Diagrammatic representation).

1, Figure 11). The life cycle passes in dogs and other canids, cattle and horses as definitive host and flies act as intermediate host as shown in Figure 15. First-stage larvae are present in the lacrimal secretions of infected humans/animals. The arthropod vectors while feeding on infected lacrimal secretions ingest these larvae, which further develop into infective third-stage larvae. The vector transmits accidentally third-stage larvae when it feeds on lacrimal secretion of other persons/animals. Within 5–6 weeks, these larvae further develop into adult form in the eye of an infected person. These parasites mainly cause infection of the anterior segment of the eye, but intraocular infections involving vitreous and retina have also been reported. It is a disease associated with poor personal hygiene.

Without treatment, worm remains in eye causing symptoms due to its presence [194]. Treatment is surgical removal of worms along with the topical application of thiabendazole. Preventive measures include use of bed nets at night, maintenance of personal hygiene and keeping surroundings clean to control the vector population responsible for the transmission of infection [8].

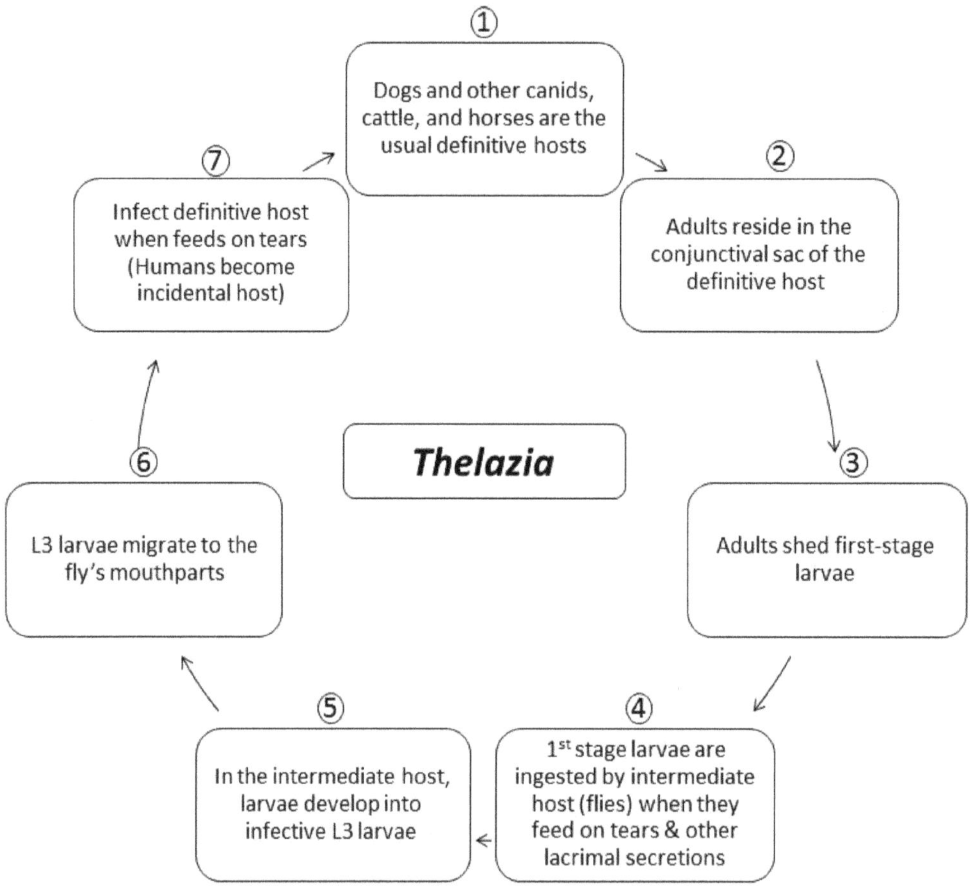

Figure 15. Life cycle of *Thelazia* (Diagrammatic representation).

5.6. Toxocariasis

Toxocariasis is caused by *Toxocara* species. *Toxocara canis* and *T. cati* are the most common species causing toxocariasis in humans worldwide, particularly in Asia, Japan, Korea, Ireland and Alabama [195–199] (Table 1, Figure 11). The life cycle of *Toxocara* involves dogs (*T. canis*)/ cats (*T. cati*) as definitive host (dog/cat). Infection is transmitted by consumption of eggs of *Toxocara* parasites, passed in the feces of definitive host (dog/cat) as shown in Figure 16. After the ingestion of eggs, larvae hatch out from the eggs in the small intestine and penetrate mucosa to migrate to different organs such as liver, lung and trachea, leading to visceral larva migrans (VLM). Sometimes, target larvae may migrate to eyes causing ocular larva migrans (OLM) [200, 201]. Host immune response is weaker in ocular larva migrans than visceral larva migrans. Various ocular clinical manifestations such as keratitis, hypopyon, iritis, uveitis, posterior pole granuloma, vitreous abscess and retinal detachment, strabismus, vision loss are attributed due to vitritis, cystoid macular edema and tractional retinal detachment [11, 202–204]. Based on clinical and physical examination, ocular toxocariasis is classified as chronic endophthalmitis, posterior granuloma and peripheral granuloma [205]. Approximately 25–50% of ocular toxocariasis patients present as posterior pole granuloma, due to lodging of the parasite in small perifoveal end-arteries, and approximately in 50% of ocular toxocariasis patients peripheral granuloma is present. Acute lesion appears as hazy, white mass in the peripheral fundus that may mimic the appearance of snowbank seen in patients with pars planitis.

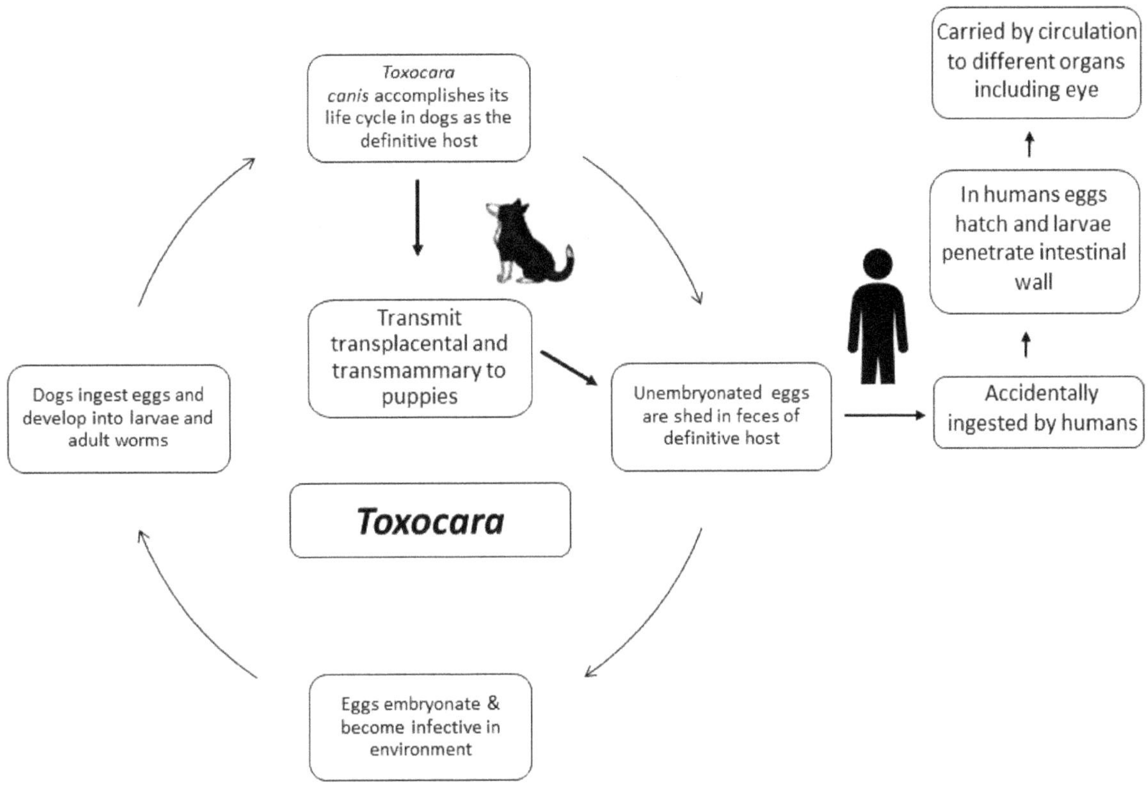

Figure 16. Life cycle of *Toxocara* (Diagrammatic representation).

High index of suspicion is required for establishing the diagnosis of OLM during ocular examination [205]. Marked eosinophilia along with positive serology by ELISA [206] helps in confirming the diagnosis [207]. Detection of specific antibodies in the vitreous fluid also helps in differentiating it from retinoblastoma [208]. ELISA based on the excretory-secretory antigens of *T. canis* reported to have a sensitivity of 78% [209]. ELISA developed by Seoul National University, using crude antigen of *Toxocara* larvae, showed a sensitivity of 92.2% and specificity of 86.6% [210]. PCR available in research laboratories [211] may help in the diagnosis of ocular toxocariasis. Nucleotide homology of 97–99% has been reported between Vietnamese *Toxocara canis* and other *Toxocara* geographical strains by comparing the nucleotide sequence of internal transcribed spacer 2 (ITS2) of ribosomal DNA of *T. canis* [212]. Although PCR has been shown to be the best diagnostic modality in animal models of ocular toxocariasis, molecular techniques are not available in hospitals of resource limiting countries [213]. Vision loss, eye inflammation or damage to the retina occurs if not treated. Prognosis is good with medical and surgical treatment [200].

Albendazole and mebendazole are the drugs of choices for the treatment of VLM [214, 215]. However, there is a limited role of antiparasitic drugs in the treatment of OLM. Photocoagulation along with steroids has been recommended for the treatment of OLM.

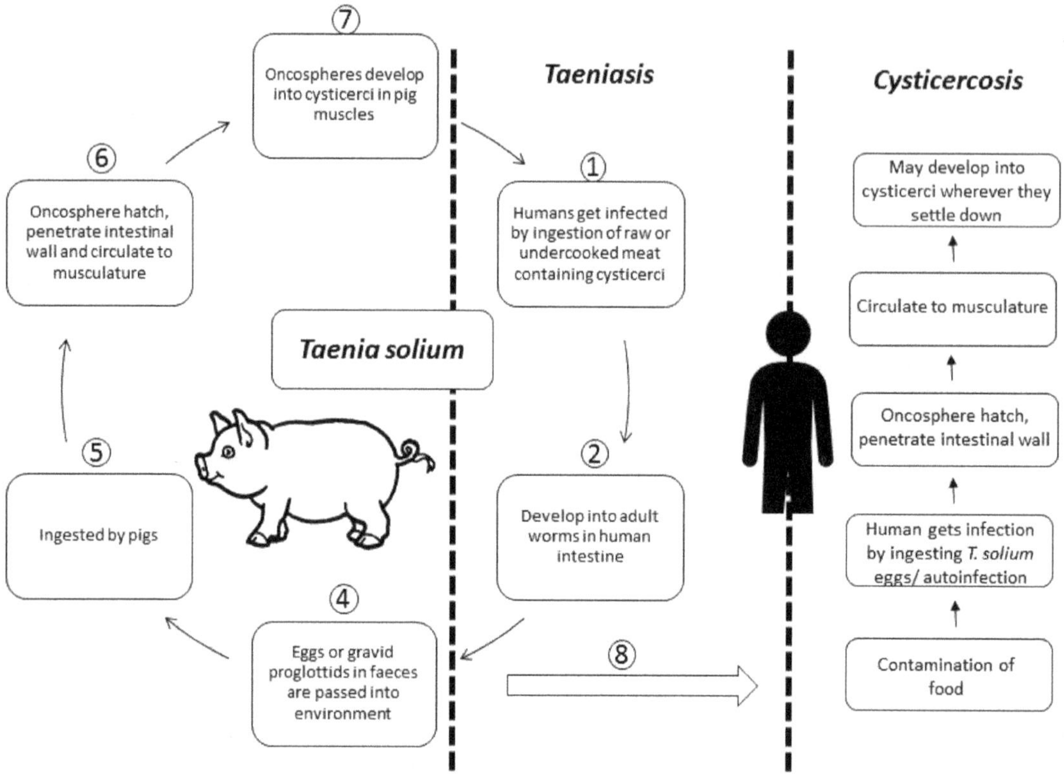

Figure 17. Life cycle of *Taenia solium* (Diagrammatic representation).

6. Cestodes infections

6.1. Cysticercosis

Cysticercosis is caused by the larval cysts of the tapeworm *Taenia solium.* Humans acquire cysticercosis infection by the consumption of food contaminated with the *Taenia solium* eggs, passed in feces of the infected humans, harboring the adult worms in their intestine as depicted in Figure 17 [216]. Autoinfection has also been reported in persons suffering from taeniasis that may result in cysticercosis. Eating of raw or uncooked pork results in adult worm infection, the taeniasis. It is considered as one of the important neglected parasitic infections (NPIs), prevalent in Asia, Africa and Latin America where poor sanitation conditions prevail (Figure 11) [217]. These larval cyst may lodge into different organs/tissues (brain, muscles, eyes or other tissues) [218], resulting in varying clinical symptoms.

Ocular involvement is well documented and several case reports have documented the orbital, intraocular, subretinal and optic nerve involvement due to cysticercosis [219, 220]. Free-floating cyst can be found in vitreous or anterior chamber of the eye. Cranial nerve or intra-ocular muscles lesions may result in gaze palsies [221–223].

Diagnosis is usually established by ophthalmoscopic examination along with imaging evidence of ultrasonography, CT scan or MRI scan. Although serology is easy to perform, it is usually negative in isolated ocular cysticercosis patient [224]. Molecular techniques such as

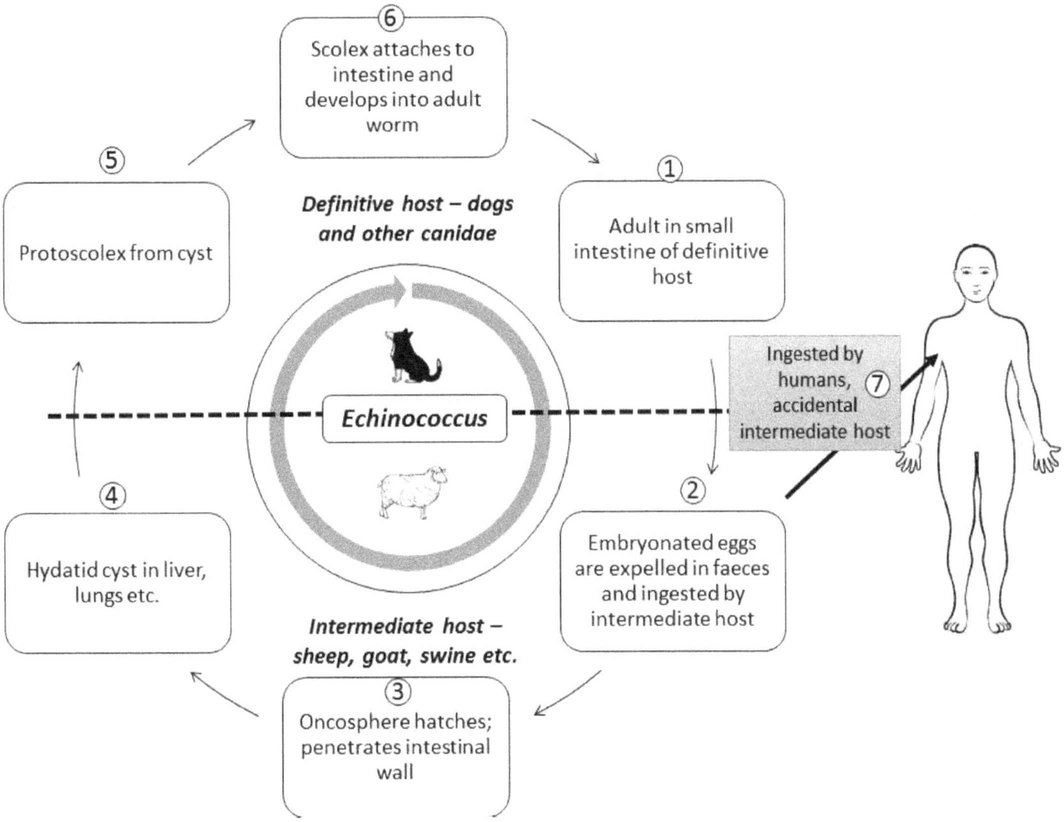

Figure 18. Life cycle of *Echinococcus* (Diagrammatic representation).

conventional PCR, real-time PCR [218] and loop-mediated isothermal amplification (LAMP) [225] can be utilized for establishing the diagnosis of ocular cysticercosis and for genotyping [30, 226]. However, it requires a sophisticated molecular laboratory setup, which is not available widely in developing nations.

Without treatment, symptoms related to visual disturbances persist. Symptoms resolve with surgical and medical treatment [227]. Albendazole along with steroids are the main drugs used in the treatment. Steroid treatment decreases the inflammatory response associated with the antihelminthic therapy around the lesions. Surgical removal of large cysts is recommended where there is an impairment of the vision [224].

6.2. Echinococcosis

Echinococcosis/hydatidosis is caused by infection of the larval stages of the *Echinococcus* spp [228], and ocular manifestations occur approximately in 1% of the cases suffering from hydatid disease [229]. Echinococcosis is mainly found in Asia, Africa, Latin America, Russia, Australia and the Mediterranean regions (Figure 11) [230]. It is acquired by the consumption of contaminated food and water with fecal matter containing eggs of *Echinococcus* parasites. The life cycle includes development of adult worms in small bowel of definitive hosts such as dogs and other canids. Eggs are passed in feces and contaminate environment as shown in Figure 18.

The symptoms and signs depend on the location of the cyst in the target organ. Most common ocular finding is the development of proptosis due to the presence of intraorbital space occupying lesion. This may further lead to exposure to keratitis and ulceration of the cornea. Other complications due to the local invasion of the expanding cyst may lead to erosion of orbital wall, optic atrophy and optic neuritis. Subretinal hydatid cyst has been reported. In severe cases, blindness may also occur [231].

The diagnosis depends on the clinical findings suggestive of hydatid cyst on ocular examination and confirmed by radiological techniques such as ultrasonography, CT scan and/or MRI [232, 233]. "Double wall" sign is a characteristic of orbital hydatid cyst seen by ultrasonography [232]. Serology may also aid in diagnosis. However, in majority of the commercially and in-house serological assays, hydatid fluid is the main antigenic component and sensitivity of IgG-ELISA reported in various studies varies from 64.8 to 100%, while specificity varies from 87.5 to 100%. Purified and recombinant antigens are also being tried for developing ELISA with high sensitivity and specificity [234]. Fine needle aspiration cytology can also be performed for establishing the diagnosis [235].

Symptoms persist if not treated [236]. Surgical removal of the cyst is the treatment of choice. Medical therapy includes administration of albendazole or mebendazole to prevent the recurrences due to the contents of the cyst leaking into the surgical sites [237]. If the cyst is accidently ruptured, in situ irrigation with hypertonic saline should be performed. However, it causes local inflammatory reaction that may lead to atrophy of optic nerve [238].

7. Trematodes infections

7.1. Fascioliasis

Fascioliasis is a food-borne parasitic infection caused by trematodes that mainly affect liver. It is acquired by eating metacercaria of *Fasciola hepatica* encysted on leaves that are eaten raw. Two important species are *Fasciola hepatica* and *F. gigantica*. The life cycle includes release of eggs from adult flukes that further develop into miracidia, sporocysts, rediae, cercariae and metacercariae as shown in Figure 19. The parasite passes its life cycle in two different hosts: sheep, goat, cattle and man act as definitive host and snails of the genus *Lymnaea* act as intermediate host. The eggs are passed out in the feces of definitive hosts that mature in water. Ciliated miracidium develops inside each egg in 2–3 weeks. Miracidium after getting released from egg finds its way to its suitable intermediate host. Inside the lymph spaces of the molluscan host, the miracidium passes through stages of sporocyst, two generations of rediae and finally to the stage of cercariae. The mature cercariae escape from the snail into the water and encyst (metacercariae) in blades of grass or water-cress, which is ingested by herbivorous animals and occasionally by man. On entering the digestive tract, the metacercariae excyst in the duodenum and migrate through intestinal wall into peritoneal cavity. It further traverses through liver capsule, parenchyma and ultimately settle in the biliary passages, where it mature into adults. The eggs are liberated in the feces through bile, completing the life cycle.

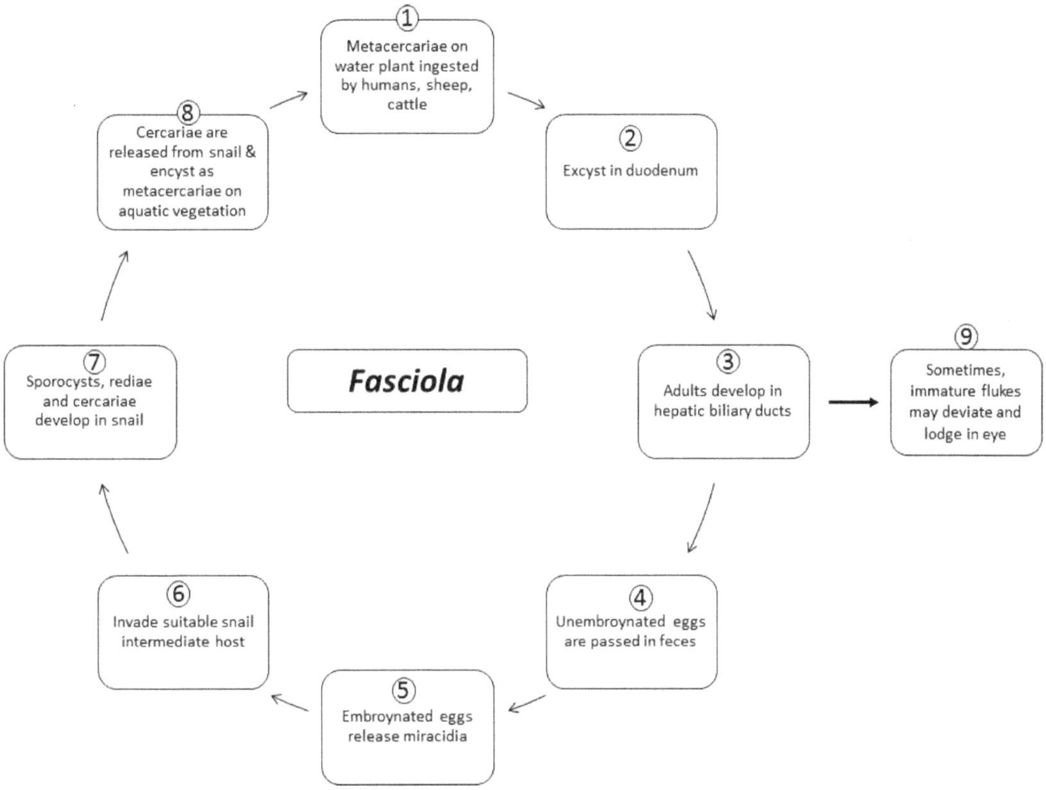

Figure 19. Life cycle of *Fasciola* (Diagrammatic representation).

Opthalmofascioliasis is the term used for those cases in which eye infection is directly caused by migrant ectopic fasciolid fluke. All other patients with ocular manifestations due to fasciolids located in liver or other organs should be classified as fascioliasis with ocular implications. Although ocular involvement in fascioliasis is rare, cases have been reported from France, Spain, Italy, Austria, Belgium, United Kingdom, Algeria, Tunisia, Iran, Uzbekistan, Korea, China, Argentina, Chile, Peru, Brazil and Guatemala (Figure 20) [239]. Symptoms and signs usually relate to the affected eye and may cause conjunctival hyperaemia, corneal oedema, dilated episcleral vessels, paralysis of extraocular muscles, decrease in perception of light, deep anterior chamber with flare, uveitis and so on. Diagnosis is established directly by visualization of leaf-shaped like organism in the eye or by studying the morphological features of the surgically removed worm. Eosinophilia, positive serology by ELISA or presence of eggs in stools may aid in diagnosis. Severe complications may occur if not treated. Early surgical intervention is associated with rapid response and reasonable final visual acuity [14]. Thus, ophthalmological manifestations have been known to be cured with surgical treatment without any antiparasitic treatment [14]. However, triclabendazole is the drug of choice if medical treatment is required.

7.2. Schistosomiasis

Schistosomiasis, or bilharziasis, is caused by trematode flatworm of the genus *Schistosoma*. Freshwater snails release the larval forms in the water, which penetrate the skin of human host

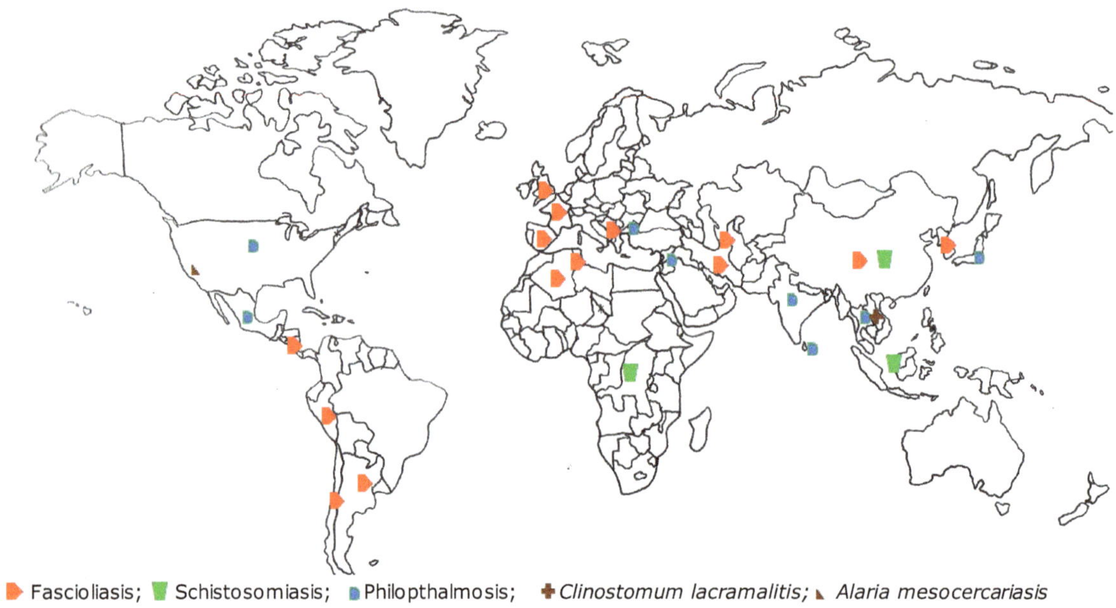

Figure 20. World map showing geographical areas endemic for ocular trematode infections.

while swimming, bathing, fishing and even domestic chores such as laundry and herding livestock. In the human body, the larvae mature into adult schistosomes, which reside in the blood vessels. Eggs released by females are passed out of the body in the urine or feces. It is prevalent in sub-Saharan Africa, China and South Asia (Figure 20) [8].

Ocular involvement is not the usual site that is involved in schistosomiasis, but cases have been reported where Schistosoma ova or even the adult worm can reach the systemic circulation and can lodge itself at ectopic sites such as eyes. Although schistosomiasis is very common, ocular cases are rare. It can cause uveitis or subretinal granuloma [240]. Diagnosis is established by direct demonstration of eggs/cercariae in the eye. Detection of eggs in the urine and feces may aid in establishing the diagnosis. Symptoms persist if not treated. Praziquantel is the drug of choice for all forms of schistosomiasis [8].

7.3. Other rare ocular infections by trematodes

The cases of acute nodular conjunctivitis and anterior chamber granuloma formation have been documented, which are caused by endemic water-borne trematode infection. The identification of the remnants of parasites aspirated from such cases revealed that these parasites belong to the genus *Philophthalmus* that are known to parasitize birds [25, 241]. Humans acquire infection accidently while bathing or playing in contaminated water. Conjunctival nodules heal spontaneously, and anterior chamber nodules can be treated with topical/oral corticosteroids. Surgical removal is recommended in cases having large nodules. First human case of *Clinostomum* lacramalitis was reported in Thailand [242]. Human cases of intraocular infection with mesocercariae of *Alaria americana* and other *Alaria* mesocercariae have been reported in patients who had ingested undercooked contaminated frogs legs [243].

8. Eye infections caused by ectoparasites

8.1. Myiasis

Myiasis is an infection caused by larvae of flies. It is common in tropical and subtropical areas. It is known as ophthalmomyiasis when ocular structures are involved. Ophthalmomyiasis is categorized into three clinical categories (ophthalmomyiasis externa, ophthalmomyiasis interna and orbital myiasis), depending on the location of larvae in the eyes. Several genera have been reported to cause myiasis such as *Dermatobia, Gasterophilus, Oestra, Cordylobia, Chrysomyia, Wohlfahrtia, Cochliomyia* and *Hypoderma* [1]. Significantly, larvae causing ophthalmomyiasis belong to the genus *Hypoderma* [16]. *Three cases of external* ophthalmomyiasis, two due to *Oestrus ovis and one due to Cochliomyia hominivorax* were reported earlier from North India [17]. *Oestra ovis* also known as sheep nasal botfly is responsible for causing ophthalmomyiasis externa in shepherding areas [244–247]. It mainly involves eyelids, conjunctiva, lacrimal sac and nasolacrimal ducts. Most common clinical feature is the foreign body sensation and may be associated with conjunctivitis and keratitis.

Diagnosis is established by the identification of the maggots. Treatment usually involves the surgical removal of the maggots. Medical treatment involves just one oral dose (150 to 200 μg/kg of body weight) of ivermectin [16]. However, the use of ivermectin for the treatment of myiasis is an off-label treatment in many countries and should be used for selected cases. The side effects such as dermal eruptions, fever, dizziness, migraines and muscular pains are common. Antibiotics and steroids may also be required to prevent the inflammation and superadded bacterial infection. Opthalmomyiasis interna [248] is caused by the invasion of the ocular structures leading to uveitis, lens dislocation and retinal detachment. Diagnosis is established by visualizing the migratory tracks along subretina by the ophthalmoscopy. Symptoms persist if not treated. Serious complications may also occur such as lens dislocation and retinal detachment due to invasion of tissue [1]. Steroid therapy is advocated if there is severe inflammation, and surgical removal is performed in severe cases. Orbital myiasis is seen in patients who are not able to maintain good personal hygiene [16]. Treatment is directed at removal of maggots and control of secondary infection. Preventive measures include maintenance of good sanitation conditions and proper disposal of waste material to control the flies in surrounding areas.

8.2. Lice

Important genera of the lice causing human infestation belong to *Pediculus* and *Phthirus*. Geographical areas where *Phthiriasis palpebrarum* is commonly found have been depicted in Table 1 and Figure 21. Eggs or nits laid down by lice glue themselves to body hairs or clothing fibers. Nymphs emerge from eggs and feed on the host, causing pruritis. Eyebrows and eyelashes are most commonly, involved. Excoriation marks along with small erythematous papules aid in diagnosis. Nits can be found at the base of eyelashes, substantiating the clinical diagnosis. Symptoms persist if not treated. Eyelid disease is treated by petrolatum and non-eyelid involvement may be treated with lindane, permethrin, pyrethrin or malathion [1].

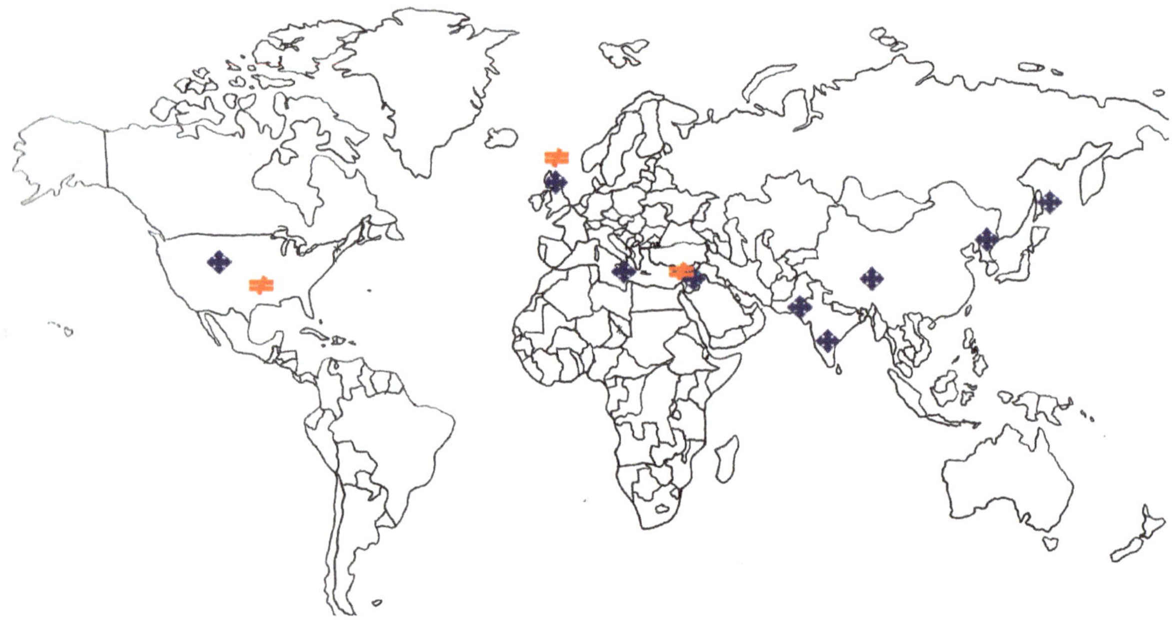

Figure 21. World map showing geographical areas endemic for ocular ectoparasites. *Phthiriasis palpebrarum*; Tick infestation.

8.3. Ticks

Ticks belonging to the class Arachnida are important vectors for the transmission of several infections to humans [1]. Geographical regions where ticks' infestation has been reported are depicted in Table 1 and Figure 21. Ticks complete their life cycle in three different stages, i.e. larva, nymph and adult, and all the life cycle stages require blood meals. Ticks have been reported to attach to ocular structures that may appear as meibomian gland mass. Symptoms persist if not treated. Treatment includes removal of ticks, and tick bite granuloma may resolve after several weeks.

9. Summary

Ocular parasitic infections are of medical importance worldwide because of significant morbidity rates, and if not diagnosed and treated on time could lead to vision loss. High index of clinical suspicion is required to establish the diagnosis for further confirmation by laboratory techniques followed by specific treatment. Direct demonstration of the parasite is possible in few ocular parasitic infections, while in few, specific clinical features such as changes in retina on direct ocular examination may point toward specific diagnosis. Serology has limited role in the diagnosis as most of the ocular parasitic infections are localized in the eye. Utility of different diagnostic techniques in various parasitic ocular infections has been summarized in Table 2. Although reports reveal that the serology for antibody detection and/or molecular techniques for parasite DNA detection, when applied directly on the ocular tissues, aqueous or vitreous humor usually confirm the diagnosis, these techniques have its own merits and demerits. IgG immunoblot technique has been applied for the diagnosis of ocular toxoplasmosis with some success, and it is suggested that local antibody production is presumed to have occurred, if immunoreactive bands are detected in the aqueous humor but not in the serum [249]. Future reports in this direction may throw further light on its utility. Moreover, application of Western blotting technique may be possible only in limited diagnostic centers.

Report on "Diagnostic Approach to Ocular Toxoplasmosis" revealed in conclusion that the clinical diagnosis of ocular toxoplasmosis may be supported by laboratory tests in 60–85% of cases, depending on the time of sampling. Analysis of the aqueous humor is particularly helpful in patients with atypical lesions or in individuals who are irresponsive to specific therapy. Even so, a laboratory confirmation of the clinical diagnosis is not achieved in 15–40% of cases [72].

In general, it can be concluded that the clinical awareness and multiple approaches/techniques for the confirmatory diagnosis of clinically suspected ocular parasitic infections may yield higher sensitivity and diagnostic efficacy, as suggested earlier [250].

Treatment depends on the causative agent and may involve surgical removal and/or medical treatment with antiparasitic drugs (Table 2). In few infections, steroids are also prescribed to prevent the damage from the inflammatory response associated with the dying parasites. Preventive strategies depend on the type of parasitic infection and mainly include control of vector population for vector borne parasitic infections, maintenance of good personal hygiene and providing awareness to people about ocular parasitic infections through information, education and communication (IEC).

The need of increased awareness and clinical suspicion of OPI for prompt and specific diagnosis followed by application of sensitive and specific diagnostic technique(s) for confirmation and effective treatment are the main challenges.

The future research priorities need to be directed to study exact host-pathogen mechanisms, local immune responses and to establish more sensitive and specific diagnostic techniques. The molecular techniques can provide rapid diagnosis of multiple ocular parasitic infections and species identification for specific therapy. Multiplex PCR assay, if developed, can add new dimensions in the diagnosis. Efforts to develop animal models are desired that may further help to study the exact host-pathogen mechanisms, local immune responses and in developing new treatment strategies.

Ocular protozoal infections	Diagnosis	Treatment
Toxoplasmosis	Serology – IgM, IgG, IgA Molecular: PCR, Real-time PCR	a. Pyrimethamine and sulfadiazine plus corticosteroids b. Trimethoprim/sulfamethoxazole plus oral prednisolone c. Intravitreal clindamycin (1-1.5mg) injection and dexamethasone d. Surgery reserved for severe complicated cases

Ocular protozoal infections	**Diagnosis**	**Treatment**
Acanthamoeba keratitis	Microscopy, culture on non-nutrient plates (coated with bacteria)/ in flasks (PBS +Bacteria), PCR, Real-time PCR	a. Biguanides – PHMB (0.02%) b. Chlorhexidine 0.02% in combination with aromatic diamidines such as 0.1% propamidine isethionate, 0.15% dibromopropamidine, hexamidine 0.1% and neomycin (Topical antimicrobials should be administered every hourly for first several days and there after frequency reduced to every 3 hours with a minimum duration of therapy of 3-4 weeks c. Surgical treatment includes keratoplasty or its variation known as DALK (Deep Anterior Lamellar Keratoplasty)
Chagas disease	Blood smear, Buffy coat, culture, xenodiagnoses and PCR	a. Benznidazole 5-10 mg/kg daily in 2-3 divided doses for 60 days b. Nifurtimox 15 mg/kg daily in 3 divided doses for 60-90 days
Malaria	Thin and thick blood film for microscopy, antigen detection, PCR	a. *Plasmodium vivax* – Chloroquine + primaquine b. *P. falciparum* – Artemisinin combination therapy (Artemisinin + sulfadoxine-pyrimethamine or artemisinin + lumefantrine) as per WHO guidelines
Leishmaniasis	Microscopy of tissue smears, culture on NNN media, PCR	Pentavalent antimonial compounds, liposomal amphotericin B, miltefosine (dose is weight dependent), paromomycin, azoles such as ketoconazole, itraconazole and fluconazole
Microsporidiosis	Microscopy, Immunofluorescence assay, PCR	Topical fumagillin bicylohexylammonium (Fumidil B) 3 mg/mL in saline (fumagillin 70 μg/mL) eye drops: two drops every 2 hours for 4 days, then two drops four times daily (investigational use only in United States) plus albendazole 400 mg orally twice daily for management of systemic infection.
Giardiasis	Confirming by intestinal infection	Metronidazole, tinidazole, and nitazoxanide. Others include paromomycin, quinacrine, and furazolidone
Ocular nematode infections		
Onchocerciasis	Slit-lamp examination, Biopsy of skin to identify larvae, skin nodules examination for identification of adult worms, PCR, antibody detection	a. Ivermectin: given every 6 months for the life span of the adult worm or as long as infected person has evidence of skin or eye infection b. New treatment: Doxycycline, before starting treatment infection with *Loa loa* has to be ruled out c. Removal of adult worms

Ocular protozoal infections	Diagnosis	Treatment
Loiasis		a. Surgical removal of the worm under the skin or across the eye b. Diethylcarbamazine (DEC) is the drug of choice c. Albendazole is given to patients not responding to DEC
Dirofilariasis		a. Surgical removal of the worm b. DEC is given for medical treatment
Gnathostomiasis	Identification of the removed worm Serology to detect antibodies	a. Surgical removal of worm
Thelaziasis	b. Identification of worm removed from conjunctival sac c. Eggs and larvae may be seen by microscopy of tears and other eye secretions	Removal of worm
Toxocariasis	Histological demonstration of toxocara larva Serology by ELISA	d. Topical and systemic corticosteroids are useful in managing intraocular inflammation e. Role of anthelmintic therapy in ocular toxocariasis remains unclear f. Recommended drugs for systemic toxocariasis are: g. Albendazole 400mg given twice daily for 7-14 days h. Diethylcarbamazine - given at 3-4 mg/kg/day for 21 days
Ocular cestode infections		
Cysticercosis	Imaging with MRI, CT scan and USG Serology	a. Antiparasitic drugs – Albendazole 15mg/kg/day for 4 weeks, Praziquantel b. Corticosteroids in tapering dose over a period of 1 month c. Surgery
Echinococcosis	Imaging	a. Surgical removal b. Albendazole is given as an anti-infective prophylaxis
Ocular trematode infections		
Fascioliasis	Detection of adult worm in the eye Other features such as eosinophilia, stool examination and serology may help	a. Surgical removal of worm b. Triclabendazole 10mg/kg body weight as a single dose

Ocular protozoal infections	Diagnosis	Treatment
Schistosomiasis	Stool and urine examination for detection of parasitic eggs or detection of eggs or cercariae in eye Serology	Praziquantel 40-60mg/kg per day in two to three divided doses for one day
Philopthalmosis	Identification of the remnants of parasites aspirated from such cases	a. Conjunctival nodules heal spontaneously and anterior chamber nodules can be treated with topical/ oral corticosteroids. b. Surgical removal is recommended in cases having large nodules
Ocular infections by ectoparasites		
Myiasis	a. Identification of the maggots b. Visualizing the migratory tracks along sub retina	a. Surgical removal of the maggots b. Ivermectin 150-200 μg/kg of body weight in single dose c. Steroid therapy
Phthiriasis palpebrum	a. Excoriation marks along with small erythematous papules b. Nits can be found at the base of eyelashes	a. Eyelid disease is treated by petrolatum b. Non-eyelid involvement may be treated with lindane, permethrin, pyrethin or malathion
Tick infestation	Biomicroscopy may reveal ticks	Removal of ticks

Table 2. Diagnosis and treatment of various ocular parasitic infections

Author details

Nancy Malla* and Kapil Goyal

*Address all correspondence to: drmallanancy@gmail.com

Department of Medical Parasitology, Postgraduate Institute of Medical Education and Research, Chandigarh, India

References

[1] Klotz SA, Penn CC, Negvesky GJ, Butrus SI. Fungal and parasitic infections of the eye. Clinical microbiology reviews. 2000;13(4):662-85.

[2] Chawla A, Armstrong M, Carley F. Acanthamoeba keratitis – an increasing incidence. Contact lens & anterior eye : the journal of the British Contact Lens Association. 2014;37(2):120.

[3] Lorenzo-Morales J, Martin-Navarro CM, Lopez-Arencibia A, Arnalich-Montiel F, Pinero JE, Valladares B. Acanthamoeba keratitis: an emerging disease gathering importance worldwide? Trends in parasitology. 2013;29(4):181-7.

[4] Montoya JG, Liesenfeld O. Toxoplasmosis. Lancet. 2004;363(9425):1965-76.

[5] Sharma S, Pasricha G, Das D, Aggarwal RK. Acanthamoeba keratitis in non-contact lens wearers in India: DNA typing-based validation and a simple detection assay. Archives of ophthalmology. 2004;122(10):1430-4.

[6] Gopinathan U, Sharma S, Garg P, Rao GN. Review of epidemiological features, microbiological diagnosis and treatment outcome of microbial keratitis: experience of over a decade. Indian journal of ophthalmology. 2009;57(4):273-9.

[7] Sharma S, Garg P, Rao GN. Patient characteristics, diagnosis, and treatment of non-contact lens related Acanthamoeba keratitis. The British journal of ophthalmology. 2000;84(10):1103-8.

[8] Nimir AR, Saliem A, Ibrahim IA. Ophthalmic parasitosis: a review article. Interdisciplinary Perspectives on Infectious Diseases. 2012;2012:587402.

[9] Joseph J, Vemuganti GK, Sharma S. Microsporidia: emerging ocular pathogens. Indian journal of medical microbiology. 2005;23(2):80-91.

[10] Malla N, Aggarwal AK, Mahajan RC. A serological study of human toxocariasis in north India. The National medical journal of India. 2002;15(3):145-7.

[11] Fomda BA, Ahmad Z, Khan NN, Tanveer S, Wani SA. Ocular toxocariasis in a child: a case report from Kashmir, north India. Indian journal of medical microbiology. 2007;25(4):411-2.

[12] Prabhakar SK, Vijaykumar GS, Mahesh BS, Shanthamallappa. Human ocular thelaziasis: a case report from Karnataka. Indian journal of medical microbiology. 2015;33(2):324-5.

[13] Sachdeva RS, Manchanda SK, Abrol S, Wadhwa SC, Ramachandran KA. Freely mobile cysticercus in the anterior chamber. Indian journal of ophthalmology. 1995;43(3): 135-6.

[14] Dalimi A, Jabarvand M. Fasciola hepatica in the human eye. Transactions of the Royal Society of Tropical Medicine and Hygiene. 2005;99(10):798-800.

[15] Joshi G, Parchand S, Dogra MR, Gupta PK, Khurana S, Gupta V, et al. Live juvenile strobilate tapeworm in the anterior chamber of the human eye. Archives of ophthalmology. 2012;130(11):1464-6.

[16] Francesconi F, Lupi O. Myiasis. Clinical microbiology reviews. 2012;25(1):79-105.

[17] Khurana S, Biswal M, Bhatti HS, Pandav SS, Gupta A, Chatterjee SS, et al. Ophthalmomyiasis: three cases from North India. Indian journal of medical microbiology. 2010;28(3):257-61.

[18] Sulyok M, Rozsa L, Bodo I, Tappe D, Hardi R. Ocular pentastomiasis in the Democratic Republic of the Congo. PLoS neglected tropical diseases. 2014;8(7):e3041.

[19] Tan SY, Liu SW, Jiang SB. HIV/AIDS and ocular complications. International Journal of Ophthalmology. 2009;2(2):95-105.

[20] Couture S, Agrawal R, Woods K, Lockwood D, Pavesio CE, Addison PKF. A case of panuveitis with hypopyon due to presumed ocular leishmaniasis in a HIV patient. Journal of Opthalmic Inflammation and Infection. 2014;4(21):1-5.

[21] Bacon AS, Dart JK, Ficker LA, Matheson MM, Wright P. Acanthamoeba keratitis. The value of early diagnosis. Ophthalmology. 1993;100(8):1238-43.

[22] Lalitha P, Lin CC, Srinivasan M, Mascarenhas J, Prajna NV, Keenan JD, et al. Acanthamoeba keratitis in South India: a longitudinal analysis of epidemics. Ophthalmic Epidemiology. 2012;19(2):111-5.

[23] Lowder CY. Ocular microsporidiosis. International ophthalmology clinics. 1993;33(1):145-51.

[24] Lim SJ, Lee SE, Kim SH, Hong SH, You YS, Kwon OW, et al. Prevalence of Toxoplasma gondii and Toxocara canis among patients with uveitis. Ocular immunology and inflammation. 2014;22(5):360-6.

[25] Otranto D, Eberhard ML. Zoonotic helminths affecting the human eye. Parasites & vectors. 2011;4:41.

[26] Hirst LW. Ocular infections – diagnosis. Australian family physician. 1991;20(2): 133-4, 7-45, 49.

[27] Rao NA. A laboratory approach to rapid diagnosis of ocular infections and prospects for the future. American journal of ophthalmology. 1989;107(3):283-91.

[28] Khurana S, Singh G, Bhatti HS, Malla N. Human subcutaneous dirofilariasis in India: a report of three cases with brief review of literature. Indian journal of medical microbiology. 2010;28(4):394-6.

[29] Cortez RT, Ramirez G, Collet L, Giuliari GP. Ocular parasitic diseases: a review on toxocariasis and diffuse unilateral subacute neuroretinitis. Journal of pediatric ophthalmology and strabismus. 2011;48(4):204-12.

[30] Sharma M, Beke N, Khurana S, Bhatti HS, Sehgal R, Malla N. An Ocular cysticercosis case: caused by Asian Genotype of Taenia solium. Indian journal of Medical Microbiology. 2015;33(4)583-585.

[31] Hogan RN, Jakobiec FA. Molecular pathological diagnosis of ocular infections. International ophthalmology clinics. 1996;36(3):223-46.

[32] Rathinam SR, Annamalai R, Biswas J. Intraocular parasitic infections. Ocular immunology and inflammation. 2011;19(5):327-36.

[33] Pasricha G, Sharma S, Garg P, Aggarwal RK. Use of 18S rRNA gene-based PCR assay for diagnosis of acanthamoeba keratitis in non-contact lens wearers in India. Journal of Clinical Microbiology. 2003;41(7):3206-11.

[34] Basu S, Sharma S, Kar S, Das T. DNA chip-assisted diagnosis of a previously unknown etiology of intermediate uveitis – Toxoplasma gondii. Indian journal of ophthalmology. 2010;58(6):535-7.

[35] Sharma S. Diagnosis of infectious diseases of the eye. Eye. 2012;26(2):177-84.

[36] Rathinam SR, Arya LK, Usha KR, Prajna L, Tandon V. Novel etiological agent: molecular evidence for trematode-induced anterior uveitis in children. Archives of ophthalmology. 2012;130(11):1481-4.

[37] Nath R, Gogoi R, Bordoloi N, Gogoi T. Ocular dirofilariasis. Indian journal of Pathology & Microbiology. 2010;53(1):157-9.

[38] Pushker N, Bajaj MS, Chandra M, Neena. Ocular and orbital cysticercosis. Acta ophthalmologica Scandinavica. 2001;79(4):408-13.

[39] Gomez Morales A, Croxatto JO, Crovetto L, Ebner R. Hydatid cysts of the orbit. A review of 35 cases. Ophthalmology. 1988;95(8):1027-32.

[40] Malla N, Goyal M, Pillai P, Ganguly NK, Mahajan RC. Experimental ocular toxoplasmosis with RH strain of Toxoplasma gondii. Japanese journal of experimental medicine. 1988;58(6):279-81.

[41] Takayanagi TH, Akao N, Suzuki R, Tomoda M, Tsukidate S, Fujita K. New animal model for human ocular toxocariasis: ophthalmoscopic observation. The British journal of ophthalmology. 1999;83(8):967-72.

[42] Malhotra A, Minja FJ, Crum A, Burrowes D. Ocular anatomy and cross-sectional imaging of the eye. Semin Ultrasound CT MR. 2011;32(1):2-13.

[43] Kaplan HJ. Anatomy and function of the eye. Chemical Immunology and Allergy. 2007;92:4-10.

[44] Paalman MH. Anatomy in the eye. Anatomical Record. 2000;261(6):221.

[45] Kolb H. Gross Anatomy of the Eye. 2005 May 1 [Updated 2007 May 1]. In: Kolb H, Fernandez E, Nelson R, editors. Webvision: The Organization of the Retina and Visual System [Internet]. Salt Lake City (UT): University of Utah Health Sciences Center; 1995. Available from: http://www.ncbi.nlm.nih.gov/books/NBK11534/

[46] Iveson-Iveson J. Anatomy and physiology: the eye. Nursing Mirror. 1979;148(8):31-3.

[47] Shitole S, Jakkal T, Khaire B. Inverse Bell's phenomenon: rare ophthalmic finding following ptosis surgery. Journal of clinical and diagnostic research: JCDR. 2015;9(3):ND01-2.

[48] Kageyama M, Nakatsuka K, Yamaguchi T, Owen RL, Shimada T. Ocular defense mechanisms with special reference to the demonstration and functional morphology of the conjunctiva-associated lymphoid tissue in Japanese monkeys. Archives of Histology and Cytology. 2006;69(5):311-22.

[49] Lerman S. Free radical damage and defense mechanisms in the ocular lens. Lens and eye toxicity research. 1992;9(1):9-24.

[50] Bito LZ. Species differences in the responses of the eye to irritation and trauma: a hypothesis of divergence in ocular defense mechanisms, and the choice of experimental animals for eye research. Experimental Eye Research. 1984;39(6):807-29.

[51] Chandler JW, Gillette TE. Immunologic defense mechanisms of the ocular surface. Ophthalmology. 1983;90(6):585-91.

[52] Lemp MA, Blackman HJ. Ocular surface defense mechanisms. Annals of ophthalmology. 1981;13(1):61-3.

[53] McDermott AM. Defensins and other antimicrobial peptides at the ocular surface. The ocular surface. 2004;2(4):229-47.

[54] Cunningham ET, Jr., Belfort R, Jr., Muccioli C, Arevalo JF, Zierhut M. Ocular toxoplasmosis. Ocular immunology and inflammation. 2015;23(3):191-3.

[55] Kijlstra A, Petersen E. Epidemiology, pathophysiology, and the future of ocular toxoplasmosis. Ocular immunology and inflammation. 2014;22(2):138-47.

[56] Robert-Gangneux F, Darde ML. Epidemiology of and diagnostic strategies for toxoplasmosis. Clinical microbiology reviews. 2012;25(2):264-96.

[57] Petersen E, Kijlstra A, Stanford M. Epidemiology of ocular toxoplasmosis. Ocular immunology and inflammation. 2012;20(2):68-75.

[58] Ho-Yen DO. Epidemiology of toxoplasmosis. Archives of pediatrics. 2003;10(Suppl 1): 3-4.

[59] Lachenmaier SM, Deli MA, Meissner M, Liesenfeld O. Intracellular transport of Toxoplasma gondii through the blood-brain barrier. Journal of neuroimmunology. 2011;232(1-2):119-30.

[60] Peixoto-Rangel AL, Miller EN, Castellucci L, Jamieson SE, Peixe RG, Elias Lde S, et al. Candidate gene analysis of ocular toxoplasmosis in Brazil: evidence for a role for toll-like receptor 9 (TLR9). Memorias do Instituto Oswaldo Cruz. 2009;104(8):1187-90.

[61] Pleyer U, Schluter D, Manz M. Ocular toxoplasmosis: recent aspects of pathophysiology and clinical implications. Ophthalmic Research. 2014;52(3):116-23.

[62] Holland GN. Ocular toxoplasmosis: a global reassessment. Part II: disease manifestations and management. American journal of ophthalmology. 2004;137(1):1-17.

[63] O'Connor GR. Manifestations and management of ocular toxoplasmosis. Bulletin of the New York Academy of Medicine. 1974;50(2):192-210.

[64] Park YH, Nam HW. Clinical features and treatment of ocular toxoplasmosis. The Korean journal of parasitology. 2013;51(4):393-9.

[65] Harper TW, Miller D, Schiffman JC, Davis JL. Polymerase chain reaction analysis of aqueous and vitreous specimens in the diagnosis of posterior segment infectious uveitis. American journal of ophthalmology. 2009;147(1):140-7 e2.

[66] Cassaing S, Bessieres MH, Berry A, Berrebi A, Fabre R, Magnaval JF. Comparison between two amplification sets for molecular diagnosis of toxoplasmosis by real-time PCR. Journal of Clinical Microbiology. 2006;44(3):720-4.

[67] Robert-Gangneux F, Sterkers Y, Yera H, Accoceberry I, Menotti J, Cassaing S, et al. Molecular diagnosis of toxoplasmosis in immunocompromised patients: a 3-year multicenter retrospective study. Journal of Clinical Microbiology. 2015;53(5):1677-84.

[68] Filisetti D, Sterkers Y, Brenier-Pinchart MP, Cassaing S, Dalle F, Delhaes L, et al. Multicentric comparative assessment of the bio-evolution Toxoplasma gondii detection kit with eight laboratory-developed PCR assays for molecular diagnosis of congenital toxoplasmosis. Journal of Clinical Microbiology. 2015;53(1):29-34.

[69] Hashoosh DA, Majeed IA. Comparison of two assays in the diagnosis of toxoplasmosis: immunological and molecular. Eastern Mediterranean Health Journal. 2014;20(1): 46-50.

[70] Remington JS, Thulliez P, Montoya JG. Recent developments for diagnosis of toxoplasmosis. Journal of Clinical Microbiology. 2004;42(3):941-5.

[71] Bou G, Figueroa MS, Marti-Belda P, Navas E, Guerrero A. Value of PCR for detection of Toxoplasma gondii in aqueous humor and blood samples from immunocompetent patients with ocular toxoplasmosis. Journal of Clinical Microbiology. 1999;37(11): 3465-8.

[72] Garweg JG, de Groot-Mijnes JD, Montoya JG. Diagnostic approach to ocular toxoplasmosis. Ocular Immunology and Inflammation. 2011;19(4):255-61.

[73] Khurana S, Bagga R, Aggarwal A, Lyngdoh V, Shivapriya, Diddi K, et al. Serological screening for antenatal toxoplasma infection in India. Indian Journal of Medical Microbiology. 2010;28(2):143-6.

[74] Singh MP, Dubey ML, Sud A, Malla N. Antibody response to Toxoplasma gondii in saliva samples from human immunodeficiency virus-infected patients. British Journal of Biomedical Science. 2005;62(2):81-4.

[75] Zargar AH, Masoodi SR, Laway BA, Sofi BA, Wani AI. Seroprevalence of toxoplasmosis in women with repeated abortions in Kashmir. Journal of Epidemiology & Community Health. 1998;52(2):135-6.

[76] Thokar MA, Malla N, Wattal C. Serological study of patients clinically suspected to have toxoplasmosis in Kashmir. Indian Journal of Medical Research. 1988;88:29-34.

[77] Delair E, Monnet D, Grabar S, Dupouy-Camet J, Yera H, Brezin AP. Respective roles of acquired and congenital infections in presumed ocular toxoplasmosis. American Journal of Ophthalmology. 2008;146(6):851-5.

[78] de Boer JH, Luyendijk L, Rothova A, Kijlstra A. Analysis of ocular fluids for local antibody production in uveitis. The British Journal of Ophthalmology. 1995;79(6):610-6.

[79] Garweg JG, Jacquier P, Boehnke M. Early aqueous humor analysis in patients with human ocular toxoplasmosis. Journal of Clinical Microbiology. 2000;38(3):996-1001.

[80] Lima GS, Saraiva PG, Saraiva FP. Current therapy of acquired ocular toxoplasmosis: a review. Journal of Ocular Pharmacology and Therapeutics : The Official Journal of the Association for Ocular Pharmacology and Therapeutics. 2015;31(9):511-7.

[81] Holland GN, Lewis KG. An update on current practices in the management of ocular toxoplasmosis. American Journal of Ophthalmology. 2002;134(1):102-14.

[82] Siddiqui R, Khan NA. Biology and pathogenesis of Acanthamoeba. Parasites & Vectors. 2012;5:6.

[83] Bharathi JM, Srinivasan M, Ramakrishnan R, Meenakshi R, Padmavathy S, Lalitha PN. A study of the spectrum of Acanthamoeba keratitis: a three-year study at a tertiary eye care referral center in South India. Indian Journal of Ophthalmology. 2007;55(1):37-42.

[84] Vaddavalli PK, Garg P, Sharma S, Sangwan VS, Rao GN, Thomas R. Role of confocal microscopy in the diagnosis of fungal and acanthamoeba keratitis. Ophthalmology. 2011;118(1):29-35.

[85] Winchester K, Mathers WD, Sutphin JE, Daley TE. Diagnosis of Acanthamoeba keratitis in vivo with confocal microscopy. Cornea. 1995;14(1):10-7.

[86] Goldschmidt P, Degorge S, Benallaoua D, Saint-Jean C, Batellier L, Alouch C, et al. New tool for the simultaneous detection of 10 different genotypes of Acanthamoeba available from the American Type Culture Collection. The British Journal of Ophthalmology. 2009;93(8):1096-100.

[87] Hauber S, Parkes H, Siddiqui R, Khan NA. The use of high-resolution (1)H nuclear magnetic resonance (NMR) spectroscopy in the clinical diagnosis of Acanthamoeba. Parasitology Research. 2011;109(6):1661-9.

[88] Lorenzo-Morales J, Khan NA, Walochnik J. An update on Acanthamoeba keratitis: diagnosis, pathogenesis and treatment. Parasite. 2015;22:10.

[89] Kumar R, Lloyd D. Recent advances in the treatment of Acanthamoeba keratitis. Clinical Infectious Diseases: An Official Publication of the Infectious Diseases Society of America. 2002;35(4):434-41.

[90] Grayson M. Chagas disease. Nature. 2010;465(7301):S3.

[91] Coura JR, Borges-Pereira J. Chagas disease: 100 years after its discovery. A systemic review. Acta Tropica. 2010;115(1-2):5-13.

[92] Frohlich SJ, Mino de Kaspar H, Peran R, Vera de Bilbao N, Schinini A, Rojas de Arias A, et al. Intraocular involvement of Chagas disease (American trypanosomiasis). Studies in Paraguay/South America. Der Ophthalmologe: Zeitschrift der Deutschen Ophthalmologischen Gesellschaft. 1997;94(3):206-10.

[93] Frohlich SJ, Mino de Kaspar H, Peran R, Rojas de Arias A, Sanchez Insfran N, Moreno Azorero R, et al. Eye involvement in Chagas disease (American trypanosomiasis). 1996/1997 studies in Paraguay. Der Ophthalmologe: Zeitschrift der Deutschen Ophthalmologischen Gesellschaft. 1998;95(3):168-71.

[94] Bern C. Chagas' disease. The New England Journal of Medicine. 2015;373(5):456-66.

[95] Morillo CA, Marin-Neto JA, Avezum A, Sosa-Estani S, Rassi A, Jr., Rosas F, et al. Randomized trial of benznidazole for chronic Chagas' cardiomyopathy. The New England Journal of Medicine. 2015;373(14):1295-306.

[96] Chagas disease. Available at http://www.nytimes.com/health/guides/disease/chagas-disease/overview.html

[97] Leishmaniasis. Available at: http://www.who.int/mediacentre/factsheets/fs375/en/

[98] Badri Prasad B, Shakya A, Poonam L, Smriti K. Caruncular Leishmaniasis – an unusual case. Orbit. 2015;34(4):232-3.

[99] Philips CA, Kalal CR, Kumar KN, Bihari C, Sarin SK. Simultaneous occurrence of ocular, disseminated mucocutaneous, and multivisceral involvement of leishmaniasis. Case Reports in Infectious Diseases. 2014;2014:837625.

[100] Khalil EA, Musa AM, Younis BM, Elfaki ME, Zijlstra EE, Elhassan AM. Blindness following visceral leishmaniasis: a neglected post-kala-azar complication. Tropical Doctor. 2011;41(3):139-40.

[101] Veraldi S, Bottini S, Curro N, Gianotti R. Leishmaniasis of the eyelid mimicking an infundibular cyst and review of the literature on ocular leishmaniasis. International Journal of Infectious Diseases: IJID: Official Publication of the International Society for Infectious Diseases. 2010;14(Suppl 3):e230-2.

[102] Salvanos P, Kabanarou SA, Xirou T, Kourentis C, Feretis E. Proliferative vitreoretinopathy in a child with visceral leishmaniasis. European Journal of Ophthalmology. 2010;20(1):231-3.

[103] Sadeghian G, Nilfroushzadeh MA, Moradi SH, Hanjani SH. Ocular leishmaniasis: a case report. Dermatology Online Journal. 2005;11(2):19.

[104] el-Hassan AM, el-Sheikh EA, Eltoum IA, Ghalib HW, Ali MS, Zijlstra E, et al. Post-kala-azar anterior uveitis: demonstration of Leishmania parasites in the lesion. Transactions of the Royal Society of Tropical Medicine and Hygiene. 1991;85(4):471-3.

[105] Dechant W, Rees PH, Kager PA, Klauss V, Adala H. Post kala-azar uveitis. The British Journal of Ophthalmology. 1980;64(9):680-3.

[106] De Cock KM, Rees PH, Klauss V, Kasili EG, Kager PA, Schattenkerk JK. Retinal hemorrhages in kala-azar. The American Journal of Tropical Medicine and Hygiene. 1982;31(5):927-30.

[107] Montero JA, Ruiz-Moreno JM, Sanchis E. Intraretinal hemorrhage associated with leishmaniasis. Ophthalmic Surgery, Lasers & Imaging: The Official Journal of the International Society for Imaging in the Eye. 2003;34(3):212-4.

[108] Biswas J, Mani B, Bhende M. Spontaneous resolution of bilateral macular haemorrhage in a patient with kala-azar. Eye. 2000;14(Pt 2):244-6.

[109] Mookerjee GC, Sen G, Chaudhuri MD, Chakraborty K. Acute kala-azar with haemorrhagic retinopathy. Journal of the Indian Medical Association. 1975;65(3):86-8.

[110] Maude RJ, Ahmed BU, Rahman AH, Rahman R, Majumder MI, Menezes DB, et al. Retinal changes in visceral leishmaniasis by retinal photography. BMC Infectious Diseases. 2014;14:527.

[111] Oliveira-Neto MP, Martins VJ, Mattos MS, Pirmez C, Brahin LR, Benchimol E. South American cutaneous leishmaniasis of the eyelids: report of five cases in Rio de Janeiro State, Brazil. Ophthalmology. 2000;107(1):169-72.

[112] Chaudhry IA, Hylton C, DesMarchais B. Bilateral ptosis and lower eyelid ectropion secondary to cutaneous leishmaniasis. Archives of Ophthalmology. 1998;116(9):1244-5.

[113] Yaghoobi R, Maraghi S, Bagherani N, Rafiei A. Cutaneous leishmaniasis of the lid: a report of nine cases. Korean Journal of Ophthalmology: KJO. 2010;24(1):40-3.

[114] Baddini-Caramelli C, Matayoshi S, Moura EM, Araf D, Santo R, Voegels R, et al. Chronic dacryocystitis in American mucocutaneous leishmaniasis. Ophthalmic Plastic and Reconstructive Surgery. 2001;17(1):48-52.

[115] Ferrari TC, Guedes AC, Orefice F, Genaro O, Pinheiro SR, Marra MA, et al. Isolation of Leishmania sp. from aqueous humor of a patient with cutaneous disseminated leishmaniasis and bilateral iridocyclitis (preliminary report). Revista do Instituto de Medicina Tropical de Sao Paulo. 1990;32(4):296-8.

[116] Petersen CA, Greenlee MH. Neurologic Manifestations of Leishmania spp. Infection. Journal of Neuroparasitology. 2011;2:N110401.

[117] Ozdemir Y, Kulacoglu S, Cosar CB, Onder F, Kural G. Ocular leishmaniasis. Eye. 1999;13(Pt 5):666-7.

[118] el Hassan AM, Khalil EA, el Sheikh EA, Zijlstra EE, Osman A, Ibrahim ME. Post kala-azar ocular leishmaniasis. Transactions of the Royal Society of Tropical Medicine and Hygiene. 1998;92(2):177-9.

[119] Leite RS, Souza NA, Barbosa AD, Ferreira AL, de Andrade AS. Evaluation of conjunctival swab as a mass-screening tool for molecular diagnosis of canine visceral leishmaniasis. Parasitology Research. 2015;114(6):2255-62.

[120] Shirian S, Oryan A, Hatam GR, Panahi S, Daneshbod Y. Comparison of conventional, molecular, and immunohistochemical methods in diagnosis of typical and atypical cutaneous leishmaniasis. Archives of Pathology & Laboratory Medicine. 2014;138(2): 235-40.

[121] Abrishami M, Soheilian M, Farahi A, Dowlati Y. Successful treatment of ocular leishmaniasis. European Journal of Dermatology: EJD. 2002;12(1):88-9.

[122] Zadeh MM, Manshai K, Shaddel M, Oormazdi H. Ocular leishmaniasis. Iranian Journal of Opthalmology. 2006;19(3):1-5.

[123] World Malaria Report. 2014 (Available at: http://www.who.int/malaria/publications/world_malaria_report_2014/en/).

[124] Sherwood JA. Progess toward understanding the pathogenesis of sequestration in falciparum malaria. Blood Cells. 1990;16(2-3):620-8.

[125] Sherwood JA, Roberts DD, Spitalnik SL, Marsh K, Harvey EB, Miller LH, et al. Parasitized erythrocyte antigens and thrombospondin adhesion in the immunology and pathogenesis of falciparum malaria. Transactions of the Association of American Physicians. 1986;99:206-13.

[126] Lagraulet J, Robet C, Bard J. The ocular complications of malaria. Bulletin de la Société de pathologie exotique. 1967;60(3):217-21.

[127] Bhattacharjya BP, Guha GS. Ocular manifestations in malaria. Indian Medical Gazette. 1946;81:79.

[128] Ross JV. Ocular complications associated with malaria. Eye Ear Nose Throat Monthly. 1953;32(12):707-11.

[129] Schemann JF, Doumbo O, Malvy D, Traore L, Kone A, Sidibe T, et al. Ocular lesions associated with malaria in children in Mali. The American Journal of Tropical Medicine and Hygiene. 2002;67(1):61-3.

[130] Maude RJ, Hassan MU, Beare NA. Severe retinal whitening in an adult with cerebral malaria. The American Journal of Tropical Medicine and Hygiene. 2009;80(6):881.

[131] Looareesuwan S, Warrell DA, White NJ, Chanthavanich P, Warrell MJ, Chantaratherakitti S, et al. Retinal hemorrhage, a common sign of prognostic significance in cere-

bral malaria. The American Journal of Tropical Medicine and Hygiene. 1983;32(5): 911-5.

[132] Beare NA, Taylor TE, Harding SP, Lewallen S, Molyneux ME. Malarial retinopathy: a newly established diagnostic sign in severe malaria. The American Journal of Tropical Medicine and Hygiene. 2006;75(5):790-7.

[133] Wongsrichanalai C, Barcus MJ, Muth S, Sutamihardja A, Wernsdorfer WH. A review of malaria diagnostic tools: microscopy and rapid diagnostic test (RDT). The American Journal of Tropical Medicine and Hygiene. 2007;77(6 Suppl):119-27.

[134] Hidayat AA, Nalbandian RM, Sammons DW, Fleischman JA, Johnson TE. The diagnostic histopathologic features of ocular malaria. Ophthalmology. 1993;100(8):1183-6.

[135] Lewallen S, Taylor TE, Molyneux ME, Wills BA, Courtright P. Ocular fundus findings in Malawian children with cerebral malaria. Ophthalmology. 1993;100(6):857-61.

[136] Nwosu S. Ocular complications of malaria treatment. Nigerian Journal of Clinical Practice. 2012;15(1):95-7.

[137] Beare NA, Southern C, Chalira C, Taylor TE, Molyneux ME, Harding SP. Prognostic significance and course of retinopathy in children with severe malaria. Archives of Ophthalmology. 2004;122(8):1141-7.

[138] Keeling P. Five questions about microsporidia. PLoS Pathogens. 2009;5(9):e1000489.

[139] Lowder CY, McMahon JT, Meisler DM, Dodds EM, Calabrese LH, Didier ES, et al. Microsporidial keratoconjunctivitis caused by Septata intestinalis in a patient with acquired immunodeficiency syndrome. American Journal of Ophthalmology. 1996;121(6):715-7.

[140] Shadduck JA, Meccoli RA, Davis R, Font RL. Isolation of a microsporidian from a human patient. The Journal of Infectious Diseases. 1990;162(3):773-6.

[141] Diesenhouse MC, Wilson LA, Corrent GF, Visvesvara GS, Grossniklaus HE, Bryan RT. Treatment of microsporidial keratoconjunctivitis with topical fumagillin. American Journal of Ophthalmology. 1993;115(3):293-8.

[142] Das S, Wallang BS, Sharma S, Bhadange YV, Balne PK, Sahu SK. The efficacy of corneal debridement in the treatment of microsporidial keratoconjunctivitis: a prospective randomized clinical trial. American Journal of Ophthalmology. 2014;157(6): 1151-5.

[143] Sanjay S. Clinical trial of 0.02% polyhexamethylene biguanide versus placebo in the treatment of microsporidial keratoconjunctivitis. American Journal of Ophthalmology. 2011;151(1):183.

[144] Savioli L, Smith H, Thompson A. Giardia and Cryptosporidium join the "Neglected Diseases Initiative'. Trends in Parasitology. 2006;22(5):203-8.

[145] Halliez MC, Buret AG. Extra-intestinal and long term consequences of Giardia duodenalis infections. World Journal of Gastroenterology. 2013;19(47):8974-85.

[146] Corsi A, Nucci C, Knafelz D, Bulgarini D, Di Iorio L, Polito A, et al. Ocular changes associated with Giardia lamblia infection in children. The British Journal of Ophthalmology. 1998;82(1):59-62.

[147] Gardner TB, Hill DR. Treatment of giardiasis. Clinical Microbiology Reviews. 2001;14(1):114-28.

[148] Onchocerciasis. (Available: http://www.who.int/mediacentre/factsheets/fs374/en/).

[149] Udall DN. Recent updates on onchocerciasis: diagnosis and treatment. Clinical Infectious Diseases: An Official Publication of the Infectious Diseases Society of America. 2007;44(1):53-60.

[150] Parasites – Onchocerciasis. (Available at: http://www.cdc.gov/parasites/onchocerciasis/epi.html).

[151] Hall LR, Pearlman E. Pathogenesis of onchocercal keratitis (River blindness). Clinical Microbiology Reviews. 1999;12(3):445-53.

[152] Higazi TB, Filiano A, Katholi CR, Dadzie Y, Remme JH, Unnasch TR. Wolbachia endosymbiont levels in severe and mild strains of Onchocerca volvulus. Molecular and Biochemical Parasitology. 2005;141(1):109-12.

[153] Brattig NW. Pathogenesis and host responses in human onchocerciasis: impact of Onchocerca filariae and Wolbachia endobacteria. Microbes and Infection. 2004;6(1): 113-28.

[154] Tamarozzi F, Halliday A, Gentil K, Hoerauf A, Pearlman E, Taylor MJ. Onchocerciasis: the role of Wolbachia bacterial endosymbionts in parasite biology, disease pathogenesis, and treatment. Clinical Microbiology Reviews. 2011;24(3):459-68.

[155] Harnett W. DNA-based detection of onchocerca volvulus. Transactions of the Royal Society of Tropical Medicine and Hygiene. 2002;96(Suppl 1):S231-4.

[156] Boatin BA, Toe L, Alley ES, Nagelkerke NJ, Borsboom G, Habbema JD. Detection of Onchocerca volvulus infection in low prevalence areas: a comparison of three diagnostic methods. Parasitology. 2002;125(Pt 6):545-52.

[157] Pischke S, Buttner DW, Liebau E, Fischer P. An internal control for the detection of Onchocerca volvulus DNA by PCR-ELISA and rapid detection of specific PCR products by DNA Detection Test Strips. Tropical Medicine & International Health. 2002;7(6):526-31.

[158] Ayong LS, Tume CB, Wembe FE, Simo G, Asonganyi T, Lando G, et al. Development and evaluation of an antigen detection dipstick assay for the diagnosis of human onchocerciasis. Tropical Medicine & International Health. 2005;10(3):228-33.

[159] Nde PN, Pogonka T, Bradley JE, Titanji VP, Lucius R. Sensitive and specific serodiagnosis of onchocerciasis with recombinant hybrid proteins. The American Journal of Tropical Medicine and Hygiene. 2002;66(5):566-71.

[160] Onchocerciasis. Available at http://www.cdc.gov/parasites/onchocerciasis/

[161] Onchocerciasis. (Available at: http://www.cdc.gov/parasites/onchocerciasis/health_professionals/).

[162] Parasites – Loiasis. (Available at: http://www.cdc.gov/parasites/loiasis/epi.html).

[163] Kelly-Hope LA, Bockarie MJ, Molyneux DH. Loa loa ecology in central Africa: role of the Congo River system. PLoS Neglected Tropical Diseases. 2012;6(6):e1605.

[164] Bhedasgaonkar S, Baile RB, Nadkarni S, Jakkula G, Gogri P. Loa loa macrofilariasis in the eyelid: case report of the first periocular subcutaneous manifestation in India. Journal of Parasitic Diseases. 2011;35(2):230-1.

[165] Cho HY, Lee YJ, Shin SY, Song HO, Ahn MH, Ryu JS. Subconjuctival Loa loa with Calabar swelling. Journal of Korean Medical Science. 2008;23(4):731-3.

[166] Dupont A, Zue-N'dong J, Pinder M. Common occurrence of amicrofilaraemic Loa loa filariasis within the endemic region. Transactions of the Royal Society of Tropical Medicine and Hygiene. 1988;82(5):730.

[167] Geldelman D, Blumberg R, Sadun A. Ocular Loa loa with cryoprobe extraction of subconjunctival worm. Ophthalmology. 1984;91(3):300-3.

[168] Klion AD, Vijaykumar A, Oei T, Martin B, Nutman TB. Serum immunoglobulin G4 antibodies to the recombinant antigen, Ll-SXP-1, are highly specific for Loa loa infection. The Journal of Infectious Diseases. 2003;187(1):128-33.

[169] Boussinesq M. Loiasis. Annals of Tropical Medicine and Parasitology. 2006;100(8):715-31.

[170] Loiasis. Available at: http://www.cdc.gov/parasites/loiasis/treatment.html (Accessed on 30 March 2016).

[171] Kalogeropoulos CD, Stefaniotou MI, Gorgoli KE, Papadopoulou CV, Pappa CN, Paschidis CA. Ocular dirofilariasis: a case series of 8 patients. Middle East African Journal of Ophthalmology. 2014;21(4):312-6.

[172] Sahdev SI, Sureka SP, Sathe PA, Agashe R. Ocular dirofilariasis: still in the dark in western India? Journal of Postgraduate Medicine. 2012;58(3):227-8.

[173] Sekhar HS, Srinivasa H, Batru RR, Mathai E, Shariff S, Macaden RS. Human ocular dirofilariasis in Kerala Southern India. Indian Journal of Pathology & Microbiology. 2000;43(1):77-9.

[174] Font RL, Neafie RC, Perry HD. Subcutaneous dirofilariasis of the eyelid and ocular adnexa. Report of six cases. Archives of Ophthalmology. 1980;98(6):1079-82.

[175] Gorezis S, Psilla M, Asproudis I, Peschos D, Papadopoulou C, Stefaniotou M. Intravitreal dirofilariasis: a rare ocular infection. Orbit. 2006;25(1):57-9.

[176] Perera L, Perez-Arellano JL, Cordero M, Simon F, Muro A. Utility of antibodies against a 22 kD molecule of Dirofilaria immitis in the diagnosis of human pulmonary dirofilariasis. Tropical Medicine & International Health. 1998;3(2):151-5.

[177] Dirofilariasis. Available at: http://www.cdc.gov/parasites/dirofilariasis/faqs.html (Accessed 0n 30 March 2016).

[178] Mittal M, Sathish KR, Bhatia PG, Chidamber BS. Ocular dirofilariasis in Dubai, UAE. Indian Journal of Ophthalmology. 2008;56(4):325-6.

[179] Diaz JH. Gnathostomiasis: an emerging infection of raw fish consumers in Gnathostoma nematode-endemic and nonendemic countries. Journal of Travel Medicine. 2015;22(5):318-24.

[180] Wiwanitkit V. Gnathostomiasis and sushi ingestion. American Journal of Dermatopathology. 2012;34(6):675.

[181] Sujata DN, Renu BS. Intraocular gnathostomiasis from coastal part of Maharashtra. Tropical Parasitology. 2013;3(1):82-4.

[182] Pillai GS, Kumar A, Radhakrishnan N, Maniyelil J, Shafi T, Dinesh KR, et al. Intraocular gnathostomiasis: report of a case and review of literature. The American Journal of Tropical Medicine and Hygiene. 2012;86(4):620-3.

[183] Bhattacharjee H, Das D, Medhi J. Intravitreal gnathostomiasis and review of literature. Retina. 2007;27(1):67-73.

[184] Buppajarntham A, Apisarnthanarak A, Khawcharoenporn T, Rutjanawech S, Mundy LM. Asymptomatic eosinophilia due to gnathostomiasis. International Journal of Infectious Diseases: IJID: Official Publication of the International Society for Infectious Diseases. 2014;23:14-5.

[185] Saksirisampant W, Chawengkiattikul R, Kraivichain K, Nuchprayoon S. Specific IgE antibody responses to somatic and excretory-secretory antigens of third stage G. spinigerum larvae in human gnathostomiasis. Journal of the Medical Association of Thailand. 2001;84(Suppl 1):S173-81.

[186] Saenseeha S, Penchom J, Yamasaki H, Laummaunwai P, Tayapiwatana C, Kitkhuandee A, et al. A dot-ELISA test using a Gnathostoma spinigerum recombinant matrix metalloproteinase protein for the serodiagnosis of human gnathostomiasis. The Southeast Asian Journal of Tropical Medicine and Public health. 2014;45(5):990-6.

[187] Laummaunwai P, Sawanyawisuth K, Intapan PM, Chotmongkol V, Wongkham C, Maleewong W. Evaluation of human IgG class and subclass antibodies to a 24 kDa antigenic component of Gnathostoma spinigerum for the serodiagnosis of gnathostomiasis. Parasitology Research. 2007;101(3):703-8.

[188] Herman JS, Chiodini PL. Gnathostomiasis, another emerging imported disease. Clinical Microbiology Reviews. 2009;22(3):484-92.

[189] Anantaphruti MT. ELISA for diagnosis of gnathostomiasis using antigens from Gnathostoma doloresi and G. spinigerum. The Southeast Asian Journal of Tropical Medicine and Public Health. 1989;20(2):297-304.

[190] Maleewong W, Morakote N, Thamasonthi W, Charuchinda K, Tesana S, Khamboonruang C. Serodiagnosis of human gnathostomiasis. The Southeast Asian Journal of Tropical Medicine and Public Health. 1988;19(2):201-5.

[191] Nawa Y, Katchanov J, Yoshikawa M, Rojekittikhun W, Dekumyoy P, Kusolusuk T, et al. Ocular Gnathostomiasis: a comprehensive review. J Trop Med Parasitol. 2010;33:77-86.

[192] Joseph A, Joseph A. Ocular thelaziasis (a case report). Indian Journal of Ophthalmology. 1985;33(2):113-4.

[193] Yospaiboon Y, Sithithavorn P, Maleewong V, Ukosanakarn U, Bhaibulaya M. Ocular thelaziasis in Thailand: a case report. Journal of the Medical Association of Thailand. 1989;72(8):469-73.

[194] Thelaziasis. Available at: http://www.cdc.gov/dpdx/thelaziasis/tx.html

[195] Jee D, Kim KS, Lee WK, Kim W, Jeon S. Clinical features of ocular toxocariasis in adult Korean patients. Ocular Immunology and Inflammation. 2016;24(2):207-16.

[196] Yokoi K, Goto H, Sakai J, Usui M. Clinical features of ocular toxocariasis in Japan. Ocular Immunology and Inflammation. 2003;11(4):269-75.

[197] Zhou M, Chang Q, Gonzales JA, Chen Q, Zhang Y, Huang X, et al. Clinical characteristics of ocular toxocariasis in Eastern China. Graefe's archive for clinical and experimental ophthalmology = Albrecht von Graefes Archiv fur klinische und experimentelle Ophthalmologie. 2012;250(9):1373-8.

[198] Woodhall D, Starr MC, Montgomery SP, Jones JL, Lum F, Read RW, et al. Ocular toxocariasis: epidemiologic, anatomic, and therapeutic variations based on a survey of ophthalmic subspecialists. Ophthalmology. 2012;119(6):1211-7.

[199] Centers for Disease C, Prevention. Ocular toxocariasis – United States, 2009-2010. MMWR Morbidity and Mortality Weekly Report. 2011;60(22):734-6.

[200] Ahn SJ, Ryoo NK, Woo SJ. Ocular toxocariasis: clinical features, diagnosis, treatment, and prevention. Asia Pacific Allergy. 2014;4(3):134-41.

[201] Arevalo JF, Espinoza JV, Arevalo FA. Ocular toxocariasis. Journal of Pediatric Ophthalmology and Strabismus. 2013;50(2):76-86.

[202] Ament CS, Young LH. Ocular manifestations of helminthic infections: onchocersiasis, cysticercosis, toxocariasis, and diffuse unilateral subacute neuroretinitis. International Ophthalmology Clinics. 2006;46(2):1-10.

[203] Teyssot N, Cassoux N, Lehoang P, Bodaghi B. Fuchs heterochromic cyclitis and ocular toxocariasis. American Journal of Ophthalmology. 2005;139(5):915-6.

[204] Stewart JM, Cubillan LD, Cunningham ET, Jr. Prevalence, clinical features, and causes of vision loss among patients with ocular toxocariasis. Retina. 2005;25(8):1005-13.

[205] Martinez-Pulgarin DF, Munoz-Urbano M, Gomez-Suta LD, Delgado OM, Rodriguez-Morales AJ. Ocular toxocariasis: new diagnostic and therapeutic perspectives. Recent Patents on Anti-Infective Drug Discovery. 2015;10(1):35-41.

[206] Lee TH, Ji YS, Lee SH. ELISA-confirmed bilateral ocular toxocariasis with different features. Optometry and Vision Science: Official Publication of the American Academy of Optometry. 2015;92(8):e176-9.

[207] Schneier AJ, Durand ML. Ocular toxocariasis: advances in diagnosis and treatment. International Ophthalmology Clinics. 2011;51(4):135-44.

[208] de Visser L, Rothova A, de Boer JH, van Loon AM, Kerkhoff FT, Canninga-van Dijk MR, et al. Diagnosis of ocular toxocariasis by establishing intraocular antibody production. American Journal of Ophthalmology. 2008;145(2):369-74.

[209] Jacquier P, Gottstein B, Stingelin Y, Eckert J. Immunodiagnosis of toxocarosis in humans: evaluation of a new enzyme-linked immunosorbent assay kit. Journal of Clinical Microbiology. 1991;29(9):1831-5.

[210] Jin Y, Shen C, Huh S, Sohn WM, Choi MH, Hong ST. Serodiagnosis of toxocariasis by ELISA using crude antigen of Toxocara canis larvae. The Korean Journal of Parasitology. 2013;51(4):433-9.

[211] Tian JX, O'Hagan S. Toxocara polymerase chain reaction on ocular fluids in bilateral granulomatous chorioretinitis. International Medical Case Reports Journal. 2015;8:107-10.

[212] Van De N, Trung NV, Duyet le V, Chai JY. Molecular diagnosis of an ocular toxocariasis patient in Vietnam. The Korean Journal of Parasitology. 2013;51(5):563-7.

[213] Zibaei M, Sadjjadi SM, Karamian M, Uga S, Oryan A, Jahadi-Hosseini SH. A comparative histopathology, serology and molecular study, on experimental ocular toxocariasis by Toxocara cati in Mongolian gerbils and Wistar rats. BioMed Research International. 2013;2013:109580.

[214] Seong S, Moon D, Lee DK, Kim HE, Oh HS, Kim SH, et al. A case of ocular toxocariasis successfully treated with albendazole and triamcinolon. The Korean Journal of Parasitology. 2014;52(5):537-40.

[215] Frazier M, Anderson ML, Sophocleous S. Treatment of ocular toxocariasis with albendezole: a case report. Optometry. 2009;80(4):175-80.

[216] Prasad KN, Prasad A, Verma A, Singh AK. Human cysticercosis and Indian scenario: a review. Journal of Biosciences. 2008;33(4):571-82.

[217] Coral-Almeida M, Gabriel S, Abatih EN, Praet N, Benitez W, Dorny P. Taenia solium Human Cysticercosis: a systematic review of sero-epidemiological data from endemic zones around the world. PLoS Neglected Tropical Diseases. 2015;9(7):e0003919.

[218] Yera H, Dupont D, Houze S, Ben M'rad M, Pilleux F, Sulahian A, et al. Confirmation and follow-up of neurocysticercosis by real-time PCR in cerebrospinal fluid samples of patients living in France. Journal of Clinical Microbiology. 2011;49(12):4338-40.

[219] Jain RS, Kumar S, Bhana I, Agarwal R. Ocular cysticercosis with vitreous hemorrhage: a rare complication of a common disease. Springerplus. 2015;4:217.

[220] Goyal S, Sandhu PS, Sharma A, Malik MA, Bansal P, Kaur J. Inferior rectus muscle ocular cysticercosis: a case report. Saudi Journal of Ophthalmology. 2015;29(2):175-7.

[221] Mohan N, Panda KG, Padhi TR. Bug inside the eye: ocular cysticercosis. JAMA Ophthalmology. 2014;132(12):1468.

[222] Sohoni CA. Neuro-ocular cysticercosis causing total retinal detachment and cataract. Journal of Family Medicine and Primary Care. 2013;2(3):300-1.

[223] Labh RK, Sharma AK. Ptosis: a rare presentation of ocular cysticercosis. Nepalese Journal of Ophthalmology. 2013;5(1):133-5.

[224] Sharma AK. Ocular cysticercosis: diagnosis and treatment. Nepalese Journal of Ophthalmology. 2014;6(2):240-1.

[225] Nkouawa A, Sako Y, Nakao M, Nakaya K, Ito A. Loop-mediated isothermal amplification method for differentiation and rapid detection of Taenia species. Journal of Clinical Microbiology. 2009;47(1):168-74.

[226] Swastika K, Dewiyani CI, Yanagida T, Sako Y, Sudarmaja M, Sutisna P, et al. An ocular cysticercosis in Bali, Indonesia caused by Taenia solium Asian genotype. Parasitology International. 2012;61(2):378-80.

[227] Ocular cysticercosis treatment and management. Available at: http://emedcine.medscape.com/article/1204683-treatment

[228] Stojkovic M, Junghanss T. Cystic and alveolar echinococcosis. Handbook of Clininical Neurology. 2013;114:327-34.

[229] Karakas HM, Tokoglu F, Kacar M, Boyacigil S. Retrobulbar hydatid cyst: assessment of two cases. Australasian Radiology. 1997;41(2):179-80.

[230] Budke CM, Carabin H, Ndimubanzi PC, Nguyen H, Rainwater E, Dickey M, et al. A systematic review of the literature on cystic echinococcosis frequency worldwide and

its associated clinical manifestations. The American Journal of Tropical Medicine and Hygiene. 2013;88(6):1011-27.

[231] Arora MM, Dhanda RP, Bhagwat AG, Kalevar VK. Intra-ocular hydatid cyst. The British Journal of Ophthalmology. 1964;48:507-9.

[232] Betharia SM, Sharma V, Pushker N. Ultrasound findings in orbital hydatid cysts. American Journal of Ophthalmology. 2003;135(4):568-70.

[233] Aksoy FG, Tanrikulu S, Kosar U. Inferiorly located retrobulbar hydatid cyst: CT and MRI features. Computerized Medical Imaging and Graphics. 2001;25(6):535-40.

[234] Manzano-Roman R, Sanchez-Ovejero C, Hernandez-Gonzalez A, Casulli A, Siles-Lucas M. Serological diagnosis and follow-up of human cystic echinococcosis: a new hope for the future? BioMed Research international. 2015;2015:428205.

[235] Mirfazaelian H, Bagheri B, Daneshbod Y. Fine needle aspiration cytology diagnosis of an ocular hydatid cyst. Cytopathology. 2014;25(6):416-7.

[236] Echinococcosis. Available at: http://www.cfsph.iastate.edu/Factsheets/pdfs/echinococcosis.pdf

[237] Al-Muala HD, Sami SM, Shukri MA, Hasson HK, Alaboudy AT. Orbital hydatid cyst. Annals of Maxillofacial Surgery. 2012;2(2):197-9.

[238] Selcuklu A, Ozturk M, Kulahli I, Dogan H. Successful surgical management of an intraorbital hydatid cyst through a transmaxillary approach: case report. Skull Base: Official Journal of North American Skull Base Society. 2003;13(2):101-5.

[239] Mas-Coma S, Agramunt VH, Valero MA. Neurological and ocular fascioliasis in humans. Advances in Parasitology. 2014;84:27-149.

[240] Dickinson AJ, Rosenthal AR, Nicholson KG. Inflammation of the retinal pigment epithelium: a unique presentation of ocular schistosomiasis. The British Journal of Ophthalmology. 1990;74(7):440-2.

[241] Mimori T, Hirai H, Kifune T, Inada K. Philophthalmus sp. (Trematoda) in a human eye. The American Journal of Tropical Medicine and Hygiene. 1982;31(4):859-61.

[242] Tiewchaloern S, Udomkijdecha S, Suvouttho S, Chunchamsri K, Waikagul J. Clinostomum trematode from human eye. The Southeast Asian Journal of Tropical Medicine and Public health. 1999;30(2):382-4.

[243] McDonald HR, Kazacos KR, Schatz H, Johnson RN. Two cases of intraocular infection with Alaria mesocercaria (Trematoda). American Journal of Ophthalmology. 1994;117(4):447-55.

[244] Dono M, Bertonati MR, Poggi R, Teneggi E, Maddalo F, Via F, et al. Three cases of ophthalmomyiasis externa by sheep botfly Oestrus ovis in Italy. New Microbiologica. 2005;28(4):365-8.

[245] Grammer J, Erb C, Kamin G, Wild M, Riedinger C, Kosmidis P, et al. Ophthalmomyiasis externa due to the sheep botfly Oestrus ovis (Diptera: Oestridae) in southwest Germany. German Journal of Ophthalmology. 1995;4(3):188-95.

[246] Gupta VP, Baveja UK. Ophthalmomyiasis externa caused by the sheep nasal botfly Oestrus ovis. Indian Journal of Ophthalmology. 1988;36(1):41-2.

[247] Harvey JT. Sheep botfly: ophthalmomyiasis externa. Canadian Journal of Ophthalmology (Journal canadien d'ophtalmologie). 1986;21(3):92-5.

[248] Mason GI. Bilateral ophthalmomyiasis interna. American Journal of Ophthalmology. 1981;91(1):65-70.

[249] Ho-Yen DO, Chapman DJ, Ashburn D. Immunoblotting can help the diagnosis of ocular toxoplasmosis. Molecular Pathology. 2000;53(3):155-8.

[250] Fekkar A, Bodaghi B, Touafek F, Le Hoang P, Mazier D, Paris L. Comparison of immunoblotting, calculation of the Goldmann-Witmer coefficient, and real-time PCR using aqueous humor samples for diagnosis of ocular toxoplasmosis. Journal of Clinical Microbiology. 2008;46(6):1965-7.

10

The Role of Renin-Angiotensin System in Ocular Inflammation and Uveitis

Ozlem Sahin and Alireza Ziaei

Abstract

The renin-angiotensin system (RAS) plays an important role in the pathogenesis of inflammation and autoimmune dysfunction. Uveitis is a sight-threatening intraocular inflammatory disorder caused by infectious agents, autoimmune mechanisms, exposure to toxins and many other unknown factors. Most components of RAS have been identified in every organ including the eye. The tissue-specific RAS is believed to exert diverse physiological effects locally independent of circulating angiotensin II (AT II) which functions as the effector arm of RAS causing potent proinflammatory responses via Angiotensin type 1 receptor (AT1R). AT II mediated stimulation of tissue factor (TF), the principal initiator of the clotting cascade and a major regulator of haemostasis and thrombosis rapidly inducible by inflammatory agents in several cell lines including monocytes. Activation of NFκB, a key redox-sensitive transcription factor encoding for the TF gene, plays a key role in that mechanism amplified by locally synthesized angiotensin I. (AT I) The second arm of RAS establishes systemic and local protective axis against inflammation and autoimmune dysfunction via angiotensin-converting enzyme 2 (ACE2) which is a zinc-metallopeptidase able to cleave AT II to form angiotensin-(1–7) [AT-(1–7)]. AT-(1–7), a biologically active peptide, binds to a G-protein coupled receptor Mas, and activates signaling pathways that counteract the effects of AT II by negatively effecting inflammatory responses and negatively modulating leukocyte migration, cytokine expression and release, and fibrogenic pathways. The purpose of this chapter is to analyze both pro-inflammatory and protective role of RAS in ocular inflammation and uveitis both in humans and experimental models.

Keywords: uveitis, renin, angiotensin, angiotensin converting enzyme, tissue factor

1. Introduction

The renin-angiotensin system (RAS) is a hormone system playing an important role in the pathogenesis of inflammation and autoimmune dysfunction [1]. RAS pathway elements are produced intrinsically in many diverse tissues, including the retina for controlling local inflammatory responses and maintaining local homeostasis [1]. While RAS is important for controlling normal inflammatory responses, hyperactivation of this pathway is disclosed to potentiate oxidative stress and inflammatory responses by the activation of nicotinamide adenine dinucleotide phosphate (NAD(P)H) oxidases [2]. The tissue-specific RAS is believed to exert diverse physiological effects locally independent of circulating angiotensin II (AT II), which functions as the effector arm of RAS causing potent pro-inflammatory responses via angiotensin type 1 receptor (AT1R) [1]. AT II is considered to stimulate tissue factor (TF), which induces synthesis of nuclear factor kappa-light-chain-enhancer of activated B cells (NF-κB) in several cell lines including monocytes [3]. The second arm of RAS is considered to establish systemic and local protective axis against inflammation and autoimmune dysfunction via angiotensin-converting enzyme 2 (ACE2), which cleaves AT II to angiotensin-(1–7) [2]. AT (1–7) is reported to counteract the effects of AT II by negatively affecting inflammatory responses, negatively modulating leukocyte migration, cytokine expression and release, and fibrogenic pathways [2].

Uveitis is considered as an intraocular inflammatory disorder caused by infectious agents or autoimmune mechanisms [4]. The purpose of this chapter is to analyze both pro-inflammatory and protective role of RAS in ocular inflammation and uveitis both in humans and experimental models.

2. RAS as an inflammatory cascade

Renin is considered to cleave angiotensinogen to AT1 that is further processed by ACE/ACE2 to different AT cleavage products including AT II, which is regarded as a principle effector molecule of the RAS [3]. The major functions of AT II are reported to be mediated by AT1R, which is considered to activate directly the key signaling pathways for cell growth and hypertrophy [4]. AT1R has been also shown to activate NF-κB and activator protein 1 (AP-1) to initiate the transcription of multiple proinflammatory genes [4]. AT II is disclosed to activate epidermal growth factor receptors (EGFR) to induce fibronectin synthesis and transforming growth factor beta (TGF-β) activity to promote fibrosis and extracellular matrix formation [3]. The effects of circulating and tissue RAS are considered to be controlled with RAS inhibitors, which prevent not only hypertension but also protect tissues against injury by limiting the potency of deleterious inflammatory responses [3].

Recently, several studies have revealed that modulators of the RAS-including ACE inhibitors or AT1R antagonists display beneficial effects in the treatment of cardiovascular diseases, atherosclerotic, neurodegenerative, autoimmune, and inflammatory diseases [5–8].

3. Angiotensin II and autoimmunity

The modulatory effect of AT II on T-cell responses in autoimmune diseases has been disclosed by a recent study [9]. The effect of AT II in the development of Th1/Th17-mediated multiple sclerosis (MS) has been disclosed in experimental autoimmune encephalomyelitis (EAE)[10]. Elevated levels of AT II, IFN-γ, and IL-17 cytokines have been shown in the peripheral CD4$^+$T cells from EAE mice [10]. AT1R is also considered to involve in experimental autoimmune uveitis (EAU) and experimental autoimmune myocarditis (EAM) through its effect on T-cell function [11]. A recent study has highlighted the role of AT1R in glomerular inflammation associated with autoimmune disease in mice leading to the inflammation resembling human systemic lupus erythematosus [12]. AT1R has also been disclosed in the pathogenesis of myelin oligodendrocyte glycoprotein-induced experimental autoimmune encephalomyelitis (MOG-EAE) [13]. The expression of renin, ACE, and AT1R has been shown to be upregulated in macrophages, DCs, and T cells during the course of the MOG-EAE [13].

4. Angiotensin II promotes inflammation and tissue injury

Inflammatory process is considered to involve activation of the endothelium of blood vessels and expression of diverse endothelial cell selectins that have been shown to lead the extravasation of specific leukocyte populations to the site of injury [14].

The expression and secretion of vascular endothelial growth factor (VEGF) by RAS and AT II have been disclosed to increase local vascular permeability [14]. AT II has also been disclosed to promote endothelial dysfunction through COX-2 activation, which generates vasoactive prostaglandins and reactive oxygen species (ROS) [15]. AT II is considered to favor the recruitment of infiltrating inflammatory cells into tissues by stimulating the production of specific cytokine/chemokines. AT II has been shown to induce the production of the potent monocyte chemoattractant MCP-1 in cultured monocytes [15]. Elevated levels of AT II associated with increased expression of MCP-1 and C–C chemokine receptor, CCR2, have been disclosed in the aorta of spontaneously hypertensive rats [16]. Modulation of MCP-1/CCR2 via AT1R blockade has been revealed to reduce vessel inflammation in hypertensive rats [16]. AT II-induced macrophage infiltration in the arterial wall was shown to be virtually absent in CCR2-deficient mice [16]. In models of progressive nephropathies, interstitial accumulation of macrophages was shown to be accompanied by increased renal expression of MCP-1, and renoprotection was provided by the ACE inhibitor lisinopril, which was considered to reduce MCP-1 expression and control inflammation [17]. Dendritic cells (DCs) and highly specialized antigen-presenting cells (APCs) were considered to mediate the pro-inflammatory activity of AT II [18]. Cultured DCs have been shown to express both AT II receptors and AT II, which were considered to enhance DCs migration, maturation, and antigen presenting ability [18]. Recent study in rats with subtotal renal ablation has disclosed blockade of AT II synthesis and its biological activity that resulted in reduction of local DC accumulation and attenuation of tubulointerstitial damage [19]. In another study considering cultured mesangial and vascular smooth muscle cells, AT II via AT1R signaling was shown to stimulate TLR-4 expression that was considered to promote cellular oxidative injury, apoptosis, and inflammation [20]. T cells were considered to show the pro-inflammatory effects of AT II via AT1R and endogenous RAS, which has been disclosed to modulate T-cell proliferation, cytoskeletal rearrangements, migration, and release of specific cytokines and chemokines [20].

5. Angiotensin II: role in immunosenesence

AT II is considered to stimulate the production of molecular oxygen species that trigger mitochondrial dysfunction and cellular injury [21]. AT II via AT1R stimulation has been shown to activate NAD(P)H oxidase to produce ROS, resulting in oxidative stress damage [21]. It has been proposed that ROSs are the most prominent molecular species involved in the aging process [22]. ROSs have been revealed to contribute significantly to various age-associated organ failures, including hypertension, cardiovascular diseases, and renal damage [22]. Hence, AT II is considered to be involved in organ senescence related to its ability to mediate the release of oxidant species [23]. Recent studies have disclosed that AT II-induced ROS production leads to functional and structural changes of blood vessels that result in vascular senescence and age-related vascular diseases [23]. Previous studies related to the long-term effects of AT II inhibition by either ACEi or ARBs disclosed protective effects on the cardiovascular system of rats and revealed the prolongation of the life span of rats [24, 25]. Another study disclosed that old mice lacking AT1R did not develop age-related cerebral circulation damage caused by the accumulation of oxygen radicals [26]. The inhibition of RAS has been disclosed to reverse age-related advanced myocardiac hypertrophy and fibrosis in old hypertensive rats, and the protective effect presumably was considered to involve the suppression of AT II-mediated oxidative stress, as disclosed by reduced expression of NAD(P)H oxidative components in the hearts of aged rats [26].

6. Further mechanisms of angiotensin II-induced inflammation: human T and natural killer cells

Co-stimulatory effects of angiotensinogen, AT I, and AT II on the proliferation of T and NK cells have been revealed [27]. T and NK cells were considered to have RAS elements, and they have been synthesizing AT II at the sites of inflammation creating a potential inflammatory amplification system [27, 28]. Th1 immune response has been disclosed to be crucial in the pathogenesis of inflammatory vascular diseases [28].

However, the interaction of AT II with Th1/Th2 cytokines during the development of inflammation is considered debatable. Recent studies have demonstrated the presence of RAS elements in human T and NK cells that they were capable to synthesize their own AT II [29]. Renin-induced inflammation has been related to the binding of AT II to the renin receptor in T cells, NK cells, and DC [29]. AT 2R which was previously considered to antagonize the actions of the AT1R and having beneficial effects in hypertension, cell growth, vascular remodeling, proliferation, and inflammation, currently, it has been thought to orchestrate the collective recruitment of leukocyte subsets to the sites of inflammation through mediating the effect of AT II [29, 30].

7. Clinical implications

New medical applications of RAS antagonists as anti-inflammatory and immunomodulatory agents without significant side-effects are being considered in the treatment of autoimmune diseases [31, 32].

7.1. Captopril suppresses inflammation in endotoxin-induced uveitis in rats

It has been suggested that ACEi captopril has a strong anti-ocular inflammatory effect in endotoxin-induced uveitis (EIU) [33]. Captopril has been shown to suppress the NF-κB activation in the iris and ciliary body cells by inhibiting the production of AT II [34]. The inhibitory effect of captopril on leucocyte infiltration, protein leakage, and other inflammatory markers in the aqueous humor including TNF-α, PGE-2, MCP-1, NO have also been revealed [35].

TNF-α is an inflammatory cytokine, which plays an important role in the recruitment of inflammatory cells, synthesis of other inflammatory cytokines, eicosanoids, and NO [35]. Anti TNF-α therapy has been used for the treatment of Behcet's disease [36]. The transcription of TNF-α was shown to be under the control of NF-κB [35, 36]. It has previously been disclosed that ACE inhibitors suppress TNF-α synthesis *in vivo* and *in vitro* and captopril was shown to successfully down regulate TNF-α in the aqueous humor by interfering the positive loop between TNF-α and NF-κB [36]. PGE2 and NO in the aqueous humor were considered to have profound effects on local inflammatory processes mainly by increasing vascular permeability and breaking down the blood-aqueous barrier in uveitis [37]. Their concentrations in the aqueous humor were disclosed to be down-regulated by captopril treatment [37]. Inhibition of both TNF-α and PGE2/NO pathways by captopril has been shown to improve EIU in rabbits [38]. Another inflammatory marker MCP-1, which is under NF-κB control, is considered as an important mediator of monocyte infiltration. MCP-1 has been shown to be over expressed in human eyes during acute anterior uveitis as well as in the rat EIU model [38]. The results of the recent studies have disclosed that captopril successfully down-regulated MCP-1 levels in anterior chamber, and it showed its anti-inflammatory properties by affecting monocyte recruitment in EIU in rats [34, 37, 38].

The beneficial effect of AT II blockers on tissue inflammation was also considered to be related to the blockage of Ang II-mediated activation of Toll-like receptors (TLRs) [39]. Drugs that limit AT II synthesis and its biological activity, ACEi lisinopril, or ARB Candesartan were disclosed to result in the suppression of Th1 and Th17 cytokine release and the induction of powerful antigen-specific regulatory T cells (Treg) through the modulation of the NF-κB pathway [40]. Administration of ARB was disclosed to suppress EAU and reduce the severity of myocardial lesions in EAM by inhibiting antigen-specific T-cell activation and contributing to the shift of Th1–Th2 immune response [41]. Chronic treatment with ACEi or ARB has been shown to reduce kidney damage associated with age, and the beneficial effect of RAS inhibition was considered to be related to the preservation of renal mitochondria [40]. Enalapril and losartan treatments have been shown to prevent the age-associated decline in the renal mitochondrial capacity for energy production and to attenuate the age-associated increase in mitochondrial oxidant production [40]. RAS inhibition was disclosed to exert a similar protective effect in the liver from aged rats through the maintenance of an adequate mitochondrial function by enhancing expression of genes responsible for mitochondrial respiration and biogenesis [41]. Aging is considered to be the result of chronic inflammation, and the use of RAS inhibitors or genetic deletion of AT1R was considered to extend the life span [41].

7.2. Oral delivery of ACE2/Ang-(1–7) bioencapsulated in plant cells protects against experimental uveitis and autoimmune uveoretinitis

Improving the systemic and local activity of the protective axis of the RAS by oral delivery of ACE2 and Ang-(1–7) bioencapsulated in plant cells has been considered as a therapeutic option for the ocular inflammation. Increased levels of ACE2 and Ang-(1–7) were observed in the retinal circulation after oral administration of ACE2 and Ang-(1–7) expressing plant cells [42]. Oral feeding of mice with bioencapsulated ACE2/Ang-(1–7) was shown significantly to reduce the incidence of EIU [42]. Treatment with bioencapsulated ACE2/Ang-(1–7) in mice disclosed dramatical decrease of cellular infiltration and retinal vasculitis in EAU [42]. It has been concluded that enhancing the protective axis of RAS by oral delivery of ACE2/Ang-(1–7) bioencapsulated in plant cells provide an innovative, highly efficient, and cost-effective therapeutic strategy for ocular inflammatory diseases [42].

8. Conclusions

Hyperactivity of the RAS resulting elevated AT II might contribute to all stages of inflammatory responses including ocular inflammation. ACE2 is more likely to establish a protective axis of RAS involving ACE2/Ang-(1–7)/Mas, which counteract the proinflammatory and hypertrophic effects of the ACE/AngII/AT1R axis. AT II might have also co-stimulatory effects on T cells, NK cells, and DC, which have specific elements of the RAS. RAS antagonists might be used in conjunction with other anti-inflammatory agents as therapy for common diseases in which inflammation plays a major pathogenic role.

Author details

Ozlem Sahin[1]* and Alireza Ziaei[2]

*Address all correspondence to: ozlem1158@yahoo.com

1 Department of Microbiology and Immunology, New York Medical College, Valhalla, New York, USA

2 Harvard Medical School, Brigham and Women's Hospital, Boston, USA

References

[1] Karnik SS, Unal H, Kemp JR, Tirupula KC, Eguchi S, et al. International Union of Basic and Clinical Pharmacology. XCIX. Angiotensin receptors: Interpreters of pathophysiological angiotensinergic stimuli. Pharmacological Reviews. 2015;**67**:754-819

[2] Marchesi C, Paradis P, Ernesto LS. Role of the renin-angiotensin system in vascular inflammation. Trends in Pharmacological Sciences. 2008;**29**:367-374

[3] Alique M, Sánchez-López E, Rayego-Mateos S, et al. Angiotensin II, via angiotensin receptor type 1/nuclear factor-κB activation, causes a synergistic effect on interleukin-1-β-induced inflammatory responses in cultured mesangial cells. J Renin Angiotensin Aldosterone Syst. 2015;**16**:23-32.

[4] Shil PK, Kwon KC, Zhu P, Verma A, Daniell H, Li Q. Oral delivery of ACE2/Ang-(1-7) bioencapsulated in plant cells protects against experimental uveitis and autoimmune uveoretinitis. Mol Ther. 2014;**22**:2069-2082.

[5] Capettini L, Monteccuco F, Mach F, Da Silva RF. Role of renin-angiotensin system in inflammation, immunity and aging. Current Pharmaceutical Design. 2012;**18**:963-970

[6] Monteccuco F, Pende A, Mach F. The renin-angiotensin system modulated inflammator processes in atheroscerosis: Evidence from basic research and clinical studies. Mediators Inflamm. 2009; **2009**: 752406.

[7] Weir MR. Effects of renin-angiotensin system inhibition end-organ protection: Can we do better? Clinical Therapeutics. 2007;**29**:1803-1824.

[8] Prisant LM. Management of hypertension in patients with cardiac disease: Use of renin-angiotensin blocking agents. The American Journal of Medicine. 2008;**121**:S8-S15.

[9] Crowley SD, Rudemiller NP. Immunologic Effects of the Renin-Angiotensin System. J Am Soc Nephrol. 2017;**28**:1350-1361.

[10] Friedrich EB, Teo KK, Böhm M. ACE inhibition in secondary prevention: Are the results controversial? Clinical Research in Cardiology. 2006;**95**:61-67.

[11] Yusuf S, Teo KK, Anderson C, et al. Effects of the angiotensin-receptor blocker telmisartan on cardiovascular events in high-risk patients intolerant to angiotensin-converting enzyme inhibitors: A randomised controlled trial. The Lancet. 2008;**372**:1174-1183.

[12] Pacurari M, Kafoury R, Tchounwou PB, et al. The renin-angiotensin-aldosterone syste in vascular inflammation ad remodelling. International Journal of Inflammation. 2014;**2014**:Article ID 689360:13

[13] Stegbauera J, Leeb DH, Seubertb S, et al. Role of the renin-angiotensin system in autoimmune inflammation of the central nervous system. Proceedings of the National Academy of Sciences. 2009;**106**:14942-14947

[14] Souza PP Fukada SY, Cunha FQ, et al. Regulation of angiotensin II receptors levels during rat induced pulpitis. Regul Pept. 2007;**140**:27-31.

[15] Luger D, et al. Either a Th17 or a Th1 effector response can drive autoimmunity: Conditions of disease induction affect dominant effector category. Journal of Experimental Medicine. 2008;**205**, 799-810.

[16] Sprovieri SR, Sens YA. Polymorphisms of the renin-angiotensin system genes in Brazilian patients with lupus nephropathy. Lupus. 2005;**14**:356-362.

[17] Valero-Esquitina V, Lucht K, Namsolleck P, et al. Direct angiotensin type 2 receptor stimulation attenuates T-cell and microglia activation and prevents demyelinization in experimental autoimmune enephalomyelitis in mice. Clincal Science. 2015;**128**:95-109.

[18] Dandona P, Dhindsa S, Ghanim H, et al. Angiotensin II and inflammation: The effect of angiotensin-converting enzyme inhibition and angiotensin II receptor blockade. Journal of Human Hypertension. 2007;**21**:20-27.

[19] Pueyo ME, Gonzalez W, Nicoletti A, et al. Angiotensin II stimulates endothelial vascular cell adhesion molecule-1 via nuclear factor-kappaB activation induced by intracellular oxidative stress. Arteriosclerosis, Thrombosis, and Vascular Biology. 2000;**20**:645-651

[20] Igase M, Strawn WB, Gallagher PE, et al. Angiotensin II AT_1 receptors regulate ACE2 and angiotensin-(1-7) expression in the aorta of spontaneously hypertensive rats. Heart and Circulatory Physiology. 2005;**289**:H1013-H1019.

[21] Remuzzi A, Fassi A, Bertani T, et al. ACE inhibition induces regression of proteinuria and halts progression of renal damage in a genetic model of progressive nephropathy. American Journal of Kidney Diseases. 1999;**34**:626-632.

[22] Nahmod KA,Vermeulen ME, Radien S, et al. Control of dendritic cell differentiation by angiotensin II. FASEB J. 2003;**17**:491-493. DOI: 10.1096:fj02-0755fje.

[23] Muller DN, Shagdarsuren E, Park JK, et al. Immunosuppressive treatment protects against angiotensin II-induced renal damage. The American Journal of Pathology. 2002;**161**:1679-1693.

[24] Griendling KK, Minieri CA, Ollerenshaw JD, et al. Angiotensin II stimulates NADH and NADPH oxidase activity in cultured vascular smooth muscle cells. Circulation Research. 1994;**74**:1141-1148.

[25] Kimura S, Zhang GX, Nishiyama A, et al. Role of NAD(P)H oxidase- and mitochondria-derived reactive oxygen species in cardioprotection of ischemic reperfusion injury by angiotensin II. Hypertension. 2005;**45**:860-866.

[26] Back P, Braeckman BP, Matthijssens F. ROS in aging Caenorhabditis elegans: Damage or signaling? Oxid Med Cell Longev. 2012;**2012**:608478.

[27] Wang JC, Bennett M. Aging and atherosclerosis mechanisms, functional consequences, and potential therapeutics for cellular senescence. Circulation Research. 2012;**111**:245-259.

[28] Tan LB, Williams SG, Goldspink DF. From CONSENSUS to CHARM – How do ACEI and ARB produce clinical benefits in chronic heart failure? International Journal of Cardiology. 2004;**94**:137-141

[29] Bai JW, Boulet G, Halpern EM, et al. Cardiovascular disease guideline adherence and self-reported statin use in longstanding type 1 diabetes: Results from the Canadian study of longevity in diabetes cohort. Cardioascular Diabetology. 2016;**15**:14.

[30] Benigni A, Cona D, Zoja C, et al. Disruption of the Ang II type 1 receptor promotes longevity in mice. Journal of Clinical Investigation. 2009;**119**:524-530.

[31] Geara AS, Azzi J, Jurewicz M, et al. The renin-angiotensin system: An old, newly discovered player in immunoregulation. Transplantation Reviews (Orlando, FL). 2009;**23**:151-158.

[32] Kossmann S, Schwenk M, Hausding M, et al. Angiotensin II-induced vascular dysfunction depends on interferon-γ-driven immune cell recruitment and mutual activation of monocytes and NK-cells. Arteriosclerosis, Thrombosis, and Vascular Biology. 2013;**33**:1313-1319.

[33] Ilieva I, Ohgami K, Jin XH, et al. Captopril suppresses inflammation in endotoxin-induced uveitis in rats. Experimental Eye Research. 2006;**83**:651-657.

[34] Di Paolo S, Schena A, Stallone G, et al. Captopril enhances transforming growth factor (TGF)-beta1 expression in peripheral blood mononuclear cells: A mechanism independent from angiotensin converting enzyme inhibition? A study in cyclosporine-treated kidney-transplanted patients. Transplantation. 2002;**74**:1710-1715.

[35] Folkersen L, Brynedal B, Diaz-Gallo LM, et al. Integration of known DNA, RNA and protein biomarkers provides prediction of anti-TNF response in rheumatoid arthritis: Results from the COMBINE study. Mol Med. 2016;**15**:22. DOI: 10.2119/molmed.2016.00078

[36] Desbois AC, Addimanda O, Bertrand A, et al. Efficacy of anti-TNF-α in severe and refractory neuro-behcet disease: An observational study. Medicine (Baltimore). 2016;**95**:e3550.

[37] Shi S, Liang D, Chen Y, et al. Gx-50 reduces β-amyloid-induced TNF-α, IL-1β, NO, and PGE2 expression and inhibits NF-κB signaling in a mouse model of Alzheimer's disease. European Journal of Immunology. 2016;**46**:665-676.

[38] Lennikov A, Kitaichi N, Noda K, et al. Amelioration of endotoxin-induced uveitis treated with an I-κB kinase β inhibitor in rats. Molecular Vision. 2012;**18**:2586-2597.

[39] Biancardi VC, Stranahan AM, Krause EG, et al. Cross talk between AT1 receptors and Toll-like receptor 4 in microglia contributes to angiotensin II-derived ROS production in the hypothalamic paraventricular nucleus. American Journal of Physiology: Heart and Circulatory Physiology. 2016;**310**:404-415.

[40] Amuchastegui SC, Azzollini N, Mister M, et al. Chronic allograft nephropathy in the rat is improved by angiotensin II receptor blockade but not by calcium channel antagonism. Journal of the American Society of Nephrology. 1998;**9**:1948-1955.

[41] El Desoky ES. Drug therapy of heart failure: An immunologic view. American Journal of Therapeutics. 2011;**18**:416-425.

[42] Shil PK, Kwon KC, Zhu P, et al. Oral delivery of ACE2/Ang-(1-7) bioencapsulated in plant cells protects against experimental uveitis and autoimmune uveoretinitis. Molecular Therapy. 2014;**22**:2069-2082.

11

Acanthamoeba Keratitis: The Emerging Vision-Threatening Corneal Disease

Lidia Chomicz, Jacek P. Szaflik, Marcin Padzik and Justyna Izdebska

Abstract

Some *Acanthamoeba* species are distributed in natural and man-made environments, in a wide range of soil and aquatic habitats, also in clinical settings. The amphizoic organisms can exist as facultative parasites - causative agents of serious human disease, *Acanthamoeba* keratitis. The vision-threatening eye disease occurring particularly in contact lens wearers is reported with increasing prevalence in different regions of the world. The amoebic keratitis is difficult to diagnose as clinical symptoms are similar to those observed in other eye diseases. Moreover, bacterial, viral, fungal, and amoebic co-infections frequently occur; also amoebae act as carriers for ~ 20 species pathogenic for humans, e.g. from *Pseudomonas, Legionella, Mycobacterium* and *Escherichia* genera; thus the corneal disease is frequently misdiagnosed. Complex etiology, late proper recognition of amoebic infections, and the exceptional resistance of *Acanthamoeba* cysts to chemicals are important factors influencing diagnostic and therapeutic difficulties. Surgical interventions are needed as an alternative treatment in refractory *Acanthamoeba* keratitis. It should be taken into consideration that the knowledge and awareness of increasing threat generated by the amphizoic amoebae are still insufficient. This compilation presents selected aspects of eye disease that is becoming the increasingly significant for human health worldwide.

Keywords: *Acanthamoeba* keratitis, risk factors, symptoms, pathogenesis, diagnostics, therapy

1. Introduction

Acanthamoeba keratitis (AK), the vision-threatening corneal disease that was first time recognized in 1973 in the United States in a Texas rancher [1], is reported with increasing prevalence in different regions and countries year after year [1- 7]. This corneal, usually acute and progressive infection is becoming increasingly significant for human health worldwide.

Eye diseases affecting the cornea are a major cause of blindness worldwide. Among different infectious agents, bacteria, fungi, viruses and protozoans may be causes of keratitis in contact lens users. At present, the epidemiology of microbial keratitis is complicated, diverse, and even controversial; the use of contact lenses is considered as the most important risk factor of corneal infections in humans [4,8]. It was emphasized in several reviews [8- 10] that the incidence rates of particular organisms causing keratitis associated with contact lens wear differ between parts of the world, from country to country and even from one population to another. Economic factors, various frequencies of contact lens wear in particular geographical locations, different availabilities and standards of eye care, and different methods of etiological agent isolation and culture in particular surveys were mentioned as factors influencing the differences and criteria taken into consideration in the studies.

The frequency of microbial keratitis cases caused by Gram-negative bacteria from genus *Pseudomonas* (as percent of total isolates from given location) varied in Europe: from 6.6% in Turkey to 72.2% in Italy and from 12% to 28.5% in various surveys from the United Kingdom [8]. Climate also influenced the incidence of bacterial keratitis: e.g.in Australia, the frequency of *P. aeruginosa* contact lens keratitis was increased in tropical zones than temperate zones.

The highest proportion of fungal corneal infections (*Aspergillus* sp., *Candida* sp.), 67% was found in India [9]; in Europe, the highest frequency of 22.2% was found in Turkey.

Correlations between the contact lens wear and percentages of bacterial and fungal keratitis were statistically significant.

The viruses from *Herpes* spp. are other agents of keratitis. There are relatively few studies on the epidemiology of *Herpes* keratitis in humans. According to review by Farooq and Shukla [11], in developed countries, *Herpes* keratitis is believed to be an important cause of infectious blindness mainly resulting from stromal opacification, e.g. it was reported from France that the incidence was 25.8 (21.2–30.4) per 100,000 person-years; 95% of the cases occurred in contact lens users. These authors found that the incidence of this keratitis is about 1.5 million, including 40,000 new cases of severe visual impairment each year, however, it is difficult to ascertain the frequency of the viral keratitis because of a lack of surveillance-based epidemiologic studies [11].

Protozoan eye disease, *Acanthamoeba* keratitis (AK), is rare in the general population (estimated incidence: 1.4 per million person- year) but much frequent in contact lens wearers. [4,12,13]. In the United States, an estimated 85% of cases occur in contact lens users. The incidence of the disease in developed countries is approximately 1-33 cases per million contact lens wearers, e.g. in England 17-21 cases per million. Currently, it is emphasized that an awareness and knowledge about AK -the serious, vision-threatening eye disease are still insufficient [12,18].

Previous and recent studies continued in many centers with a participation of practicing researchers and other scientists are crucial for a better understanding of *Acanthamoeba* keratitis [4,14-18]. Advances in the field are expected by both laboratory and clinical practitioners; particularly, an improvement in duration from first symptoms until suitable diagnosis as well as in efficacy of the therapeutic management and prophylaxis is the urgent need. Here, we present selected aspects of this multi-factorial human disease, including the results of our studies and own experiences in the topic.

1.1. Possible environmental sources of *Acanthamoeba* spp.

Free-living amoebae belonging to *Acanthamoeba* genus are ubiquitous and widely distributed in natural and man-made environments of many parts of the world [4,19-25]. The amoebae have been isolated from a wide range of soil and aquatic habitats; they occur in sea, fresh- chlorinated- and tap- water, drinking water systems, bottled mineral water, thermal recreational waters, swimming pools, air, air-conditioning systems including humidifiers, soil and dust, and sewage. The amoeboid protists have been found in fruits, vegetables, and also healthy, diseased or dead animals [12,18]. The amoebae have been isolated also from clinical settings and the hospital environment: on surfaces of different equipment and accessories, in water and air-conditioning systems, on surgical instruments, in dental irrigation units, in contact lenses and their cases, and in dialyzers [7,26,27].

1.2. The developmental forms and classification of *Acanthamoeba* spp.

The amoeboid, mitochondria-bearing protist is known as free-living organism that exists in two morphologic forms: trophozoite and cyst [4,12,18]. The life cycle of *Acanthamoeba* is asexual; the reproduction of trophozoite is by binary fission. This active vegetative stage contains one nucleus with large, central nucleolus (endosome), ectoplasm and granular endoplasm, with a large contractile vacuole as well as numerous mitochondria and digestive vacuoles. The trophozoite is changing in shape, 15–45μm in size and moving by cytoplasmic-transparent pseudopodia that create characteristic protrusions: spine-like acanthopodia. The dormant stage, cyst is smaller, 8-24μm in size, rounded or polygonal in shape, and double - walled, with wrinkled or rippled outer layer; the form indicates minimal metabolic activity. The outer wall of the cyst, the so-called ectocyst, contains lipids and proteins; the inner cyst wall, endocyst contains cellulose that is not present in trophozoite stage. The two cyst walls are separated by a space, except of points in that both walls meet; in these points - pores, i.e. ostioles occur that are covered by plugs, so-called opercula. The plugs are removed when trophozoites emerge from cysts during excystation [4,12]. Trophozoites transform into cyst stages after the growth developmental phase of amoeba population, in which high cell density occurs as well as under harmful environmental conditions (e.g. extremes in temperature and pH, increased or decreased osmolarity, lack of nutrients). The therapeutic experience and many *in vitro* studies showed that the cysts are highly resistant to antimicrobial drugs and a variety of chemical and physical agents [reviewed in 4,12]; they can remain viable under prolonged desiccation, starvation, heat and cold. Also, they can survive *in vitro* in distilled water as long as 25 years [28] and maintain their viability and virulence.

Following the recognition of the amoebae and increasing number of isolates belonging to the genus *Acanthamoeba*, for years they were classified using morphological criteria. In this classification, a size of cysts and the number of characteristic arm -like structures visible within a single cyst in light microscope were mainly taken into consideration [4,12,18,29,30]. At the time, 18 species have been determined and placed in three morphological groups I, II and III.

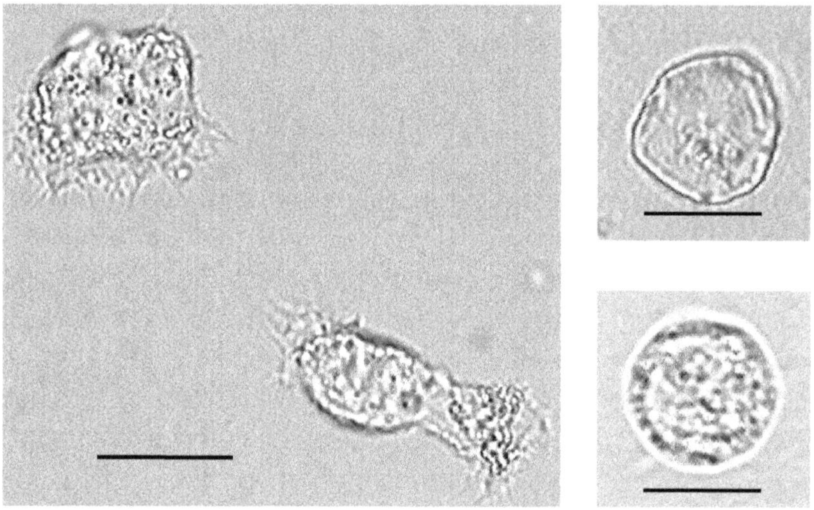

Figure 1. *Acanthamoeba* sp. - wet-mount slides from corneal scrapings; note characteristic spine-like acanthopodia in trophozoites and the double-walled cysts; light micrographs; scale bar = 10μm

The classification of *Acanthamoeba* species /isolates changed with the advances in molecular methods. Recently, it is based on genotype associations - the 18S rRNA gene sequence [5,20,31-33]. The modern approach differs from morphology solely: the species identification is based on combination of the morphological and molecular characterization [3,5,15,20]. At present, 18 or19 genotypes are distinguished for diagnostics and for the characterization of clinical and environmental *Acanthamoeba* isolates [12,15,18,31-33].

2. *Acanthamoeba* spp. as potential agents of human diseases

The protozoans belonging to *Acanthamoeba* spp. complete their life cycles in different outer environments as free-living organisms. Trophozoite forms are able to feed on various micro-organisms dwelling in soil and water (on bacteria, algae, and yeasts as well as on other protozoans) and on small organic particles. In natural, and even in man-made environments, the amoebae develop without entering human or animal organisms. However, in predisposing circumstances, the amoebae may enter the human body. According to literature [34,35], there are evidences from various regions that humans are exposed frequently to the amoebae: it has been confirmed by 50–100% of the healthy populations having specific anti- *Acanthamoeba* antibodies. The protists may permeate into the human body without pathogenic consequences. Investigations in which serological, biochemical and molecular methods were applied showed that people may be exposed both, to pathogenic as well as non-pathogenic *Acanthamoeba* strains [reviewed in 12,13,18]. In immunocompetent individuals, infections with these amoebae may be asymptomatic and/or self-limited.

Nevertheless, several amoebic strains belonging to this genus are able to enter, and colonize human organs and multiply within them, indicating pathogenic effects [4,12,26,27,36].

For this reason, these amoebae are called amphizoic amoebae, because they are able to exist in two different modes: as free-living-exozoic organisms and as endozoic parasitic organisms, within host tissues; thus, the free-living protozoans are also believed as facultative parasites.

Trophozoites and cysts of *Acanthamoeba* were detected during infections of various human cavities and tissues: in paranasal sinuses in rhino-sinusitis, in skin inflammation and skin ulceration, and in pneumonia [7,37,38]. We also found trophozoites and numerous cysts of *Acanthamoeba* among the oral cavity microbiota in 4% somatically and mentally disordered patients. The amoebae accompanied infections with other amoebae, *Entamoeba gingivalis*, the oral amoebae associated with a prolonged deterioration of the periodontium and gingiva [39].

Developmental stages of the amphizoic species may be causative agents of an systemic opportunistic disease developing in immunocompromised individuals. This is rare but almost always fatal granulomatous *Acanthamoeba* encephalitis (GAE) [6,12,18,40]. Other infection caused by the amphizoic amoebae may result in a sight-threatening *Acanthamoeba* keratitis (AK), a non-opportunistic disease occurring mainly in immunocompetent persons, mostly in contact lens wearers [1-3,7,14].

3. Pathogenesis in AK

In the early phase of AK, there are nonspecific symptoms variable in their intensity starting with redness, photophobia, and excessive tearing. Most commonly, only one eye is involved. Active epithelial inflammations usually progress from the outermost layer of the cornea deeper, to the stroma. Symptoms of the devastating eye disease include loss of the visual acuity. In many cases of AK, excruciating eye pain occurs, in which the intensity is often incommensurate with relatively small degree of corneal deterioration. There are clinical and histopathological evidences that the severe pain is associated with *Acanthamoeba* trophozoite activeness that result in the inflammation of the corneal nerves -radial keratoneuritis [4,27]. It is also emphasized that a characteristic ring-like corneal infiltration may occur in some patients. This amoebic eye infection may develop from a few days to several months, as a severe, prolonged disease, which, without suitable treatment may lead to blindness.

A pathogenesis of *Acanthamoeba* keratitis is a multi-factorial process connected with some factors contributing directly and indirectly in production of diseases in humans [12].

Among the direct contributing factors, the following are listed: adhesion of *Acanthamoeba* trophozoites to host cells, phagocytosis to take up food particles, neuraminidase activity, and secretion of toxins. The neuraminidase enzyme, which is active at 25-30 ºC, is believed to be important in a damaging of corneal epithelial cells [12,41]. Recently, the first toxin, acanthaporin, with pore-forming activity, cytotoxic for human neuronal cells was isolated from *Acanthamoeba*, which activation mechanism remains under investigations [12,42].

Among the indirectly contributing factors, there are amoebic and host determinants. Morpho-physiological features: the amoeboid motion and spine-like acanthopodia allow protozoans to modulate binding to biological and inert surfaces. Also, changes in the overall numbers of the amoebae as well as in the proportion of trophozoites and cysts dependent on the environmental conditions are also listed as the amoebic pathogenesis determinants. The temperature tolerance, osmotolerance and growth at different pH allow the amphizoic *Acanthamoeba* to exist in different environments and simultaneously easy adapt to different human organ and tissues, including the human cornea. Moreover, it has been shown that both, clinical and environmental *Acanthamoeba* strains/isolates vary in their among the oral cavity microbiota pathogenicity. The thermal tolerance and ability to grow at high temperature are considered to be indirect markers of the pathogenicity of *Acanthamoeba* strains [12,17,18,43-45].

4. Predisposing/ risk factors sufficient to contract AK

In several studies it is underlined that the initiating of AK is a multi-factorial process, in which both host and environmental determinants are likely involved, apart connected with *Acanthamoeba* pathogenic strains [4,12].

It is considered that *Acanthamoeba* keratitis is mainly related to contact lens wear, although, *Acanthamoeba* corneal infections are also detected in persons not using contact lenses [7,12-14, 46]. After the first case of AK associated with contact lenses in Central Europe was reported from Germany, more than 85% of all incidences of the disease have been recognized in different countries in wearers of contact lenses [12,17,18,47-50].

The estimation of AK findings in several countries showed various, generally relatively low, but constantly increasing number of the cornel disease incidents during the last few decades i.e. 1.36 cases per million contact lens wears in the United States, 17 to 21 cases per million in England, 1 per 30,000 contact lens wears in France, 0.05 per 10,000 in Holland [4,12,13]. However, "it is noteworthy", as Khan [4] concluded "that variations in the incidence rate of *Acanthamoeba* keratitis do not reflect the geographical distribution of *Acanthamoeba*, and are most likely due to variations in the extended wear of soft contact lenses, varied awareness of the potential risk associated with the contact lens wear, enhanced detection, and/or local conditions that promote growth of pathogenic *Acanthamoeba* only e.g.. water hardness or salinity, or conditions that suppress growth of non-pathogenic *Acanthamoeba*." Interestingly, in Austria, women and men were affected almost equally; the highest AK incidences occurred in the 21-30-years-old patients; simultaneously, poor contact lens hygiene is indicated as the most important risk factor of AK in this country [46].

Some micro-traumas occurring earlier or appearing in connection with the use of the lenses predispose to contract AK; a human organism's susceptibility, tissue specificity, tear factors, and secretory immunoglobulin A (sIgA), important in the specific immune defense mechanism, are among other host factors influencing development of this corneal disease. Environmental conditions such as temperature, osmolarity, and pH may be important in initiating AK.

Simultaneously, the amoebae were found in contact lens and in storage cases that may be potential sources and reservoirs of the facultative parasites [12,18,47-53]. In spite of this, the incidence rate of AK in wearers of contact lenses is remarkably low in comparison with the contact lens storage cases contaminated with *Acanthamoeba*.

Additionally, it has been confirmed for various *Acanthamoeba* strains that a swimming in recreational pools while contact lenses wearing promotes the infection; it is because of some human corneal micro-defects caused by lenses and extremely high resistance of the amoebae to chlorine disinfectants [12,17, 49-53].

In persons not using contact lenses, other circumstances influence as important for contract AK [4,47]. The different *Acanthamoeba* strains are ubiquitous in natural and man-made environments thus, an exposure of the eye especially to dust, water or moist soil, as well as to any foreign particle, on which trophozoites and cyst of the amoebae can occur, is considered as an AK predisposing factor. Also, if corneal epithelial injuries appear, and also during eye surgery, circumstances promoting the infection may occur.

There have been no reports of *Acanthamoeba* keratitis being spread from one person to another.

5. When the clinician should suspect *Acanthamoeba* keratitis?

It is known, that the emerging vision-threatening AK is difficult to diagnose because clinical manifestations are similar to those observed in the course of other infectious eye diseases.

In anamnesis, in the early stage of this eye disease - patients are complaining of photophobia, excessive tearing, and reduced visual acuity; the clinical manifestations of this keratitis may also include redness and eyelid edema [13,17,50,54].

Particularly, if a presence of any foreign particles will be excluded, appearing of excruciating eye pain with intensity incommensurate with degree of corneal deterioration may suggest that *Acanthamoeba* infection develops; however, the pain not always occurs. As a rule, AK should be suspected if, in anamnesis, the contact lens wear, a history of swimming in a lake, and in recreational pools while contact lenses wearing, exposure to soil, any case of corneal trauma, surgical procedures are reported to clinician [12,18]. However, according to different reports and own experience, the amoebic etiology of the keratitis cannot be excluded in patients with above mentioned symptoms and history, previously unsuccessfully treated in ophthalmic units with antiviral, antibacterial and/or antifungal medications that delayed proper diagnosis and the suitable therapeutic management [17,50,55].

6. Differential diagnosis of AK

6.1. A tentative diagnosis of AK

The non-invasive methods are useful for the tentative diagnosis of AK, in which the slit-lamp that provides magnification from 10 to 25 times and *in vivo* confocal microscopy (Figures 2 and 3) are applied [4,12,44,50,56].

The use of a slit lamp is indicated in any acute situation that requires magnification to inspect the anterior segment of the eye. Active epithelial inflammations and hyper reflective tissues in the affected eye may be visualized by the slit lamp; a corneal ulcer and characteristic, ring-like corneal infiltration may occur in some patients. However it should be underlined that the characteristic ring infiltrate is seen in approximately 50% of AK cases.

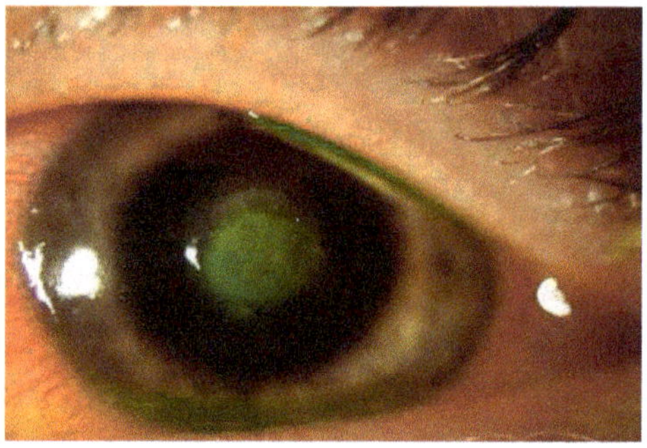

Figure 2. Slit-lamp photograph of corneal ulceration of severe *Acanthamoeba* keratitis case.

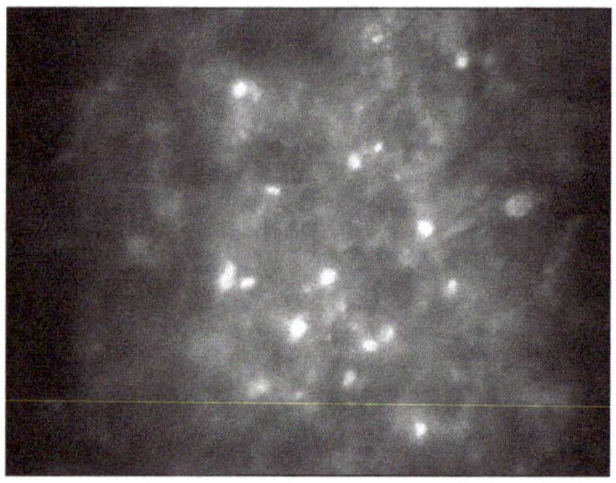

Figure 3. Hyper reflective objects - *Acanthamoeba* cysts in the affected eye with the late diagnosed severe keratitis; *in vivo* confocal microscopy; scale bar = 50μm

Different clinical presentations may occur in various causes of keratitis. However, in clinical AK practice there are nonspecific signs variable in their intensity starting with photophobia, redness, and excessive tearing that present with similar symptoms as viral, bacterial and fungal keratitis (4,7, 9-12].

In the slit lamp, corneal epithelial disease caused by *Herpes simplex* virus may be seen as dendritic keratitis or the geographic ulcer. The edges of these lesions with swollen epithelial cell stain with rose bengal while the central part stains with fluorescein [11,12,18].

Bacterial corneal infection appears typically as a one gray-white stromal infiltrate with well-demarked borders. Critical sings for fungal keratitis, e.g. *Fusarium* keratitis, are stromal gray-white or yellow-white infiltrate with a feathery border, satellite lesions surrounding the primary lesion; co-infections with fungi and bacteria can complicate the fungal keratitis [9,10,12].

In the early epithelial stage of *Acanthamoeba* keratitis, this infection can be misdiagnosed as a *Herpes simplex* keratitis because of irregular grayish lesions and pseudodendrites that are frequently observed in the epithelium. In advanced stage, AK can be mistaken as a fungal keratitis [9,11,12].

Active epithelial inflammations usually progresses from the outermost layer of the cornea -a superficial keratitis -to deeper stroma -the stromal or interstitial keratitis.

In the initial epithelial phase, typical signs of AK include epithelial or sub-epithelial infiltrates, pseudodendrites resembling these observed in *Herpes* keratitis, radial keratoneuritis (infiltrates along corneal nerves) and recurrent puncture staining of the corneal epithelium. Perineural infiltrates -a radial keratoneuritis are described as pathognomonic for the diagnosis of *Acanthamoeba* keratitis [12,18]; they are evoked by tropism of the amoebic organism for corneal nerves. Radial keratoneuritis is the reason for the extreme pain and is usually seen during the first one to four weeks of disease. Anterior stromal infiltrates are another common sing of AK. They gradually enlarge and coalesce to form a ring abscess, commonly located in the center of the cornea. Less specific signs of AK are satellite stromal infiltrates, diffuse stromal infiltrates and endothelial plaques observed in many of the patients.

Later signs of AK develop in 3-8 weeks and include a deep inflammation of the cornea consisting of a central stromal thinning and melting, anterior chamber cells and flare, hypopyon and extension of inflammation into sclera. The latter is generally reactive reaction rather than extension of infection; later in the disease course, the slowly progressive stromal opacifications and neovascularization may occur.

Etiological agents of infectious keratitis can be differing using *in vivo* confocal microscopy that is confirmed as useful tool for rapid diagnosis with high sensitivity [4,12,18,56,57].

Common findings in viral keratitis are: highly reflective, desquamating epithelial cells in superficial epithelial layer, multiple dendritic cells in basal epithelial layer, the absence of subepithelial nerve plexus, and hyperreflective keratocytes in the anterior stroma.

In bacterial keratitis, confocal micrographs typically reveal leucocytes infiltrating the corneal stroma and adherent to vessel walls. In some cases, the dendritic cells are present intrastromally; the bacteria themselves cannot be detected with the confocal microscopy.

Filamentous fungi and bacteria (e.g. *Nocardia*) can form filamentous structures that are large enough to be distinguished by confocal microscopy [57]. Another characteristics sing of filamentous fungal infection is hyphae branching, in a case of *Aspergillus* at 45° and in a case of *Fusarium* at 90°.

The examination of affected eyes by *in vivo* confocal microscopy make possible to distinguish AK from the aforementioned infectious keratitis. Lately, confocal scan features of cysts and trophozoites as well as associated corneal epithelial and stromal findings were described as criteria to specify AK in clinical diagnosis [57]. Presumable *Acanthamoeba* cysts can be visible as numerous hyper reflective, double-walled ovoid or spherical objects, 10-25μm in diameter, localized typically in deeper parts of epithelium and in anterior layers of the corneal stroma [4,18,57]. These findings should be distinguished from the well-delineated individual epithelial cell nuclei or leucocytes; the latter are larger and more regular than *Acanthamoeba* cysts. The outer wall of the cyst is more reflective than internal wall; with time, some cysts are not seen and the others become calcified. Trophozoites are also described as visible in confocal scan images, however, false results can occur because the forms are difficult to distinguish from nuclei of leukocytes and keratocytes [4,12,18]. Although confocal microscopy, if available, is non-invasive, high- sensitive tool for rapid *in vivo* diagnosis, examiners have to be familiar with morphology of *Acanthamoeba* forms. Also, differences in strain pathogenicity and viability can be taken into consideration.

It was evident also in our studies on monitoring of *in vitro* dynamics of *Acanthamoeba* strains isolated from infected eyes [17,50]; the presence of hyper reflective objects/cysts was revealed by this non-invasive *in vivo* confocal microscopy mainly for severe, late diagnosed infections with strains of which strong viability was indicated by intensive multiplying of trophozoites *in vitro* and their long survival time (42 months) in culture medium. Contrary to this, no cysts were detected by the confocal technique in material from corneal scraping if infections with weak viability strains occurred; a low amoeba number in the exponential growth phase and short (10 days) survival time of such amoeba strains were manifested *in vitro* in the culture medium. Also, no cyst was found in confocal microscopy images when mixed infections occurred, although finally the infection with *Acanthamoeba* was confirmed by laboratory methods.

Negative results of the *in vivo* confocal microscopy were reported if patients have already been pre-treated, thus the amoeba density was very low [12,50].

6.2. Why clinical manifestations are not sufficient to indicate a causative agent of keratitis

Knowledge and awareness of threat are necessary as the most important step in proper AK diagnosis as it is underlined by J. Lorenzo-Morales et al. [12].

The careful anamnesis is very important and helpful. Most of the clinical symptoms of *Acanthamoeba* keratitis are nonspecific and frequently a variability in their intensity is observed and reported from different world regions. AK is often misdiagnosed as viral infection with *Herpes simplex,* bacterial with *Pseudomonas aeruginosa* or keratitis caused by fungi of genera *Fusarium* or *Candida*; moreover, bacterial, viral, and fungal co-infections with *Acanthamoeba* may occur [2,4,46]. This is why the clinical symptoms alone, as non- pathognomonic, are not sufficient to indicate an etiological agent of human keratitis.

Undoubtedly, the non-invasive *in vivo* confocal microscopy is a valuable technique, however usefulness of it is limited if bacterial or viral keratitis occurs, thus it should be applied for the tentative diagnosis.

Also, in our several studies we analyzed serious keratitis cases regarding patients who were under suspicion of *Acanthamoeba* etiology of the infections. Although, in our hospital, finally AK was determined, there were mistakes in results of earlier diagnostics. The mixed amoebic, bacterial (*P. aeruginosa, E. faecalis*), and fungal (*Candida* sp.) infections have been revealed by us in more than 50% cases regarding persons previously unsuccessfully treated only with antibacterial and antifungal medications in other ophthalmic units [17,50].

It has been reported that *Acanthamoeba* protozoans may carry more than 20 species pathogenic for humans, among others bacteria belonging to genera *Legionella, Pseudomonas, Mycobacterium,*

Listeria and *Escherichia*, protozoa *Cryptosporidium* sp., and fungi *Cyrptococcus neoformans*. The microorganisms are able not only to survive within cells but even proliferate inside the amoebae; thus, secondary infections can occur and influence diagnostic difficulties [4,12, 18].

6.3. Laboratory evaluation

Literature data as well as results of our studies indicated that microscopic visualization of amoebae in unstained or stained slides prepared directly from corneal scraping is usefulness for AK diagnostics. Also, laboratory examinations of specimens from *in vitro* cultivated corneal isolates allow to identify directly the facultative pathogens and to verify previous misdiagnoses [4,12,46,50].

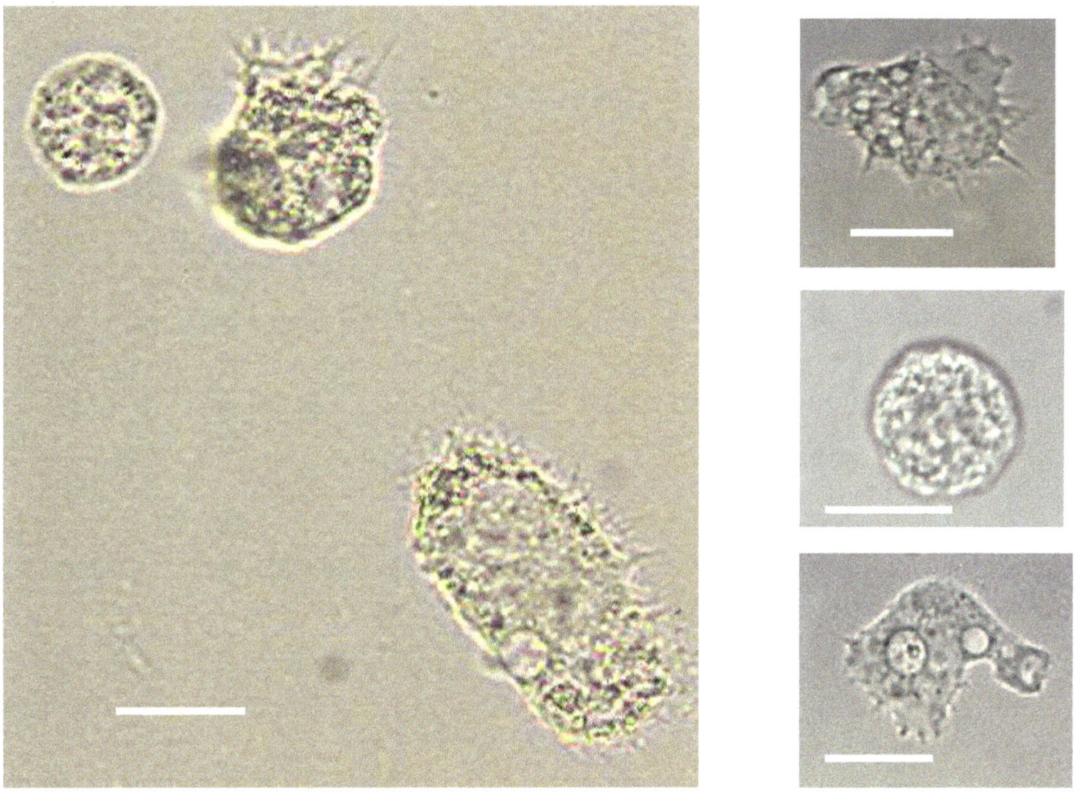

Figure 4. Live *Acanthamoeba* trophozoites and cysts in unstained preparations from corneal isolates cultured *in vitro*; light micrographs. Scale bars = 10μm

Moreover, culture methods are considered as the gold standard of diagnosis, which needs, however, collaboration between clinicians and laboratory staff and, also, the familiarization with a morphological characteristic of *Acanthamoeba* stages [12,14,18,55,58-60]. Non-nutrient (NN) agar plates seeded with Gram- negative, non-mucous bacteria: *Escherichia coli* or *Enterobacter aerogenes* are applied for isolation/growth of *Acanthamoeba* trophozoites both from environmental and clinical samples (corneal scrapings, biopsies, swabs). The incubation of the plates at 30ºC promotes a transformation of amoeba trophozoites into cysts within approximately 1 week. Also, the cultivation of amoebae in bacteria-free (axenic) conditions in a modified enriched culture medium containing antibiotics (penicillin, streptomycin) is useful for classification cysts to the morphological level.

Simultaneously, molecular methods of classification of *Acanthamoeba* isolates, with the use of sensitive PCR techniques, basing on genotype associations are distinguishing for diagnostics and for the characterization of clinical and environmental *Acanthamoeba* isolate [12,18,27,32,33,59]. In this modern approach, the species identification is based on the combination of morphological and molecular characteristics of amoebae. Additionally, our experiences gave convincing evidences of an importance of a clinical examination of the affected eyes and laboratory differentiations/identification of amoebic forms in material deriving from infected corneas.

7. Treatment options in AK

7.1. Factors complicating effective pharmacotherapy in AK

AK treatment is difficult and often unsuccessful despite of advances in pharmacotherapy. There are several factors that are listed as influencing difficulties and still not fully effective of applied therapy [12,18].

AK is often incorrect diagnosed due to nonspecific clinical symptoms; similar clinical pictures to this observed in the amoebic keratitis may give a wide range of agents e.g. viral *Herpes simplex*, bacterial -mostly *Pseudomonas aeruginosa* or fungi of *Fusarium* spp.

Additionally, mixed amoebic, fungal viral and bacterial keratitis may occur that complicate therapeutic management.

Acanthamoeba strains vary in their pathogenicity: they may be virulent, weakly virulent or non-virulent; they show different susceptibilities to chemicals and answer to pharmacotherapy.

It is also underlined that extremely high resistance of *Acanthamoeba* cysts to different chemicals, disinfectants as well as anti-microbial and anti-parasitic drugs result in disappointing therapeutic management [12,18,54,59-64].

Among the abovementioned facts, diagnostic mistakes that cause delayed in a beginning of an efficient treatment may result in a prolonged, severe course of AK and vision deterioration.

It is also emphasized that some chemicals can induce amoebic encystment that subsequently, by excystment, may lead to repeated development of trophozoites, thus an activation of the dormant cysts can lead to recurrence of the disease. It is why not only amoebicidal effects but also the cysticidal efficacy of applied therapeutics is very important [43-46].

In some research works, also in our experimental studies it has been reported that higher concentrations of drugs and some new-synthesized imidazole derivatives may be *in vitro* efficacious against *Acanthamoeba* strains and result not only in amoebostatic but also in amoebicidal effects. However, many of these chemicals cannot be applied *in vivo* in such concentrations due to their toxicity for human tissues [44-50].

7.2. Treatment recommended in management in AK

Currently, there are not known single-treatment methods effective against both trophozoites and cysts of *Acanthamoeba*; generally, AK is difficult to treat. *Acanthamoeba* stages differ in their susceptibility to various drugs. Trophozoite form is highly responsive to the treatment, while cysts are highly resistant as the cystic form protects the amoebic organism from unfavorable environmental factors, including drugs. The therapeutic approach recommended in AK consists of antimicrobial agent's combination [4,12,18,36].

The mainstay agents that are used as a first-line treatment for *Acanthamoeba* keratitis are diamidines (propamidine, hexamidine) and biguanides (polyhexamethylene biguanide (–PHMB), chlorhexidine), which were found to be cysticidal anti-amoebics *in vitro*. PHMB is the most preferred agent in monotherapy or in combinations with other drugs. Chlorhexidine can also be used in monotherapy, but it is much more effective in combined treatment. Propamidine is used in combination with one of biguanides, as the latter are more effective against cysts of *Acanthamoeba* [65]. Although neomycin was used widely, it is ineffective against cysts *in vitro*; thus, it is no longer used by most ophthalmologists.

However, particularly after earlier improper treatment in other centers, the combination drug therapy with the antimicrobial agents is used more or less successfully. Additionally, such factors as human organism status, a virulence of amoeba strains, phase of infection, and kind and concentration of the chemicals applied may determine variability in effects of drugs on trophozoites and cysts of several *Acanthamoeba* strains [12,16,22,45,50,64-67].

The most frequently used agents that achieve sufficient high concentrations at the site of infection and are effective against trophozoites and cysts of *Acanthamoeba* are cationic disinfectants: chlorhexidine 0.02–0.2% (200–2000 g/ml), polyhexamethylene biguanide (PHMB) 0.02–0.06% (200–600g/ml), and propamidine isethionate (Brolene 0.1%). These topical antimicrobials should be administered immediately to the infected eye one to two drops on the surface of the cornea at the first several days, every hour, minimum nine times/day, and, next, every 3h. The therapy duration is depending on clinical response. The amoebae may persist in the encysted stage for months and reactivate after therapy discontinuation. It was indicated in many earlier and current studies that a therapy continuation is very important to avoid an activation of the dormant cysts that may lead to repeated trophozoite development and thus to recurrence of the disease [4,12,13]. Some authors advise the treatment for 3- 4 months in order to preclude recurrence; however, the treatment for 6–12 months is also recommended. Nevertheless, it is reported that *Acanthamoeba* strains/cysts resistance to drug may occur, which is the main difficulty in AK treating [12,18,43,63,66]; particularly, resistance to propamidine and, also toxicity effect are observed in the course of AK. Corneal epithelial toxicity has been minimal for both chlorhexidine 0.02% and PHMB 0.02%. The greatest frequency of ocular toxicity has been reported with propamidine; the most common side effect is the superficial punctate keratopathy [65]. Pain can be relieved by topical cycloplegics (e.g. atropine 0.5-1.0%, scopolamine 0.25% t.i.d.), agents and oral non-steroidal anti-inflammatory medications (e.g. naproxen 250-500mg p.o. b.i.d.).

It should be also taken into consideration that co-infections with other microorganisms may complicate the course and treatment of the severe amoebic disease [18,49-51].

Although the low doses of topical steroids can be useful to diminish inflammation in cases of controlled infection but the use of topical corticosteroids is controversial.

Systemic corticosteroids are preferred over topical ones in cases of severe inflammation. This route of administration provides better ocular safety profile (less concentration in the cornea) but less body safety profile. However there are some suggestions that steroid use may result in increased pathogenicity of the amoebae [68].

If the topical pharmacotherapy fails, surgical interventions are needed [12,44,64,67]. Cross-linking and cryopreserved amniotic membrane graft (AMG) have been reported to be effective in AK.

The corneal transplantation can be performed for therapeutic or optical indications. Therapeutic, usually penetrating, keratoplasty is applied when the infectious process spreads to the corneal stroma, causing corneal melting and thinning despite of aggressive prolonged anti-amoebic therapy [4,12,18]. In a case of threatening or completed perforation of the cornea, the surgery must be performed urgently. Some authors recommend systemic steroids prior to surgery if concomitant limbitis or scleritis is present [69].

Sacher et al.[70] show that pretreatment of *Acanthamoeba* keratitis with intravenous pentamidine before therapeutic keratoplasty may assist with the achievement of microbiological cure, clear graft, and good visual outcome in a majority of eyes with AK.

The size of corneal graft should be minimum to excise an inflamed and necrotic tissue. Although remaining clinically healthy cornea is frequently also infected, this tissue should be saved because of the higher risk of rejection with large/decentrated grafts and because the possibility of repeat grafting should be kept in mind in the event of recurrence; a further graft represents a new food source for the organism and can be used to attract residual amoebae [69].

In a case of therapeutic keratoplasty for AK, the topical steroids in combination with anti-amoebic drugs are applied for 6-12 months following keratoplasty, to relieve pain, lessen the inflammation, and prevent graft rejection and recurrence of infection. Corneal grafts performed in the eyes with active inflammation are the high-risk transplants and they required systemic immunosuppression similar to this given in organ transplants (cyclosporine and/or mycophenolate mofetil). Apart from a poor graft survival, the postoperative glaucoma is a frequent complication.

In optical keratoplasty performed after resolution of active keratitis there is an excellent prognosis for both graft survival and visual outcome [71].

Promising clinical results were reported from amoebicidal effect of combined riboflavin and UV-A (ultraviolet light A, 365nm wavelength) exposure -corneal cross-linking (CXL) that was used for stabilization of corneal melting which can delay surgical treatment [12,72,73]. CXL has also an antimicrobial effect that is due to the effect of UV light interacting with riboflavin as the chromophore. It damages both the DNA and RNA of pathogens. Photoactivated chromophore for infectious keratitis (PACK)-CXL is an alternative to standard antibiotic therapy in treating infectious corneal disorders, and may help reduce the microbial resistance to antibiotics and avoid therapeutic keratoplasty in some cases [74].

Many chemicals and antimicrobials were examined and are still tested *in vitro* for their potential activity against different species, strains and isolates of *Acanthamoeba* [45,54,61-63,67]. Due to the toxicity of high concentrations of agents tested and a drug resistance, an optimal strategy for anti-acanthamoebic treatment is not yet defined. Further studies in this field are needed, particularly, in terms of cysticidal effects of the chemicals tested.

8. Prevention and prognosis of AK

The *Acanthamoeba* species are ubiquitous and widely distributed in natural and man-made environments. In various regions, humans were exposed frequently to the amoebae, that has been confirmed when in healthy populations specific anti- *Acanthamoeba* antibodies have been detected. For this reason, knowledge and awareness of threat are important to avoid the infection [6,12,18].

The contact lens wearers must be well educated as for the proper use and care of their lenses; do not use saline solution for lens storage, and do not to swim wearing contact lenses or use the swimming goggles. It is also very important to educate the ophthalmologist to be aware of signs and symptoms of AK and be able to early diagnose and initiate suitable treatment.

The prognosis for visual recovery with only mild residual stromal involvement is very good; in other cases, the visual prognosis is poor. Generally, a prediction depends on inflammation status at the time of diagnosis and the prompt initiation of proper treatment.

A retrospective review indicates that early diagnosis (less than 18 days) results in better final visual acuity and less likely needs keratoplasty [75]. In the early stage of infection, trophozoite forms are predominated, and the infection is confined to the superficial corneal layers. With time as the process progresses, the microorganisms enter to the deeper corneal stroma and encyst. Cysts are much more resistant to anti-protozoan drugs compared to trophozoites. Severe inflammation, scleral involvement, late diagnosis, and retardation of the therapy initialization are associated with poor clinical outcomes. In 10% of cases, there is associated scleritis. *Acanthamoeba* sclerokeratitis is associated with poor clinical outcomes [12,13,75].

9. Conclusions

Complex infective etiology and late recognition of amoebic infections were the important factors influencing diagnostic and therapeutic difficulties in AK. Laboratory examinations including *in vitro* cultivation of the isolates, acquired from corneal scrapings, allow directly to identify the facultative pathogens -the causative agents of the keratitis and to verify previous misdiagnoses. Early proper diagnosis in *Acanthamoeba* keratitis, confirmed by detection of live trophozoites in corneal scraping cultures are decisive for the treatment efficacy, particularly in contact lens wearers. The pharmacotherapy of the infectious eye disease is often unsuccessful; among others, it is if chemicals induce amoebic encystment; subsequently, an activation of the cysts can lead to repeated development of trophozoites and recurrence of the disease.

In some severe cases, keratoplasty and prolonged application of a mixture of drugs may be an appropriate option for visual rehabilitation.

Moreover, as our studies and experience show, *in vitro* monitoring of dynamics of *Acanthamoeba* strains isolated from affected eyes may be useful tool for proper diagnosis, therapeutic management and treatment prognosis.

Human infections with facultative parasitic *Acanthamoeba* strains are serious medical problem that should be taken into consideration as emerging threats of the public health worldwide.

Therefore, further educational efforts directed first of all to contact lens users are desirable for the prevention of this vision-threatening corneal disease.

Author details

Lidia Chomicz[1*], Jacek P. Szaflik[2], Marcin Padzik[1] and Justyna Izdebska[2]

*Address all correspondence to: lidia.chomicz@wum.edu.pl

1 Department of Medical Biology, Medical University of Warsaw, Warsaw, Poland

2 Department of Ophthalmology, Medical University of Warsaw, SPKSO Ophthalmic University Hospital, Warsaw, Poland

References

[1] Nagington J, Watson PG, Playfair TJ, McGill J, Jones BR, Steele ADM: Amoebic infection of the eye. Lancet. 1974;304:1537–540.

[2] Ibrahim YW, Boase DL, Cree IA: Factors affecting the epidemiology of *Acanthamoeba* keratitis. Ophthalmic Epidemiology. 2007;14:53–60.

[3] Lorenzo-Morales J, Martín-Navarro CM, López-Arencibia A, Arnalich-Montiel F, Piñero JE, Valladares B: *Acanthamoeba* keratitis: an emerging disease gathering importance worldwide? Trends in Parasitology. 2013;29(4):181–187.

[4] Khan NA: Acanthamoeba: Biology and Pathogenesis. Caister Academic Press, Norfolk, UK. 2009;290.

[5] Schroeder M, Booton GC, Hay J: Use of subgenic 18S ribosomal DNA PCR and sequencing for genus and genotype identification of *Acanthamoebae* from humans with keratitis and from sewage sludge, Journal of Clinical Microbiology. 2001;39:1903–1911.

[6] Schuster FL, Visvesvara GS: Amebic encephalitides and amebic keratitis caused by pathogenic and opportunistic free-living amebas. Current Treatment Options in Infectious Diseases. 2003;5:273–282.

[7] Marciano-Cabral F, Cabral G: *Acanthamoeba* spp. as agents of disease in humans. Clinical Microbiology Reviews. 2003;16(2):273-307.

[8] Giese MJ, Weissman BA: Contact lens associated corneal infections. Where do we go from here? Clinical & Experimental Optometry. 2002;85(3):141-148.

[9] Shah A, Sachdev A, Coggon D, Hossain P: Geographic variations in microbial keratitis: an analysis of the peer-reviewed literature. British Journal of Ophthalmology. 2011;95:762-767. doi:10.1136/bjo.2009.169607.

[10] Willcox M DP: Management and treatment of contact lens-related *Pseudomonas* keratitis. Clinical Ophthalmology. 2012: 6:919- 924. http://dx.doi.org/10.2147/OPTH.S25168.

[11] Farooq AV, Shukla D: *Herpes simplex* epithelial and stromal keratitis: an epidemiologic update. Survey of Ophthalmology. 2012;57(5):448-462. doi:10.1016/jsurvophthal.2012.01.005.

[12] Lorenzo-Morales J, Khan NA, Walochnik J: An update on *Acanthamoeba* keratitis: diagnosis, pathogenesis and treatment. Parasite. 2015;22:1-20.

[13] Trabelsi H, Dendana F, Sellami A, Sellami H, Cheikhrouhou F, Neji S, Makni F, Ayadi A: Pathogenic free-living amoebae: Epidemiology and clinical review. Pathologie Biologie. 2012;60:399–405.

[14] Khan NA: *Acanthamoeba*: biology and increasing importance in human health. FEMS Microbiology Reviews. 2006;30:564–595.

[15] Booton GC, Joslin CE, Shoff M: Genotypic identification of *Acanthamoeba* sp. isolates associated with an outbreak of *Acanthamoeba* keratitis. Cornea. 2009;28(6):673–676.

[16] Alizadeh H, Apte S, El-Agha MS: Tear IgA and serum IgG antibodies against *Acanthamoeba* in patient with *Acanthamoeba* keratitis. Cornea. 2001;20:622–627.

[17] Chomicz L, Conn DB, Padzik M, Szaflik JP, Walochnik J, Zawadzki PJ, Pawłowski W, Dybicz M: Emerging threats for human health in Poland: pathogenic isolates from drug resistant *Acanthamoeba* keratitis monitored in terms of their *in vitro* dynamics and temperature adaptability. BioMed Research International. 2015:Article ID 231285, 8pages, doi:10.1155/2015/231285.

[18] Khan NA: Acanthamoeba: Biology and Pathogenesis 2nd ed, Caister Academic Press. Norfolk, UK. 2015;295.

[19] Rodriguez-Zaragoza S, Magana-Becerra A: Prevalence of pathogenic *Acanthamoeba* (Protozoa: Amoebidae) in the atmosphere of the city of San Luis Potosi, Mexico. Toxicology & Industrial Health. 1997;13:519–526.

[20] Kilic A, Tanyuksel M, Sissons J, Jayasekera S, Khan NA: Isolation of *Acanthamoeba* isolates belonging to T2, T3, T4 and T7 genotypes from environmental samples in Ankara, Turkey. Acta Parasitologica. 2004;49(246):252.

[21] Martinez AJ, Visvesvara GS: Free-living, amphizoic and opportunistic amebas. Brain Pathology. 1997;7:583–598.

[22] Łanocha N, Kosik-Bogacka D, Maciejewska A, Sawczuk M, Wilk A, Kuźna-Grygiel W: The occurrence *Acanthamoeba* (free living amoeba) in environmental and respiratory samples in Poland. Acta Protozoologica. 2009;48(3):271–279.

[23] Nagyová V, Nagy A, Jane ček Š, Timko J: Morphological,physiological, molecular and phylogenetic characterization of new environmental isolates of *Acanthamoeba* spp. from the region of Bratislava, Slovakia. Biologia. 2010;65(1):81–91.

[24] Mahmoudi MR, Taghipour N, Eftekhar M, Haghighi A, Karanis P: Isolation of *Acanthamoeba* species in surface waters of Gilan province-north of Iran. Parasitology Research. 2012;110(1):473–477.

[25] Visvesvara GS, Moura H, Shuster FL: Pathogenic and opportunistic free-living amoebae: *Acanthamoeba* spp., *Balamuthia mandrillaris, Naegleria fowleri* and *Sappinia diploidea.* FEMS Immunology and Medical Microbiology. 2007;50:1–26.

[26] Schuster FL, Visvesvara GS: Free-living amoebae as opportunistic and non-opportunistic pathogens of humans and animals. International Journal for Parasitology. 2004a;34:1001–1027.

[27] Trabelsi H, Sellami A, Dendena F, Sellami H, Cheikh-rouhou F, Makni F, S. Ben Dhiaa·Ayadi A: Free-living amoebae (FLA): morphological and molecular identification of *Acanthamoeba* in dental unit water. Amibes libres : identification morphologique et moléculaire d'*Acanthamoeba* dans l'eau des unités dentaires. Parasite. 2010;17:67–70.

[28] Mazur T, Hadas E, Iwanicka I: The duration of the cyst stage and the viability and virulence of *Acanthamoeba* isolates. Tropical Medicine and Parasitology. 1995;46:106–108.

[29] Poussard M, Pons R: Morphologies de la paroi kystique et taxonomie du genre *Acanthamoeba* (Protozoa, Amoebida). Protistologica. 1997;13:557-610.

[30] Page FC: A New Key to Fresh Water and Soil Gymnamoebae, Freshwater Biological Association Scientific Publications, Ambleside. 1988;122.

[31] Khan NA, Jarroll EL, Paget TA: Molecular and physiological differentiation between pathogenic and nonpathogenic *Acanthamoeba*, Current Microbiology. 2002;45:197-202.

[32] Rivière D, Szczebara FM, Berjeaud JM, Frère J, Héchard Y: Development of a realtime PCR assay for quantification of *Acanthamoeba* trophozoites and cysts. Journal of Microbiological Methods. 2006; 64(1):78–83.

[33] Risler A, Coupat-Goutaland B, Pelandakis M: Genotyping and phylogenetic analysis of *Acanthamoeba* isolates associated with keratitis. Parasitology Research. 2013;112(11):3807-3816.

[34] Chappell CL, Wright JA, Coletta M, Newsome AL: Standardized method of measuring *Acanthamoeba* antibodies in sera from healthy human subjects. Clinical and Diagnostic Laboratory Immunology. 2001;8:724–730.

[35] Brindley N, Matin A, Khan NA: *Acanthamoeba castellanii*: high antibody prevalence in racially and ethnically diverse populations. Experimental Parasitology. 2009;121:254–256.

[36] Schuster FL, Visvesvara GS: Opportunistic amoebae: challenges in prophylaxis and treatment. Drug Resistance Updates. 2004b;7:41–51.

[37] Teknos TN, Poulin MD, Laruentano AM, Li KK: *Acanthamoeba* rhinosinusitis: characterization, diagnosis and treatment. American Journal of Rhinology. 2000;14:387–391.

[38] van Hamme C, Dumont M, Delos M, Lachapelle JM: Cutaneous acanthamoebiasis in a lung transplant patient. Annales de Dermatologie et de Vénéréologie. 2001;128:1237–1240.

[39] Chomicz L, Piekarczyk J, Starościak B, Fiedor P, Piekarczyk B, Szubińska D, Zawadzki PJ, Walski M: Comparative studies on the occurrence of protozoans, bacteria and fungi in the oral cavity of patients with systemic disorders. Acta Parasitologica. 2002;47:147–153.

[40] Jones B, Visvesvara GS and Robinson NM: *Acanthamoeba polyphaga* keratitis and *Acanthamoeba* uveitis associated with fatal meningoencephalitis, Transactions of the Ophthalmological Societies of the United Kingdom. 1975;95:221-232.

[41] Pellegrin JL, Ortega-Barria E, Barza M, Baum J, Pereira ME: Neuraminidase activity in *Acanthamoeba* species trophozoites and cysts. Investigative Ophthalmology and Visual Science. 1991;32:3061–3066.

[42] Michalek M, Sönnichsen FD, Wechselberger R, Dingley AJ, Hung CW, Kopp A,Wienk H, Simanski M, Herbst R, Lorenzen I, Marciano-Cabral F, Gelhaus C, Gutsmann T, Tholey A, Grötzinger J, Leippe M: Structure and function of a unique pore-forming protein from a pathogenic *Acanthamoeba*. Nature Chemical Biology. 2013;9:37–42.

[43] Aksozek A, McClellan K, Howard K: Resistance of *Acanthamoeba castellanii* cysts to physical, chemical and radiological conditions. Journal of Parasitology. 2002;88:621-623.

[44] Szaflik JP, Padzik M, Chomicz L, Oledzka G, Izdebska J: Usefulness of *in vitro* diagnostics in difficult incidences of *Acanthamoeba* keratitis requiring pharmacotherapy and surgical management. Okulistyka. 2012;3:28–32.

[45] Chomicz L, Padzik M, Graczyk Z, Starociak B, Graczyk T., Naprawska A, Olędzka G, Szostakowska B: *Acanthamoeba castellanii*: *in vitro* effects of selected biological, physical and chemical factors. Experimental Parasitology. 2010;126,103–105.

[46] Walochnik J, Scheikl U, Haller-Schober EM: Twenty years of *Acanthamoeba* diagnostics in Austria. Journal of Eukaryotic Microbiology. 2015;62(1),3–11.

[47] Padzik M, Chomicz L, Szaflik JP, Chruscikowska A, Perkowski K, Szaflik J: *In vitro* effects of selected contact lens care solutions on *Acanthamoeba castellanii* strains in Poland. Experimental Parasitology. 2014;145:98–101.

[48] Witschel H, Sundmacher R, Seitz HM: Amebic keratitis: clinico-histopathologic case report. Klinische Monatsblatter fur Augenheilkunde: 1984;185:46–49.

[49] Moore MB, McCulley JB, Luckenbach M: *Acanthamoeba* keratitis associated with soft contact lenses. American Journal of Ophthalmology. 1985;100:396–403.

[50] Chomicz L, Padzik M, Szaflik JP, Nahorski WL, Kryczka T, Szaflik J: Monitoring of *in vitro* dynamics of *Acanthamoeba* strains isolated from infected eyes as a useful tool in keratitis management. Experimental Parasitology. 2014;145:73-77.

[51] Larkin DFP, Kilvington S, Easty L: Contamination of contact lens storage cases by *Acanthamoeba* and bacteria. British Journal of Ophthalmology. 1990;74:133–135.

[52] Hiti K, Walochnik J, Haller-Schober EM, Faschinger C, Aspock H: Viability of *Acanthamoeba* after exposure to a multipurpose disinfecting contact lens solution and two hydrogen peroxide systems. British Journal of Ophthalmology. 2002;86:144–146.

[53] Hiti K, Walochnik J, Faschinger C, Haller-Schober EM, Aspock H: One- and two-step hydrogen peroxide contact lens disinfection solutions against *Acanthamoeba*: how effective are they? Eye. 2005;19:1301–1305.

[54] Chomicz L, Zebrowska J, Piekarczyk J, Starosciak B, Myjak P, Walski M, Kazimierczuk Z: *In vitro* studies on susceptibility of *Acanthamoeba castellanii* to selected chemical agents. Acta Parasitologica. 2005;50:25–31.

[55] da Rocha-Azevedo B, Tanowitz HB, Marciano-Cabral F: Diagnosis of infections caused by pathogenic free-living amoebae. Hindawi Publishing Corporation. Interdisciplinary Perspectives on Infectious Diseases. 2009:1–14. ID 251406.

[56] Winchester K, Mathers WD, Sutphin JE, Daley TE: Diagnosis of *Acanthamoeba* keratitis *in vivo* with confocal microscopy. Cornea. 1995;14(1):10-17.

[57] Rezaei Kanavi M, Naghshgar N, Javadi MA, Sadat Hashemi M: Various confocal scan features of cysts and trophozoites in cases with *Acanthamoeba* keratitis. European Journal of Ophthalmology. 2012; 22:46-50.

[58] Schuster FL: Cultivation of pathogenic and opportunistic free-living amebas. Clinical Microbiology Reviews. 2002;15(3):342–354.

[59] Lass A, Szostakowska B, Idzińska A, Chomicz L: The first genotype determination of *Acanthamoeba* potential threat to human health, isolated from natural water reservoirs in Poland. Parasitology Research. 2014;113(7):2693-2699.

[60] Walochnik J, Obwaller A, Aspock H: Correlations between morphological, molecular biological, and physiological characteristics in clinical and nonclinical isolates of *Acanthamoeba* spp. Applied and Environmental Microbiology. 2000;66:4408–4413.

[61] Lloyd D, Turner NA, Khunkitti W, Hann AC, Furr JR, Russell AD: Encystation in *Acanthamoeba castellanii*: development of biocide resistance. Journal of Eukaryotic Microbiology. 2001;48:11–16.

[62] Kopanska K, Najda A, Zebrowska J, Chomicz L, Piekarczyk J, Myjak P, Bretner M: Synthesis and activity of 1H-benzimidazole and 1H-benzotriazole derivatives as inhibitors of *Acanthamoeba castellanii.* Bioorganic & Medicinal Chemistry. 2004;12:2617-2624.

[63] Turner NA, Russell AD, Furr JR, Lloyd D: Emergence of resistance to biocides during differentiation of *A. castellanii.* Journal of Antimicrobial Chemotherapy. 2000;46:27–34.

[64] Chomicz L, Szaflik JP, Padzik M, Oledzka G, Iwanczyk B, Szaflik J: Anti-amoebic chemotherapeutics and surgical procedures in *Acanthamoeba* keratitis difficult to diagnose. In: Proceedings of 47th Congress of the European Society for Surgical Research, 6-9 June, 2012, Lille, France. Medimond International Proceedings. 2012;55–57.

[65] Yolton DP, Haesaert SP: Anti-infective drugs. Bartlett JD, Jaanus SD. Clinical Ocular Pharmacology. 5th ed. Elsevier. Butterworth Heinemann. 2008

[66] Ficker L, Seal D, Warhurst D, Wright P: *Acanthamoeba* keratitis- resistance to medical therapy. Eye. 1990;4:835–838.

[67] Chomicz L, Padzik M, Izdebska J, Baltaza W, Wroczynski P, Szaflik JP: *In vitro* activity of toyocamycin and novel thioinozine derivative as potential drugs against amphizoic amoebae -the causative agents of *Acanthamoeba* keratitis. The International Symposium on Ocular Pharmacology and Therapeutics. 12th ISOPT Clinical, Berlin, Germany, July 9-12. Session: Inflammation and Infection, Abstracts. 2015;732.

[68] Robaei D, Carnt N, Minassian DC, Dart JK: The impact of topical corticosteroid use before diagnosis on the outcome of *Acanthamoeba* keratitis. Ophthalmology. 2014;121(7):1383–1388.

[69] Graffi S, Peretz A, Jabaly H Naftali M: *Acanthamoeba* Keratitis. Israel Medical Association Journal. 2013; 15:182–185.

[70] Sacher BA, Wagoner MD, Goins KM, Sutphin JE, Greiner MA, Kitzmann AS: Treatment of *Acanthamoeba* keratitis with intravenous pentamidine before therapeutic keratoplasty. Cornea. 2015;34(1):49-53.

[71] Kitzmann AS, Goins KM, Sutphin JE, Wagoner MD: Keratoplasty for treatment of *Acanthamoeba* keratitis. Ophthalmology. 2009;116(5):864-869. doi:10.1016/j.ophtha.2008.12.029.

[72] Garduño-Vieyra L, González-Sánchez CR, Hernández-Da Mota SE: Ultraviolet-A light and riboflavin therapy for *Acanthamoeba* keratitis: a case report. Case Reports in Ophthalmology. 2011;2(2):291–295.

[73] Khan YA, Kashiwabuchi RT, Martins SA, Castro-Combs JM, Kalyani S, Stanley P, Flikier D, Behrens A: Riboflavin and ultraviolet light a therapy as an adjuvant treatment for medically refractive *Acanthamoeba* keratitis: report of 3 cases. Ophthalmology. 2011;118(2),324–331.

[74] Tabibian D, Richoz O, Hafezi F: PACK-CXL: Corneal cross-linking for treatment of infectious keratitis. Journal Ophthalmic and Vision Research. 2015;10(1):77-80.

[75] Claerhout I, Goegebuer A, Van Den Broecke C., Kestelyn P:Delay in diagnosis and outcome of *Acanthamoeba* keratitis. Graefes Archive for Clinical and Experimental Ophthalmology. 2004;242(8):648-653.

Permissions

All chapters in this book were first published in ACEI, by InTech Open; hereby published with permission under the Creative Commons Attribution License or equivalent. Every chapter published in this book has been scrutinized by our experts. Their significance has been extensively debated. The topics covered herein carry significant findings which will fuel the growth of the discipline. They may even be implemented as practical applications or may be referred to as a beginning point for another development.

The contributors of this book come from diverse backgrounds, making this book a truly international effort. This book will bring forth new frontiers with its revolutionizing research information and detailed analysis of the nascent developments around the world.

We would like to thank all the contributing authors for lending their expertise to make the book truly unique. They have played a crucial role in the development of this book. Without their invaluable contributions this book wouldn't have been possible. They have made vital efforts to compile up to date information on the varied aspects of this subject to make this book a valuable addition to the collection of many professionals and students.

This book was conceptualized with the vision of imparting up-to-date information and advanced data in this field. To ensure the same, a matchless editorial board was set up. Every individual on the board went through rigorous rounds of assessment to prove their worth. After which they invested a large part of their time researching and compiling the most relevant data for our readers.

The editorial board has been involved in producing this book since its inception. They have spent rigorous hours researching and exploring the diverse topics which have resulted in the successful publishing of this book. They have passed on their knowledge of decades through this book. To expedite this challenging task, the publisher supported the team at every step. A small team of assistant editors was also appointed to further simplify the editing procedure and attain best results for the readers.

Apart from the editorial board, the designing team has also invested a significant amount of their time in understanding the subject and creating the most relevant covers. They scrutinized every image to scout for the most suitable representation of the subject and create an appropriate cover for the book.

The publishing team has been an ardent support to the editorial, designing and production team. Their endless efforts to recruit the best for this project, has resulted in the accomplishment of this book. They are a veteran in the field of academics and their pool of knowledge is as vast as their experience in printing. Their expertise and guidance has proved useful at every step. Their uncompromising quality standards have made this book an exceptional effort. Their encouragement from time to time has been an inspiration for everyone.

The publisher and the editorial board hope that this book will prove to be a valuable piece of knowledge for researchers, students, practitioners and scholars across the globe.

List of Contributors

Lawan Abdu
Department of Ophthalmology, Faculty of Clinical Sciences, College of Health Sciences, Bayero University Kano, Nigeria

Maria Maślińska and Brygida Kwiatkowska
Early Arthritis Clinic, National Institute of Geriatrics, Rheumatology and Rehabilitation the name of Prof. Eleonora Reicher, Warsaw, Poland

Humberto D. Silva and Eduardo D. Silva
Universidade Federal de Pernambuco, Recife, Brazil

Maria Tamires D. Silva, Cristiana P. Dória and Cristiane P. Dória
Independent Professional, Recife, Brazil

S. Malhotra, S. Sharma, N. J. K. Bhatia, and C. Hans and P. Kumar
Department of Microbiology, Dr. Ram Manohar Lohia Hospital and PGIMER, New Delhi, India

Alejandro Rodriguez-Garcia
Tecnológico de Monterrey, Escuela de Medicina y Ciencias de la Salud, Institute of Ophthalmology and Visual Sciences, Ocular Immunology and Uveitis Service, Monterrey, Mexico

C. Stephen Foster
Massachusetts Eye Research and Surgery Institute, Waltham, MA, USA
Ocular Immunology and Uveitis Foundation, Weston, MA, USA
Department of Ophthalmology, Harvard Medical School, Boston, MA, USA

Victor M. Bautista-de Lucio, Mariana Ortiz-Casas,Jonathan Quevedo-Martínez and Herlinda Mejía-López
Institute of Opthalmology Conde de Valenciana, Mexico

Carlos Alberto Pantoja-Meléndez
Institute of Opthalmology Conde de Valenciana, Mexico
National Autonomous University of Mexico, School of Medicine, Public Health Department, Mexico

Shimon Rumelt
Western Galilee, Nahariya Medical Center, Nahariya, Israel
Faculty of Medicine, Bar Ilan University, Zefat, Israel

Parul Ichhpujani
Department of Ophthalmology, Glaucoma Services, Government Medical College and Hospital, Chandigarh, India

Nancy Malla and Kapil Goyal
Department of Medical Parasitology, Postgraduate Institute of Medical Education and Research, Chandigarh, India

Ozlem Sahin
Department of Microbiology and Immunology, New York Medical College, Valhalla, New York, USA

Alireza Ziaei
Harvard Medical School, Brigham and Women's Hospital, Boston, USA

Lidia Chomicz and Marcin Padzik
Department of Medical Biology, Medical University of Warsaw, Warsaw, Poland

Justyna Izdebska and Jacek P. Szaflik
Department of Ophthalmology, Medical University of Warsaw, SPKSO Ophthalmic University Hospital, Warsaw, Poland

Index

www.ingramcontent.com/pod-product-compliance
Lightning Source LLC
LaVergne TN
LVHW081039210926
848485LV00004B/1060
* 9 7 8 1 6 3 9 8 7 4 1 1 8 *